COVID Chronicles

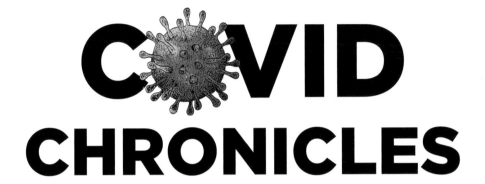

COVID CHRONICLES

A Comics Anthology

EDITED BY KENDRA BOILEAU AND RICH JOHNSON

Graphic Mundi

This book is dedicated to

our frontline workers

and to those who lost their

lives to COVID-19.

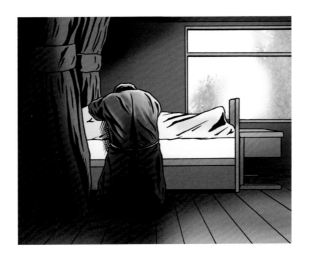

CONTENTS

PREFACE

What can we draw out of this moment, when words fail us? In early April, when COVID-19 cases spiked in the US and life as we knew it slipped quietly from view, I sent out a call for short comics to see how comics creators were responding to the pandemic. COVID comics have gone viral these past months on Facebook, Twitter, and Instagram. Digital publications like *The Nib* and anthologies such as *Heroes Need Masks* have collected and published pandemic-themed comics.[1] It turns out that comics creators have had a lot to say in these exceptional times. This volume, *COVID Chronicles,* was compiled over the course of six months, from mid-April 2020 to mid-October 2020. It comprises sixty-four short comics that were sent in response to the call or were solicited expressly for this anthology, and in some cases, we have included comics we discovered online. The comics here run the gamut in perspective and style. Some are true, deeply personal stories; others are invented ones, either based on real events or inspired by a vivid imagination. They are documentary, memoiristic, meditative, lyrical, fantastic, and speculative, offering a view onto the countless ways the COVID-19 pandemic has changed lives.

There are comics here about getting COVID-19 and recovering from it, about losing someone to it, adjusting to home schooling, being furloughed, working the front lines, getting evicted, reliving past trauma, witnessing police brutality, and protesting for social justice. We see how world leaders measure up (or not) in their efforts to manage the pandemic. As a character in Kay Sohini's "Pandemic Precarities" says, "this pandemic has exposed and amplified everything that is wrong with our world." It has exacerbated economic inequalities, inadequate healthcare systems, social injustice, racism, xenophobia, and political hegemony, all of which are pervasive themes in these comics. In short, these comics reveal the pure fear, anxiety, and grief so many of us are experiencing these days—feelings that will no doubt be with us for years to come.

Strange, perhaps, for these emotions to resonate so clearly in a medium that people often assume is either directed toward children or there for our amusement. But comics have a history of tackling weighty and mature subjects—and doing it well. Comics expert Hillary Chute reminds us that disaster is deeply rooted in comics, whether it's in the superhero comics of the Silver Age (from the late 1950s through the '60s), where the plot often revolves around some calamitous ordeal for the protagonist, or in the themes of more recent nonfiction comics—a classic example being Art Spiegelman's *Maus,* which retells his father's experience in the Holocaust. With the underground movement of the 1960s and '70s and the rise of alternative comics that took on controversial and taboo topics, the medium has shown itself to be particularly well suited to expressing difficult subject matter. As Chute points out, comics "[make] readers aware of limits, and also possibilities for expression in which disaster, or trauma, breaks the boundaries of communication, finding shape in a hybrid medium."[2]

Fast-forwarding to the twenty-first-century comics scene, a more recent movement known as "graphic medicine" has looked to comics to articulate complex or unsettling ideas, especially as they relate to important issues surrounding illness, disability, and healthcare. The term was coined in 2007 by UK physician and comics artist Ian Williams (also a contributor to this volume). Graphic medicine began as an area of study for scholars, educators, practitioners, and artists who saw in the subversive power of comics the ability to challenge prevailing attitudes toward the disabled, the ill, the dying, and those who care for them. In time, and quite rapidly, graphic medicine grew into a movement and a diverse community that includes not only scholars, educators, and practitioners but also people who create comics, people with illness and disabilities, family caregivers, medical students, librarians, and publishers. The movement became as much about the creation and dissemination of comics as about the study of comics, about "merging the personal with the pedagogical, the subjective with the objective," with the goal of making and using comics to effect cultural change.[3]

Penn State University Press brought graphic medicine to its list when Susan Squier, now Brill Professor Emerita of English and Women's, Gender, and Sexuality Studies at Penn State University, introduced me to the cross-disciplinary intersection of comics and medicine. Over the course of a distinguished career in the medical and health humanities, Squier made space for comics in her scholarship and teaching, because they "enable us to enter, imaginatively, a number of complex, ambiguous debates."[4] She joined with other pioneers of graphic medicine to organize an annual conference and to develop the Graphic Medicine book series at Penn State University Press, which she edits with Ian Williams. We launched the series with the *Graphic Medicine Manifesto* in 2015 and since then have published more than twenty graphic novels in the graphic medicine genre.[5]

This book, *COVID Chronicles,* now launches a trade graphic novel imprint at Penn State University Press called Graphic Mundi.[6] With the tagline "Drawing Our Worlds Together," Graphic Mundi will continue the tradition of graphic medicine by giving voice to storytellers who challenge the status quo, enlighten, and inspire in an ever-changing, complex world. Following Squier's lead, graphic novels published in Graphic Mundi will "'scale up' the concept of health," taking into account the intersecting worlds not only of humans but also of microbes, plants, and non-human animals to highlight our myriad connections.[7] In fact, a book like *COVID Chronicles* is a great example of how graphic medicine so effectively conveys ideas of scale and connection. Documenting what people have experienced for more than half of 2020, it is, to date, the most comprehensive collection of comics about the pandemic. It reveals the shifting scale of the pandemic over time, illustrating how the actions of an invisible microbe have led, in the space of just months, to systemic upheaval, such that we find ourselves now struggling to comprehend the greatest medical, economic, political, and social challenges many of us have had to face in our lifetimes.

COVID Chronicles also demonstrates the power of comics to make connections, whether it's helping people connect their own thoughts in difficult circumstances or helping them connect with one another. Characters in these comics use drawing as a "way to think and feel on the page[, to] try and make some sense of all this," or they imagine themselves as a comic superhero in an attempt to feel less helpless. One family draws graffiti art to cheer up a neighbor, while another one comes together over a jigsaw puzzle when there's not much else to do. A whimsical character in these comics embodies the very idea of comics forging community: the Japanese mythical creature Amabie says, "Drawing my picture and sharing it makes people feel connected with each other. A global connection through art!"[8] This kind of connection inspires hope.

And there is hope in these pages. In the figure of Amabie and in all the ways these comics show people managing to stay connected during lockdown, keeping businesses open, keeping kids busy, maintaining rituals, starting families, supporting one another—in short, responding in very creative ways to a world out of control. I want to thank the artists, writers, letterers, colorists, and translator who donated their time and talents to this project. We will be donating a portion of the proceeds from the sale of this book to the Book Industry Charitable Foundation in support of bookstores and their employees whose livelihoods have been upended by COVID-19. Thanks also to Rich Johnson and my wonderful colleagues at Penn State University Press for the unfailing expertise and care they brought to the publication of this book. Finally, I want to thank Susan Squier and my graphic medicine friends, who have drawn me along this path with them, on this remarkable voyage of discovery through comics.

Kendra Boileau
Publisher, Graphic Mundi

Notes

1. *The Nib,* https://thenib.com/; Eddy Hedlington and Greg Smith, *Heroes Need Masks* (Tacoma, WA: Grit City Comics, 2020).

2. Hillary Chute, *Why Comics? From Underground to Everywhere* (New York: Harper, 2017), 34.

3. MK Czerwiec et al., *Graphic Medicine Manifesto* (University Park: Penn State University Press, 2015), 2–3.

4. Susan Squier, "Comics and Graphic Medicine as a Third Space for the Health Humanities," in *Routledge Companion to the Health Humanities*, ed. Paul Crawford et al. (New York: Routledge, 2020), 61–62.

5. See more on this at https://www.graphicmedicine.org/ and https://www.psupress.org/books/series/book_SeriesGM.html.

6. See https://www.graphicmundi.org.

7. Squier, "Comics and Graphic Medicine," 64.

8. For these examples, see the contributions to this volume by Sarah Firth, Justin LaRocca Hansen, Stephanie Nina Pitsirilos and Seth Martel, Kelly Latham, and Zack Davisson and Lili Chin.

COVID Chronicles

COVID-19 DIARY

I GOT THE VIRUS. IF YOU GET IT, HERE'S WHAT YOU <u>MIGHT</u> EXPECT TO HAPPEN.

BY

JASON CHATFIELD

Please Note:

WHAT FOLLOWS
IS <u>NOT</u> PROFESSIONAL
MEDICAL ADVICE.

Please
call your doctor if you're
experiencing symptoms.

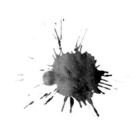

DAY 1 : DENIAL

You're sitting at the
kitchen table researching covid-19
(watching French bulldog puppy
videos on YouTube) when you
get that tingle in your joints.

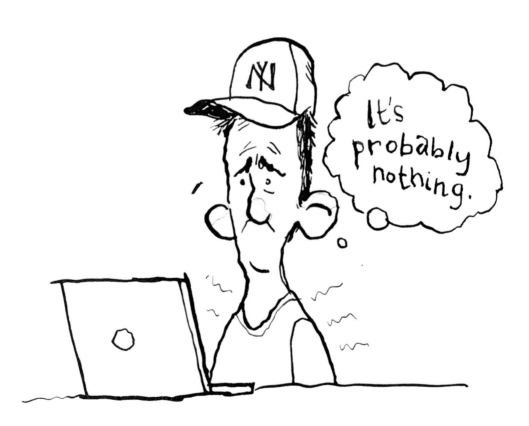

DAY 2: STILL DENIAL

You're lying in bed...
with a fever of 105°
but you convince yourself
only <u>other</u> people get
"the virus."

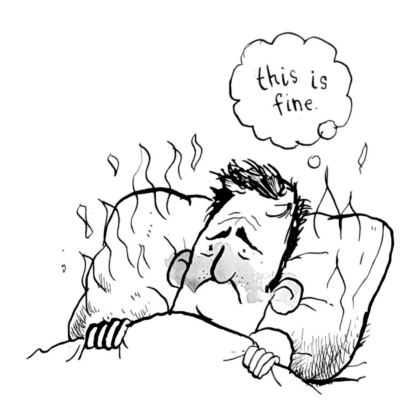

DAY 3: NETFLIX AND THE CHILLS

You isolate yourself from humanity. You walk outside.

You can **not** stop shaking.

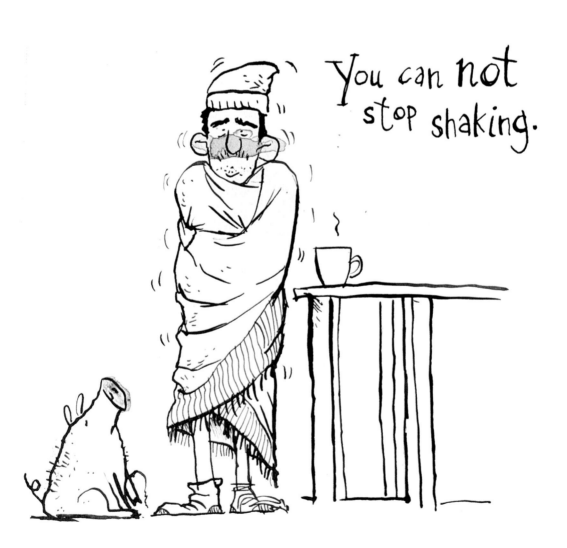

DAY 4 : HORIZONTAL IS YOUR FRIEND.

You can't stand up without feeling like you're going to pass out. No more showers. (But wash your hands.)

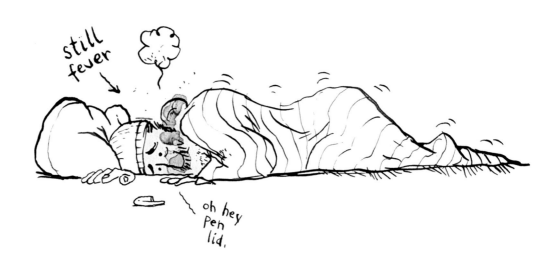

still fever

oh hey pen lid.

DAY 5: IT COMES IN WAVES.

You feel <u>fine</u> for like a while-ish, then out of nowhere you get PUNCHED in the FACE with diarrhea and fever and chills and more pooing.

(sorry)

You realize you lost your sense of smell three days ago.

Also taste.

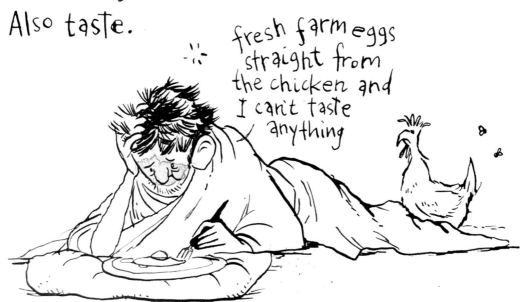

fresh farm eggs straight from the chicken and I can't taste anything

DAY 6: GATORADE AND MORE GATORADE

You drink lots of fluids because you have the world's driest mouth.

This is about the time your chest starts to feel like it's slowly filling with flour...

You now look like
Tom Hanks in CastAway.
You haven't showered
in four days.

COVID-19
SURVIVOR

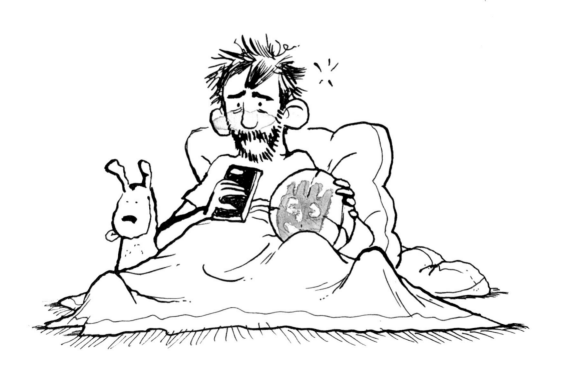

DAY 7: TRY TO FINISH A SENTENCE

It might just be the f
It might just be the f
It might just be th

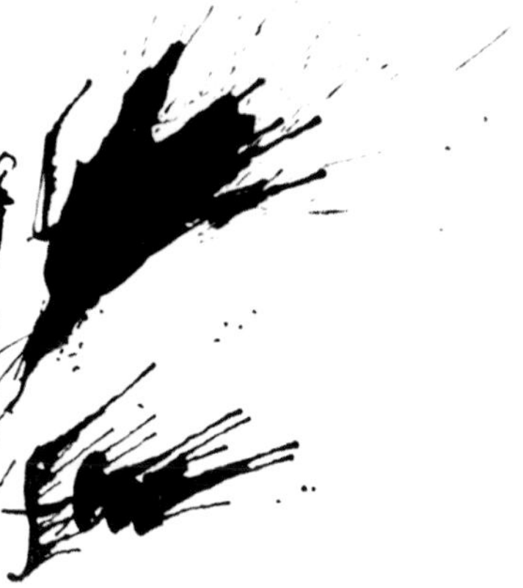

You breathe in and it sounds like the sound Coco Pops make when you pour milk on them.

You call your local HEALTH DEPT. You ask them for a test for COVID-19.

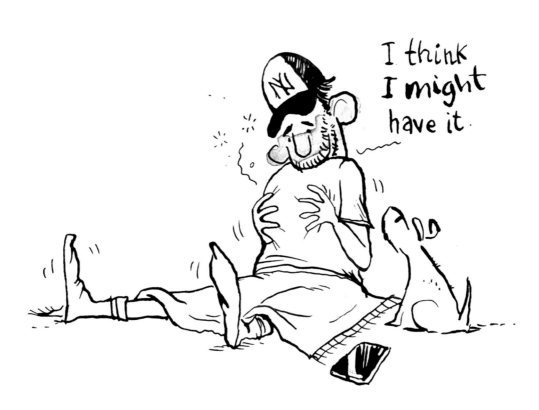

I think I might have it

DAY 8 : PASS OUT IN THE SHOWER

You're still waiting on the results from the test where they shoved a swab up your nostril and into your BRAIN.
You still have vain hope that this is just the flu. (cough)

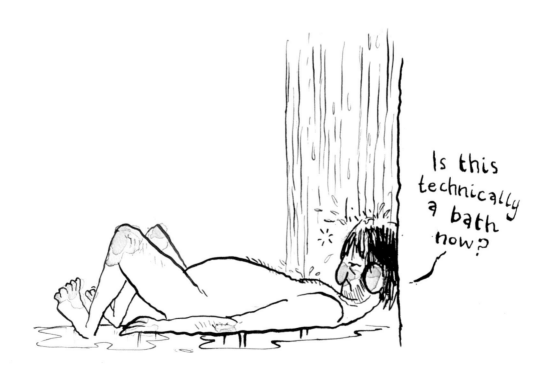

Is this technically a bath now?

DAY 9: PAN(DEM)IC

You get confirmation from the HEALTH DEPT. that you do indeed have the virus.

You already knew deep down.

Your mind immediately runs to Kate Winslet in *Contagion*.

YOU HAVE IT.
I'm going to die in a local basketball stadium.

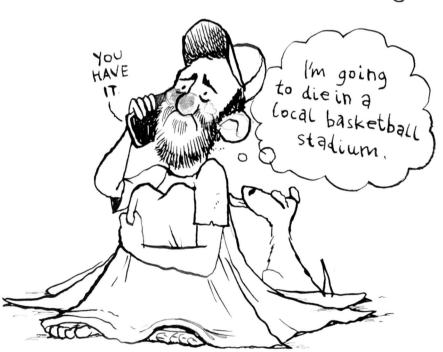

Time to tell your parents.

DAY 10: HOWARD HUGHES

You completely isolate yourself from the world and think about every single object you touched in the last month.

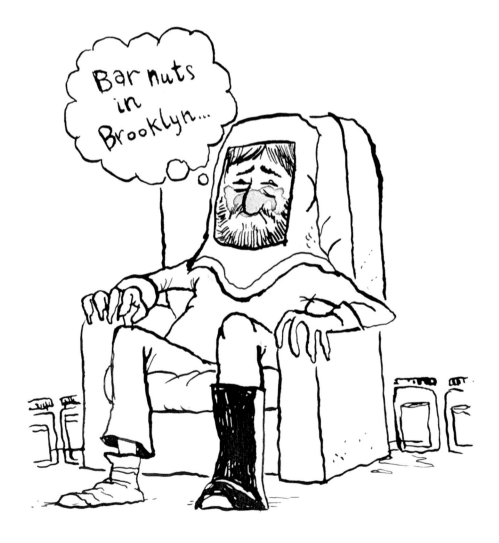

DAY 11: COUGH INTO YOUR ELBOW.

You cannot stop coughing.*
It rules your life.
You get sent videos of
old, matronly nurses tapping
patients on the back to
loosen mucus in the lungs.

You haven't taken a solid
poop for a week.

(sorry).

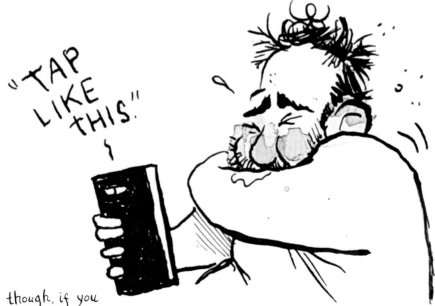

"TAP LIKE THIS!"

* Seriously though, if you
have trouble breathing,
call your doctor immediately.

DAY 12: NOW YOUR WIFE HAS IT...

It's probably nothing

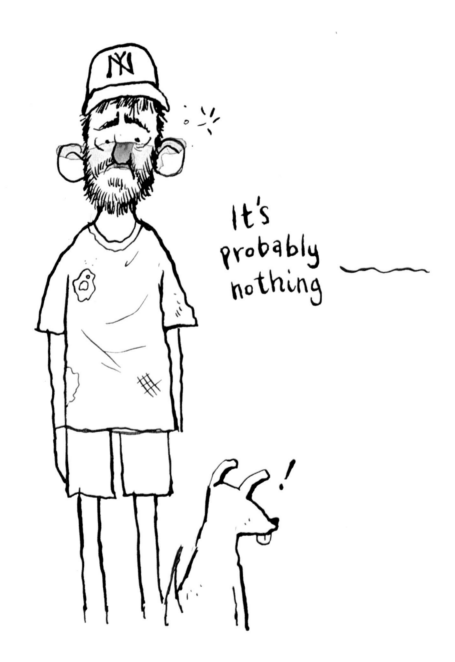

Footnote:

MY WIFE AND I HAVE
SINCE MADE A FULL
RECOVERY. WE WENT
INTO FULL ISOLATION
WHILE WE WERE
BOTH SICK.

PLEASE
STAY SAFE!

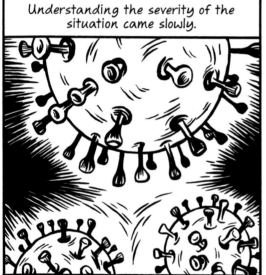

COVID DAWN
JESSE LAMBERT

Covid-19 came from afar.

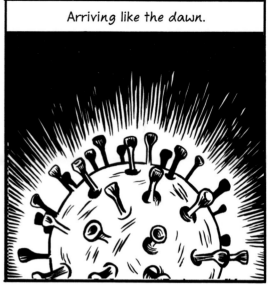

Arriving like the dawn.

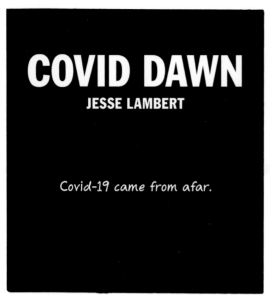

Understanding the severity of the situation came slowly.

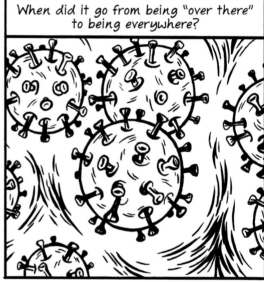

When did it go from being "over there" to being everywhere?

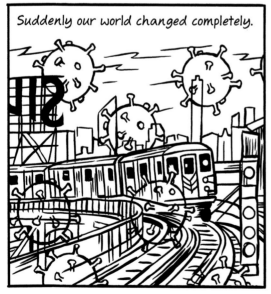

Suddenly our world changed completely.

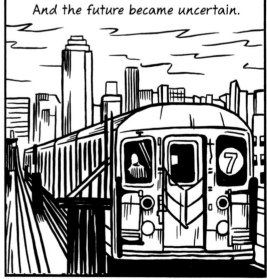

And the future became uncertain.

Time is so strange now. It's lost its edges.
I tried to backtrack and reconstruct a timeline of how things have changed. Then I gave up.
Boost
10:22 AM
40%
Mar 2020
S M T W T F S
1 2 3 4 5 6 7
8 9 10 11 12 13 14
15 16 17 18 19 20 21
22 23 24 25 26 27 28
29 30 31
What was that movie where the protagonist had only 15 minutes of short term memory?
MEMENTO
JOE PANTOLIANO
Do I really need to watch 12 Monkeys again?
Memes are funny and comforting when they expose your own foibles.
Time spent looking at exponential graphs
January
February
March
Facing reality is much more frightening.
COVID-19 total and daily cases in New York City
35,000
30,000
25,000
20,000
15,000
10,000
5,000
Total case count
New daily cases
March 10 13 16 19 22 25 28

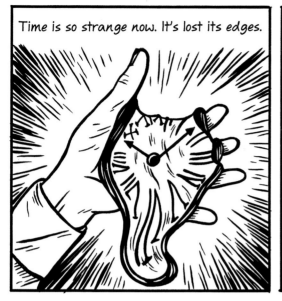

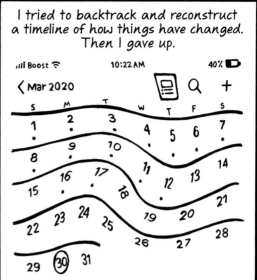

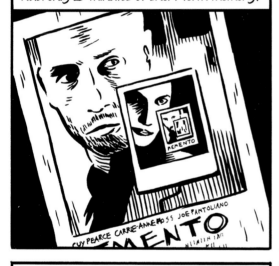

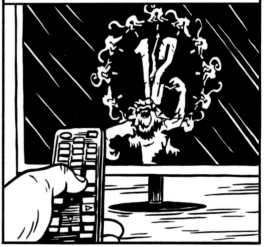

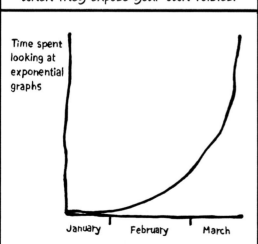

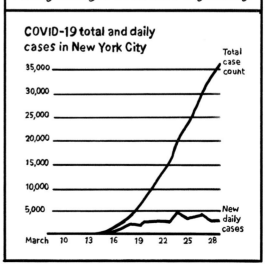

We live in Jackson Heights in Central Queens, NYC, the epicenter of the epicenter.
East Elmhurst
Jackson Heights
North Corona
Woodside
Elmhurst
Corona
Our home is 5 blocks from Elmhurst Hospital.
We've had to go to the emergency room there a couple of times over the years.
Elmhurst
Emergency & Trauma Center
It's surreal to see it on the news, now described as coronavirus "Ground Zero."
Elmhurst TRAUMA CENTER
FD NY
To see local residents, my neighbors, lining up to be tested in tents.
Elmhurst TRAUMA CENTER

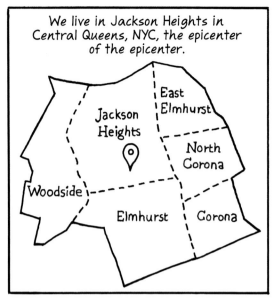

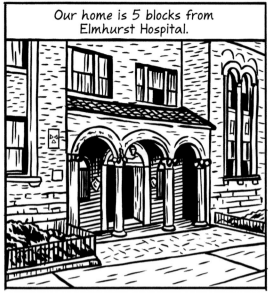

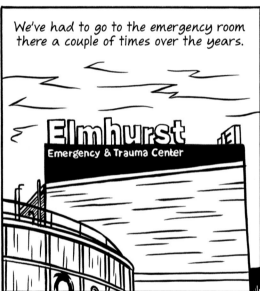

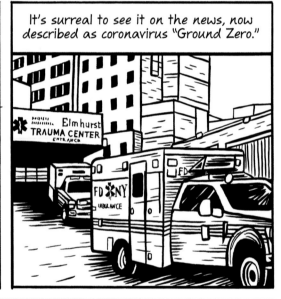

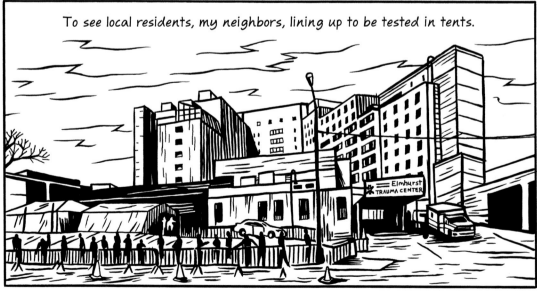

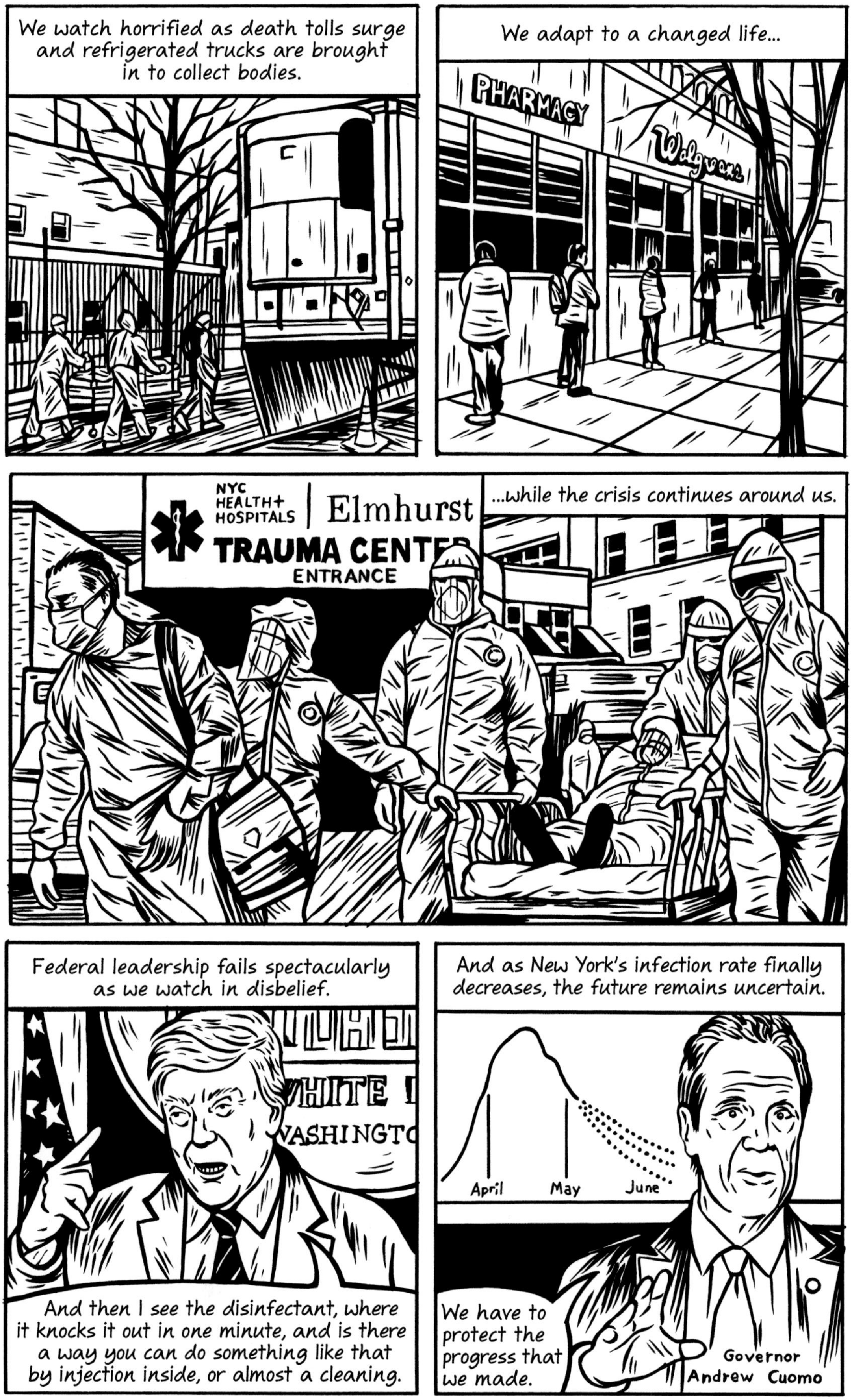
We watch horrified as death tolls surge and refrigerated trucks are brought in to collect bodies.
We adapt to a changed life...
PHARMACY
Walgreens
NYC HEALTH+ HOSPITALS
Elmhurst
TRAUMA CENTER
ENTRANCE
...while the crisis continues around us.
Federal leadership fails spectacularly as we watch in disbelief.
WHITE
WASHINGT
And then I see the disinfectant, where it knocks it out in one minute, and is there a way you can do something like that by injection inside, or almost a cleaning.
And as New York's infection rate finally decreases, the future remains uncertain.
April
May
June
We have to protect the progress that we made.
Governor Andrew Cuomo

RING THE BELLS

EMILY STEINBERG

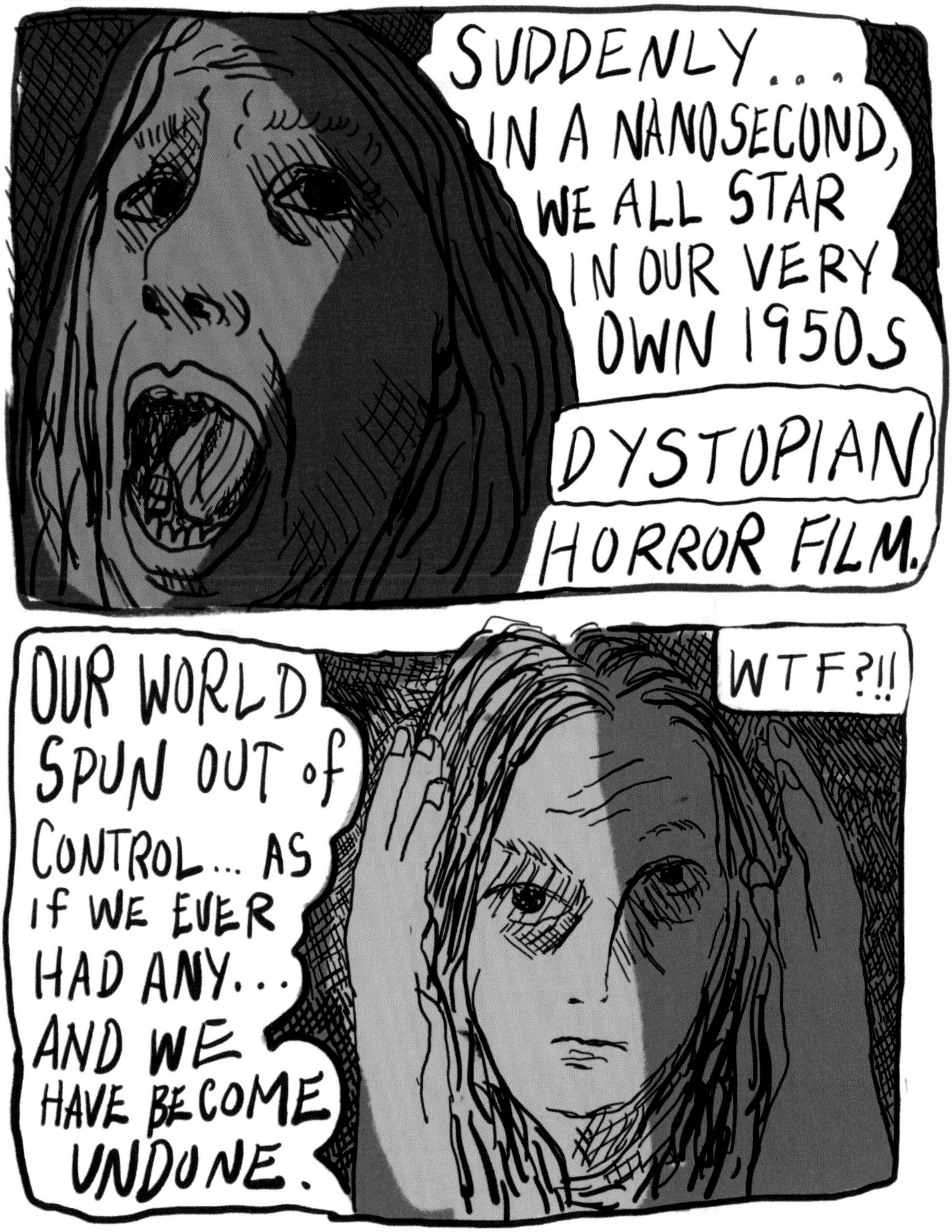
SUDDENLY... IN A NANOSECOND, WE ALL STAR IN OUR VERY OWN 1950s
DYSTOPIAN
HORROR FILM.
OUR WORLD SPUN OUT of CONTROL... AS if WE EVER HAD ANY... AND WE HAVE BECOME UNDONE.
WTF?!!

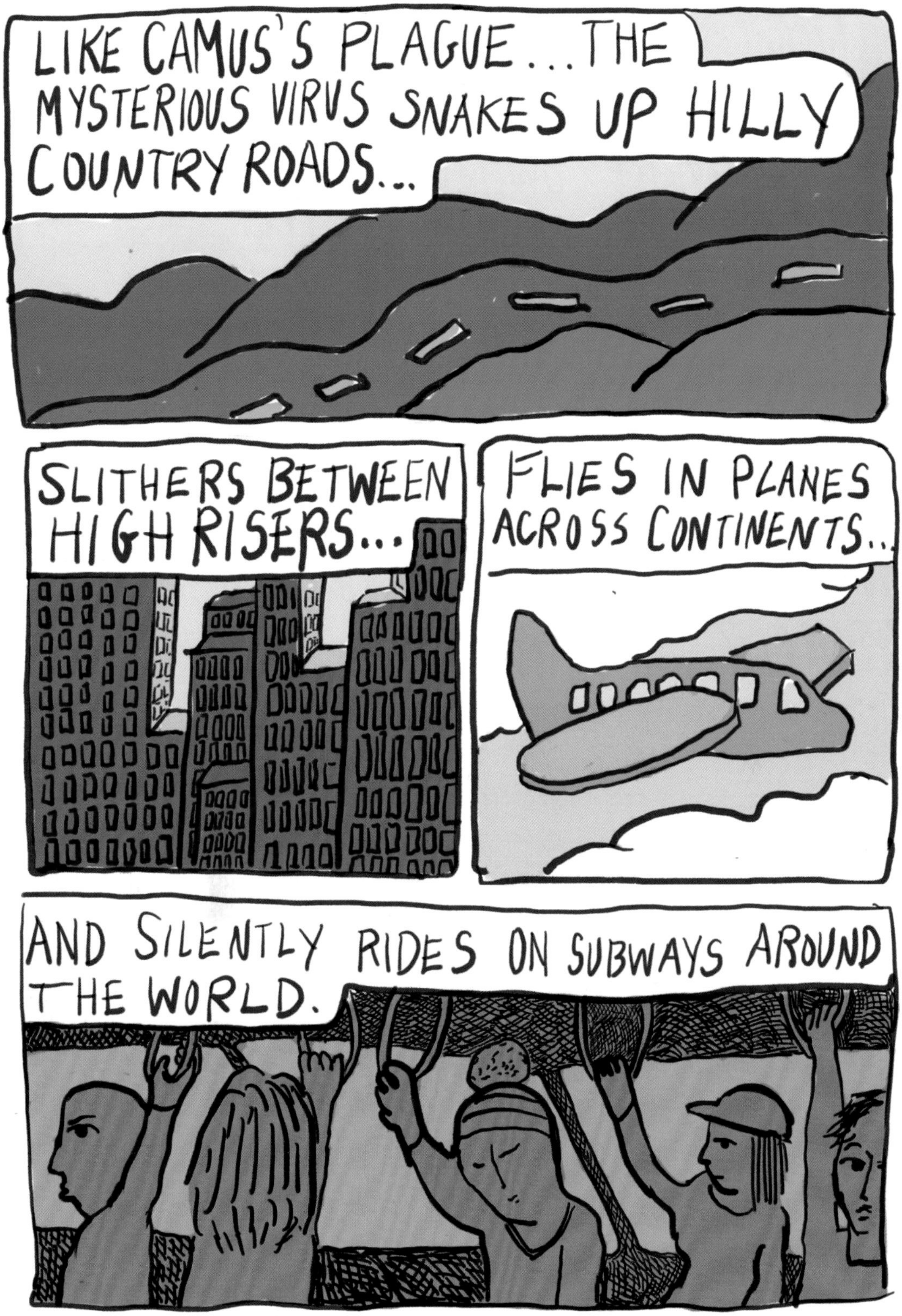
LIKE CAMUS'S PLAGUE... THE MYSTERIOUS VIRUS SNAKES UP HILLY COUNTRY ROADS...
SLITHERS BETWEEN HIGH RISERS...
FLIES IN PLANES ACROSS CONTINENTS...
AND SILENTLY RIDES ON SUBWAYS AROUND THE WORLD.

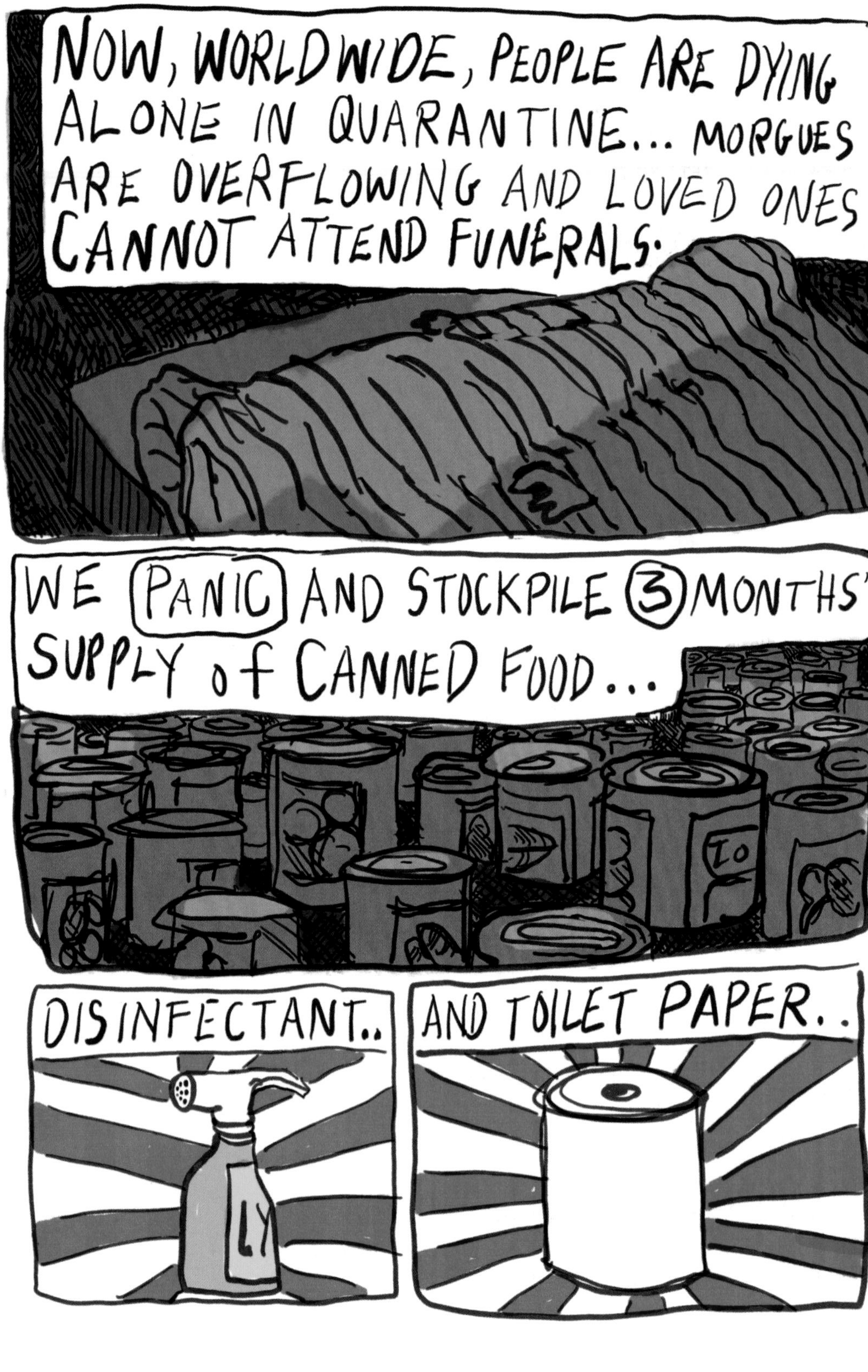
NOW, WORLDWIDE, PEOPLE ARE DYING ALONE IN QUARANTINE... MORGUES ARE OVERFLOWING AND LOVED ONES CANNOT ATTEND FUNERALS.
WE PANIC AND STOCKPILE 3 MONTHS' SUPPLY of CANNED FOOD...
DISINFECTANT..
AND TOILET PAPER..

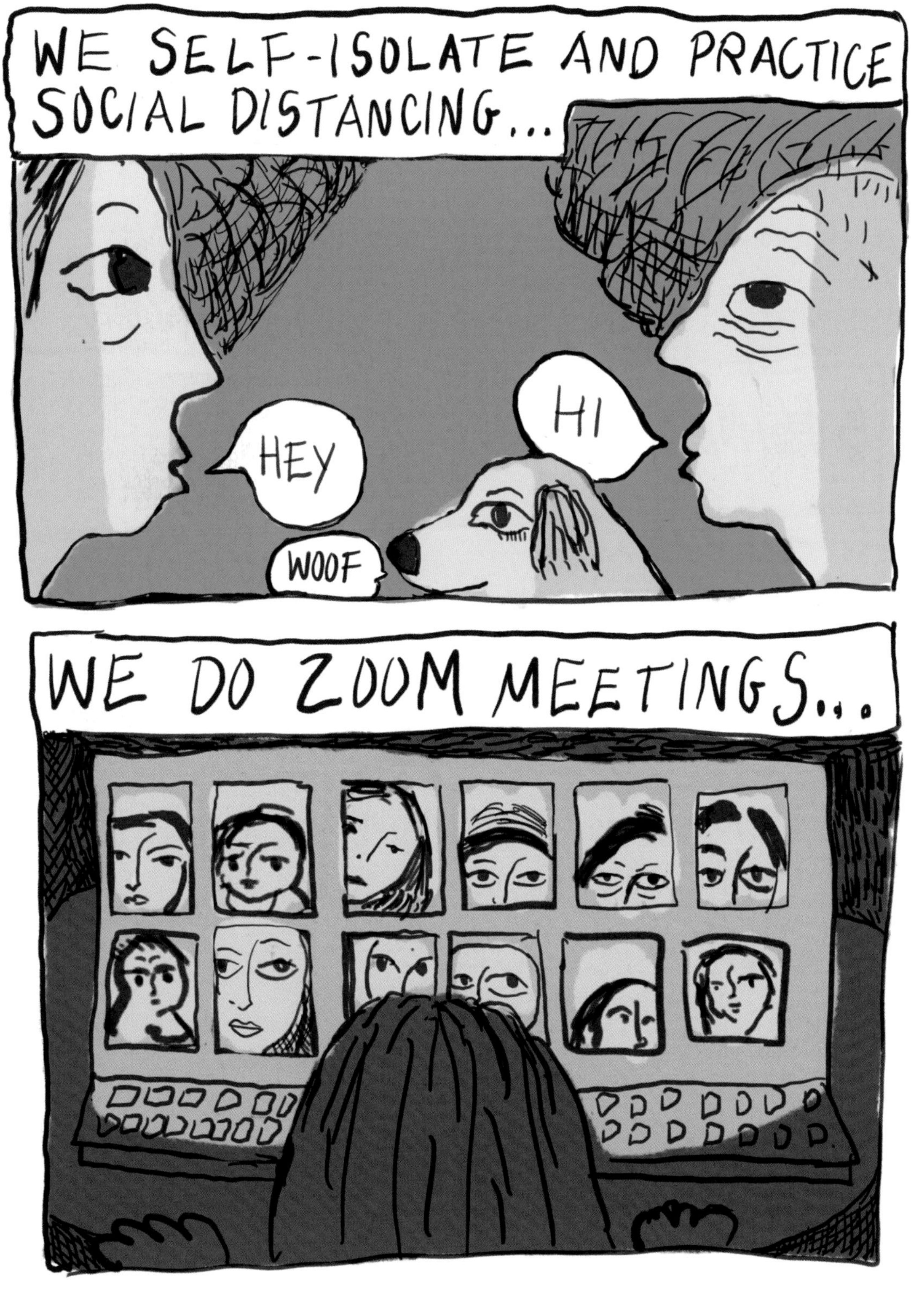
WE SELF-ISOLATE AND PRACTICE SOCIAL DISTANCING...
HEY
HI
WOOF
WE DO ZOOM MEETINGS...

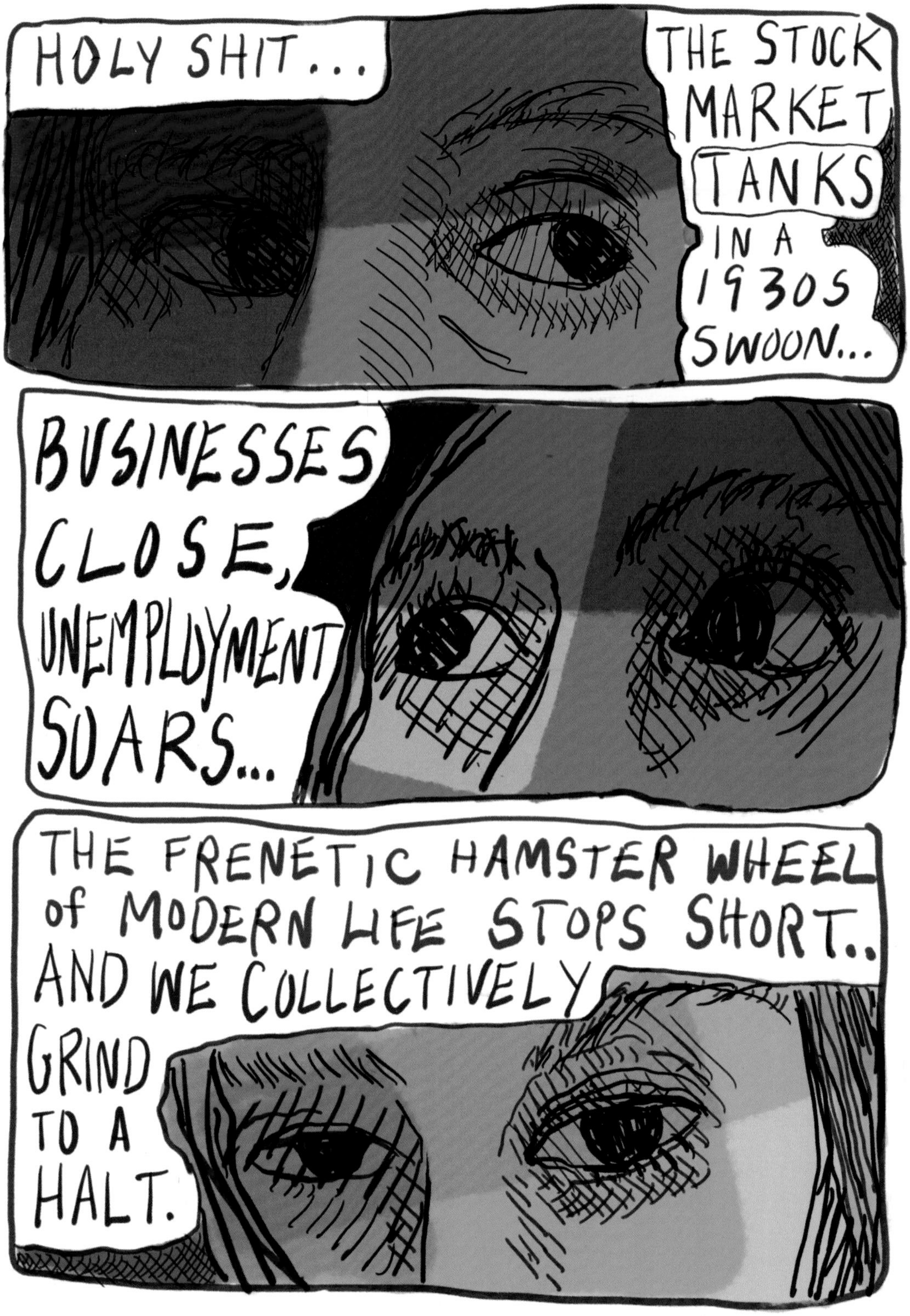
HOLY SHIT...
THE STOCK MARKET TANKS IN A 1930S SWOON...
BUSINESSES CLOSE, UNEMPLOYMENT SOARS...
THE FRENETIC HAMSTER WHEEL of MODERN LIFE STOPS SHORT.. AND WE COLLECTIVELY GRIND TO A HALT.

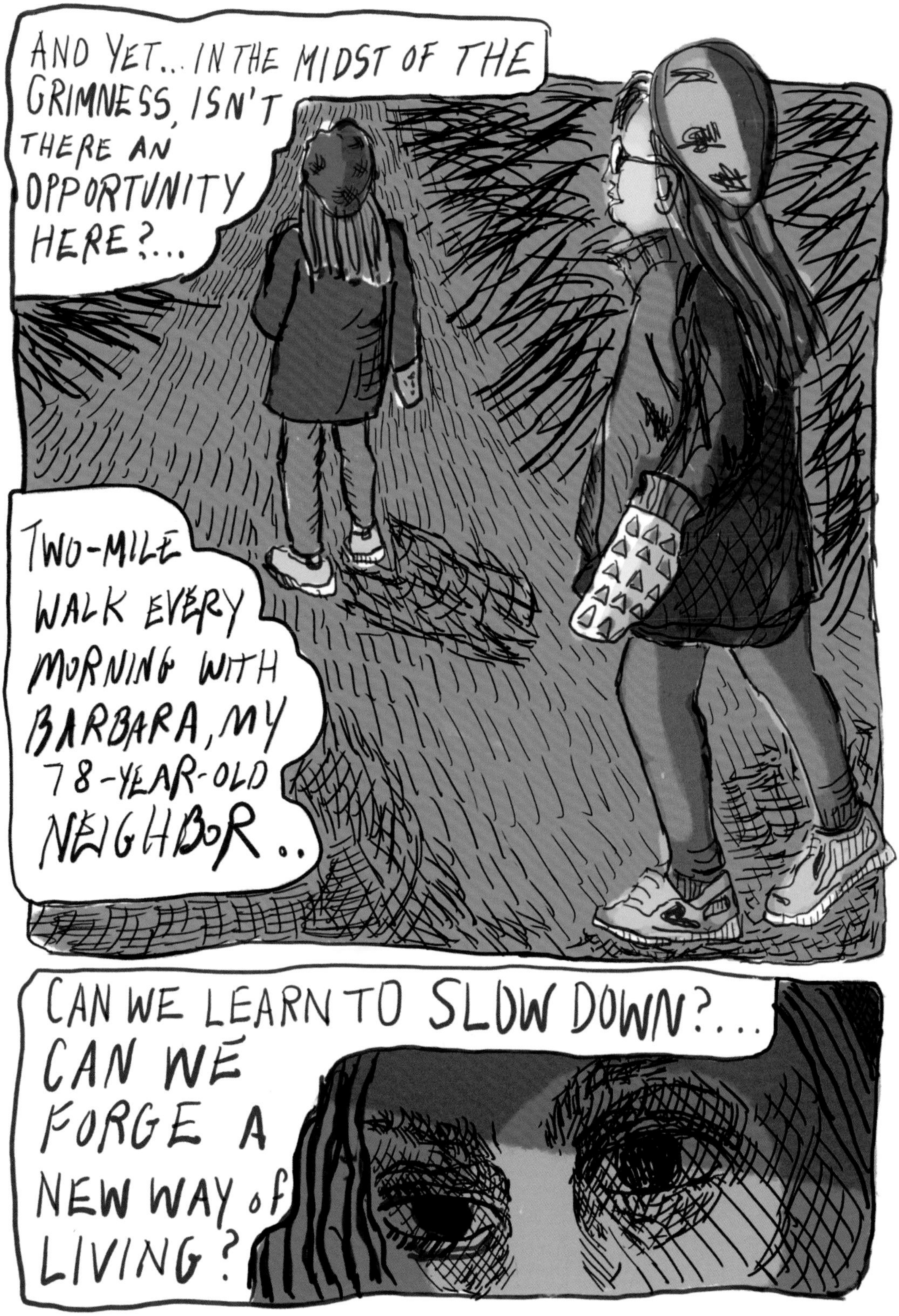
AND YET... IN THE MIDST OF THE GRIMNESS, ISN'T THERE AN OPPORTUNITY HERE?...
TWO-MILE WALK EVERY MORNING WITH BARBARA, MY 78-YEAR-OLD NEIGHBOR..
CAN WE LEARN TO SLOW DOWN?... CAN WE FORGE A NEW WAY of LIVING?

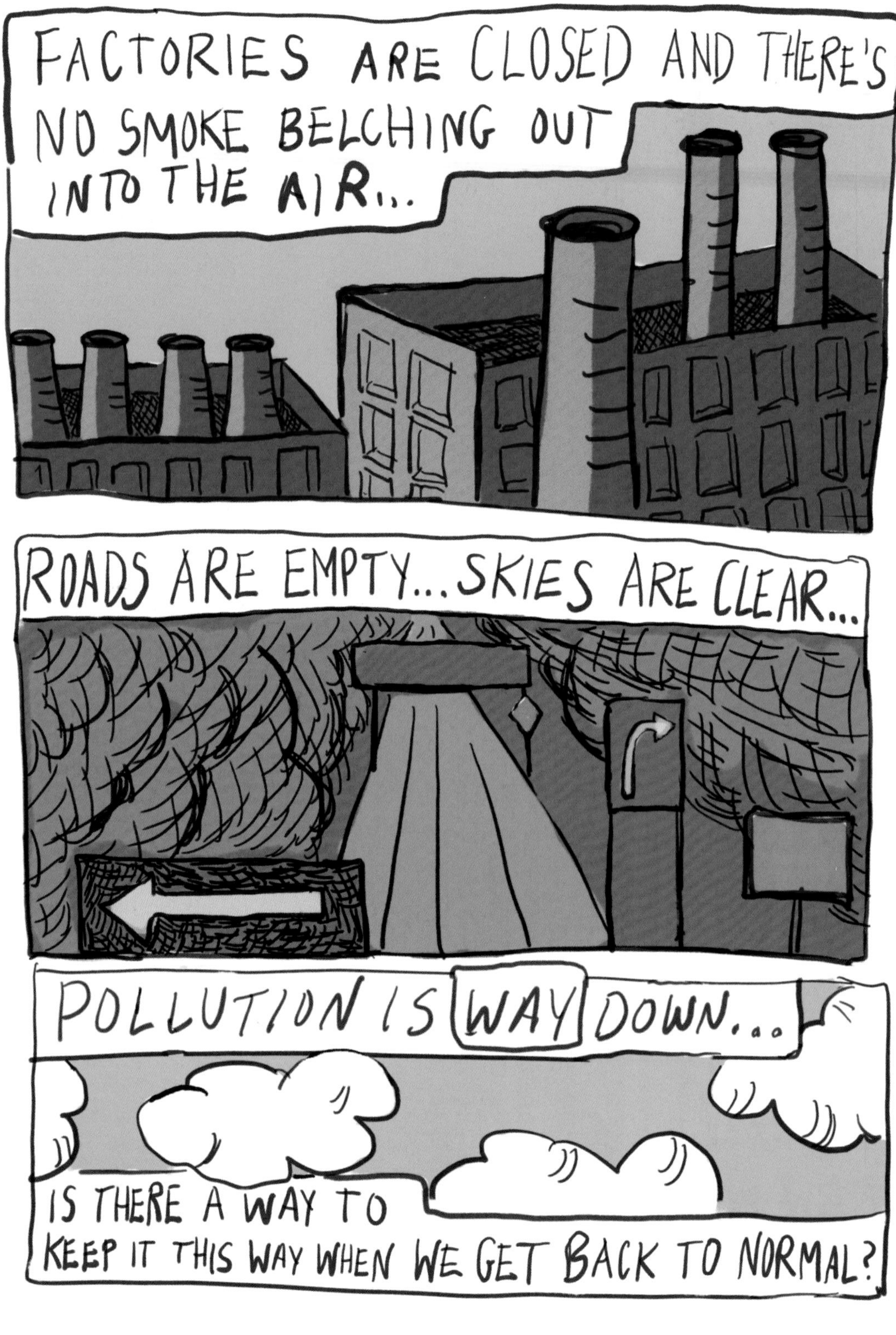
FACTORIES ARE CLOSED AND THERE'S NO SMOKE BELCHING OUT INTO THE AIR...
ROADS ARE EMPTY... SKIES ARE CLEAR...
POLLUTION IS WAY DOWN...
IS THERE A WAY TO KEEP IT THIS WAY WHEN WE GET BACK TO NORMAL?

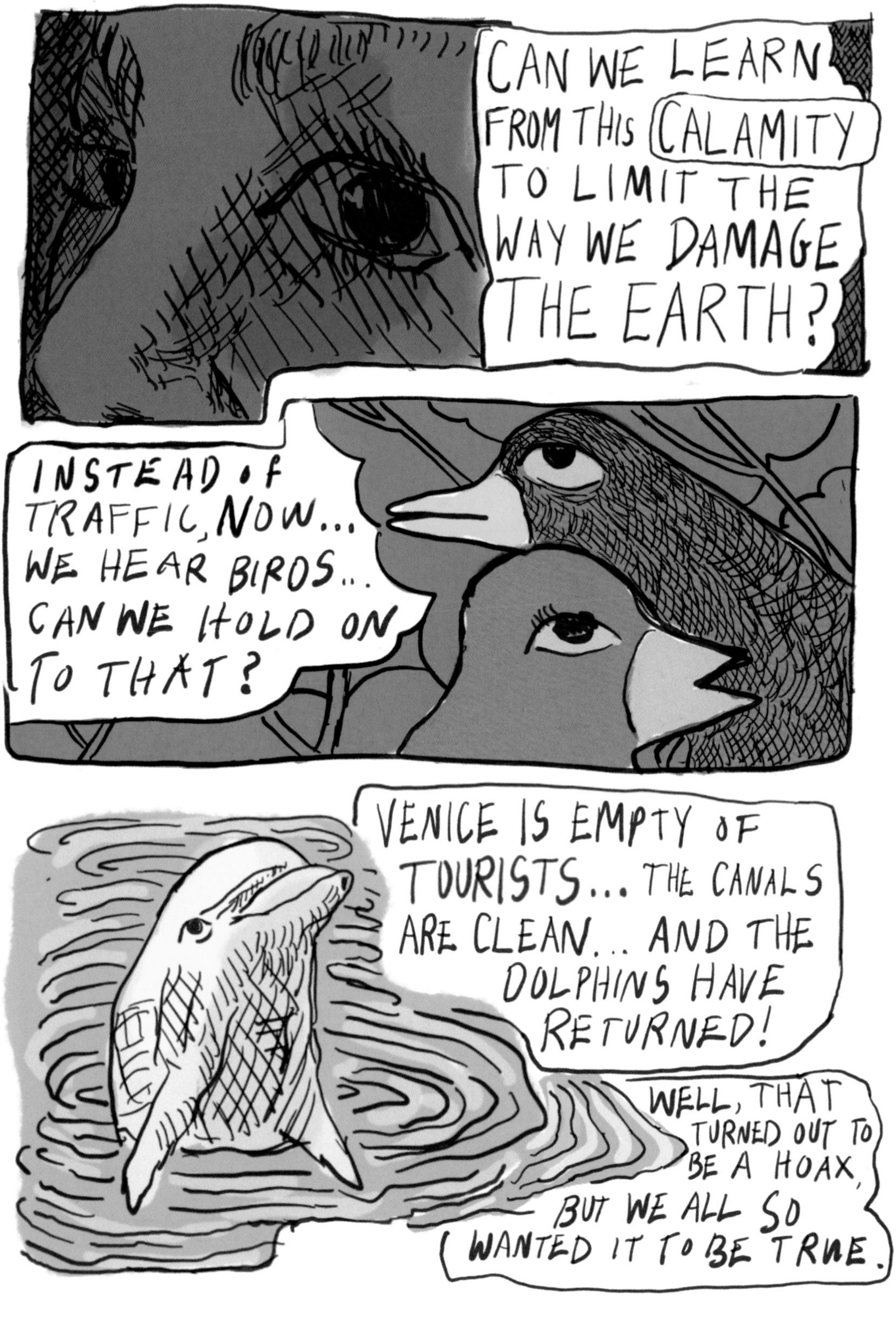
CAN WE LEARN FROM THIS CALAMITY TO LIMIT THE WAY WE DAMAGE THE EARTH?
INSTEAD OF TRAFFIC, NOW... WE HEAR BIRDS... CAN WE HOLD ON TO THAT?
VENICE IS EMPTY OF TOURISTS... THE CANALS ARE CLEAN... AND THE DOLPHINS HAVE RETURNED!
WELL, THAT TURNED OUT TO BE A HOAX, BUT WE ALL SO WANTED IT TO BE TRUE.

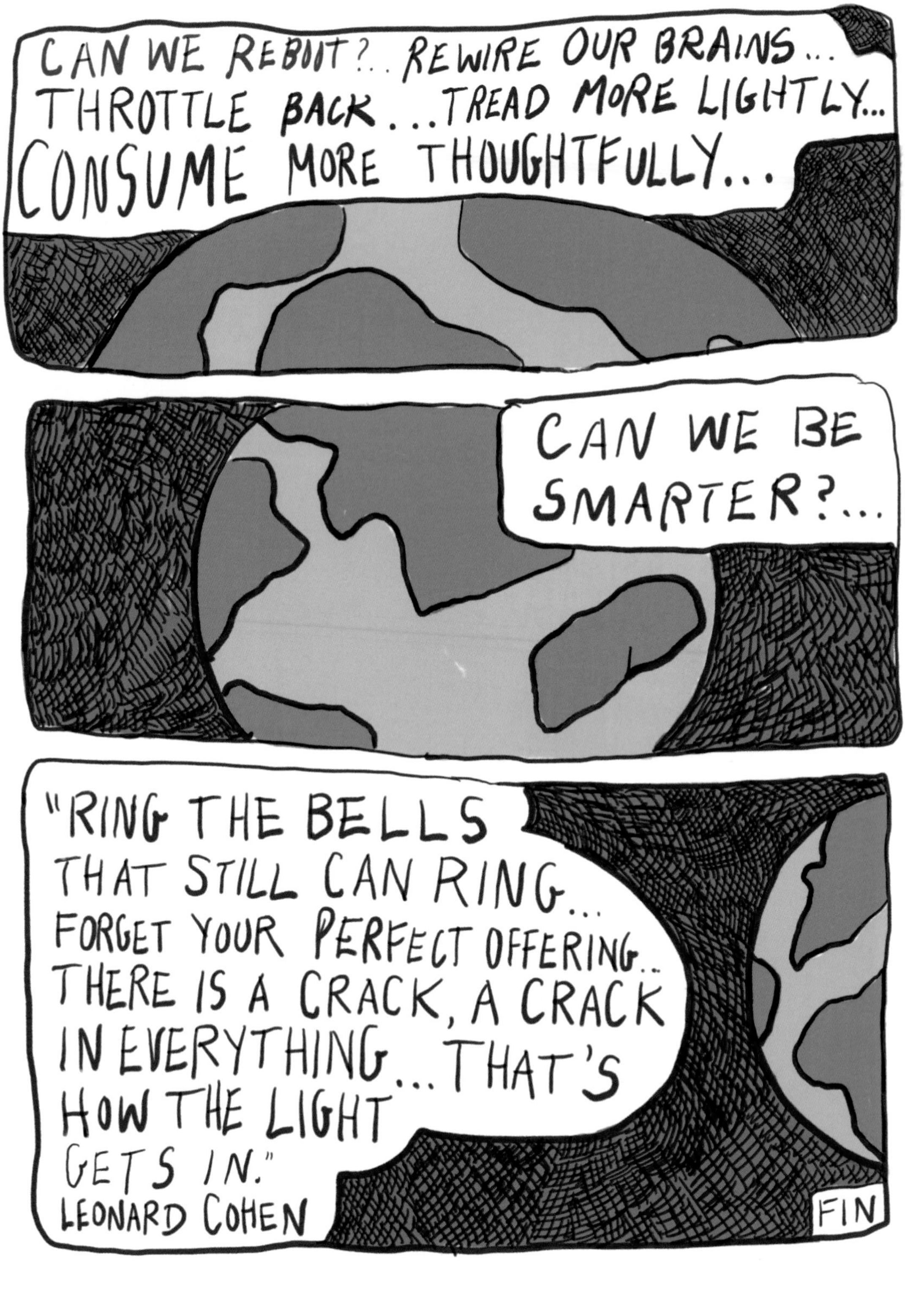
CAN WE REBOOT?.. REWIRE OUR BRAINS... THROTTLE BACK... TREAD MORE LIGHTLY... CONSUME MORE THOUGHTFULLY...
CAN WE BE SMARTER?...
"RING THE BELLS THAT STILL CAN RING... FORGET YOUR PERFECT OFFERING... THERE IS A CRACK, A CRACK IN EVERYTHING... THAT'S HOW THE LIGHT GETS IN."
LEONARD COHEN
FIN

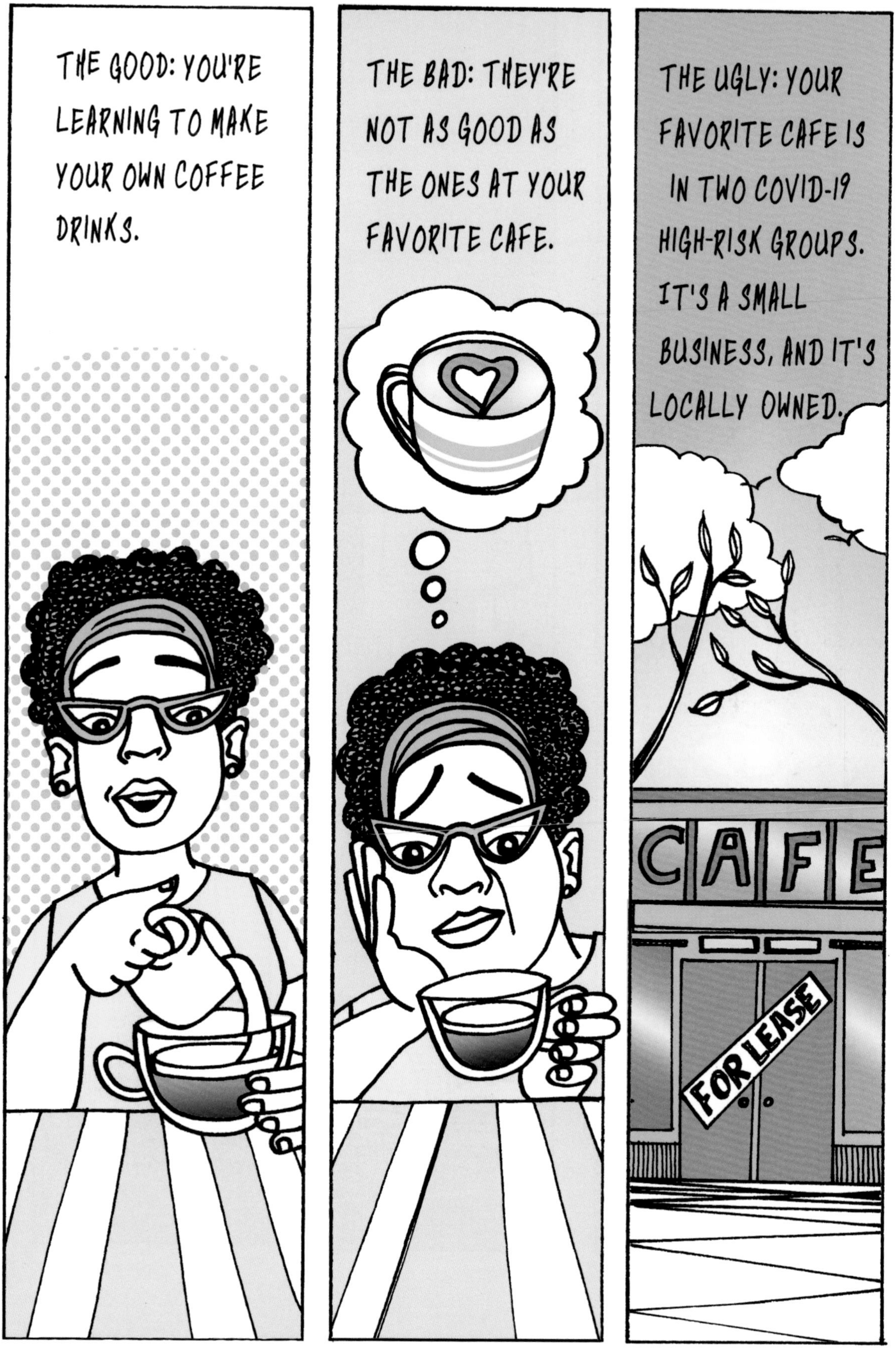
THE GOOD: YOU'RE LEARNING TO MAKE YOUR OWN COFFEE DRINKS.
THE BAD: THEY'RE NOT AS GOOD AS THE ONES AT YOUR FAVORITE CAFE.
THE UGLY: YOUR FAVORITE CAFE IS IN TWO COVID-19 HIGH-RISK GROUPS. IT'S A SMALL BUSINESS, AND IT'S LOCALLY OWNED.
CAFE
FOR LEASE

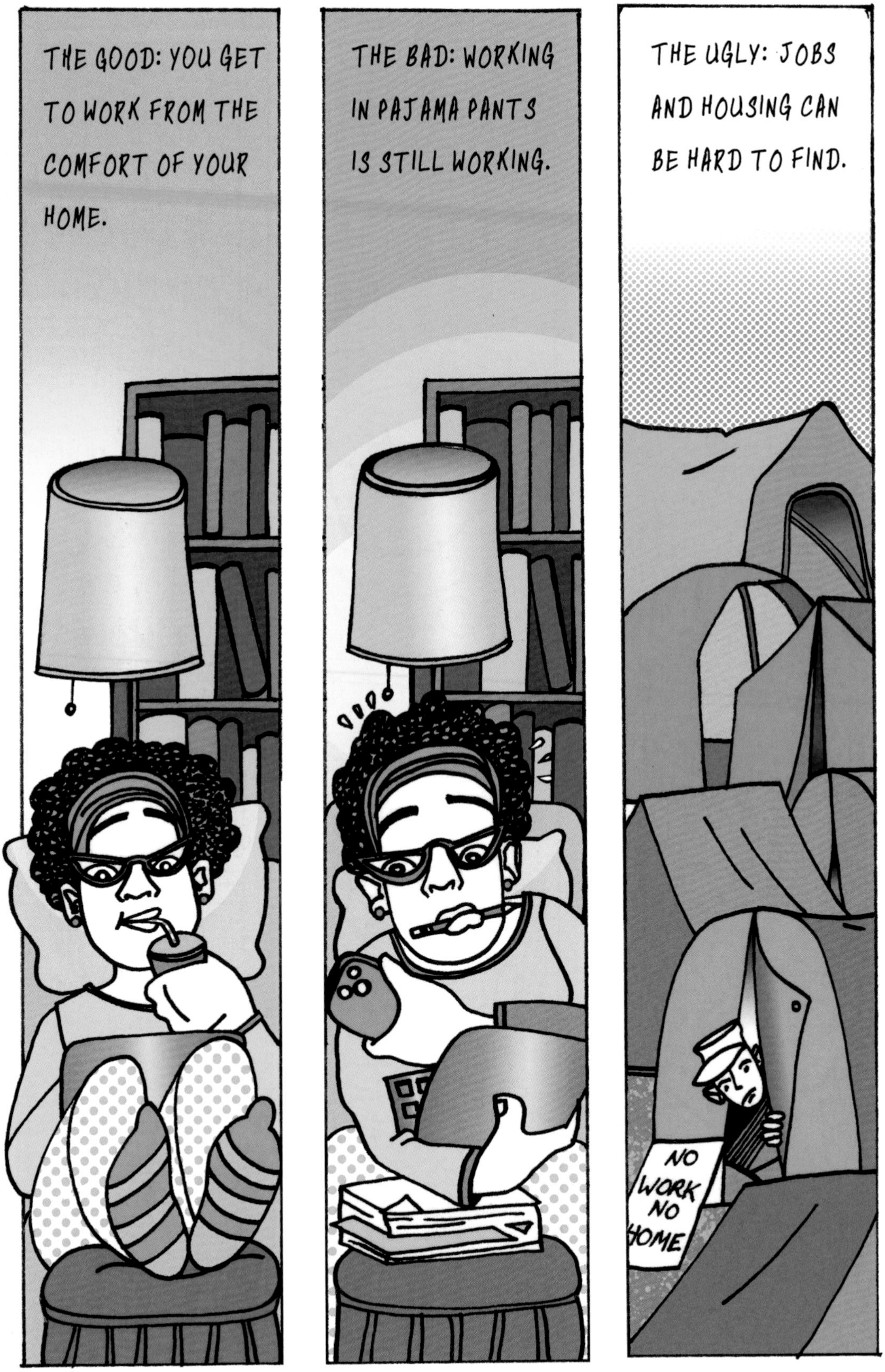
THE GOOD: YOU GET TO WORK FROM THE COMFORT OF YOUR HOME.
THE BAD: WORKING IN PAJAMA PANTS IS STILL WORKING.
THE UGLY: JOBS AND HOUSING CAN BE HARD TO FIND.
NO WORK NO HOME

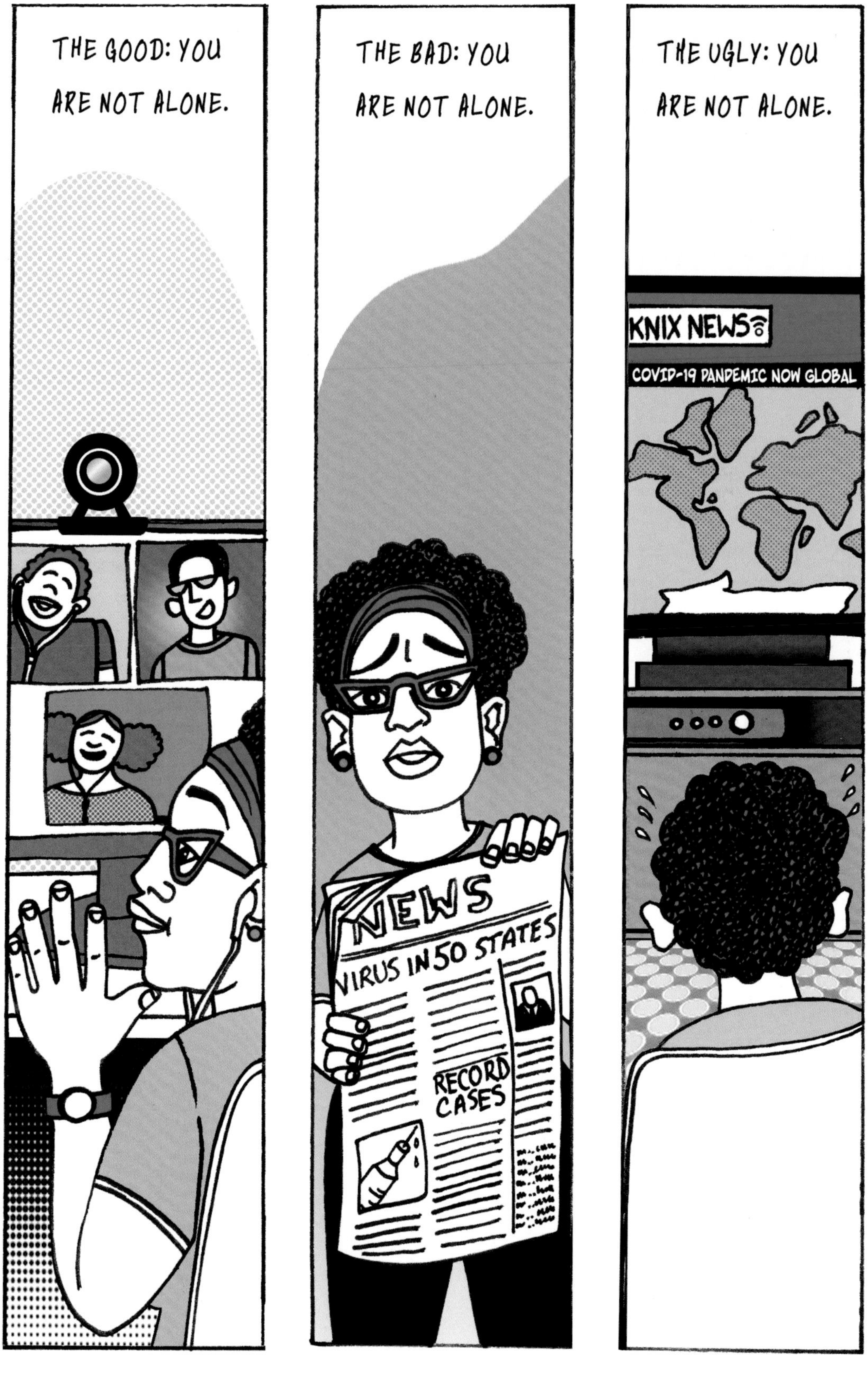
THE GOOD: YOU ARE NOT ALONE.
THE BAD: YOU ARE NOT ALONE.
NEWS
VIRUS IN 50 STATES
RECORD CASES
THE UGLY: YOU ARE NOT ALONE.
KNIX NEWS
COVID-19 PANDEMIC NOW GLOBAL

morning commute
Ria

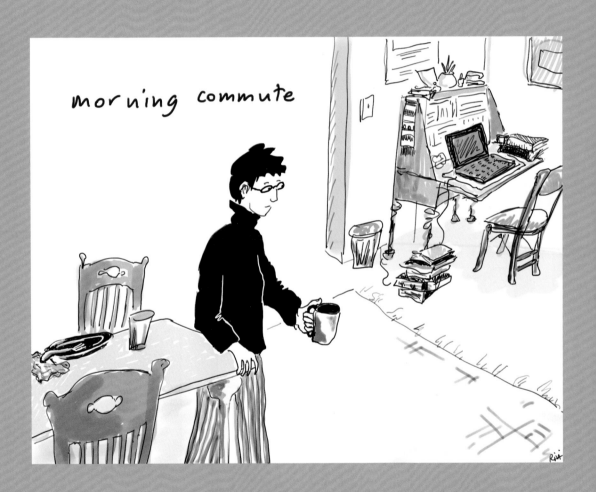

The IRON LUNG in the ENDERS LAB

by Katy Doughty

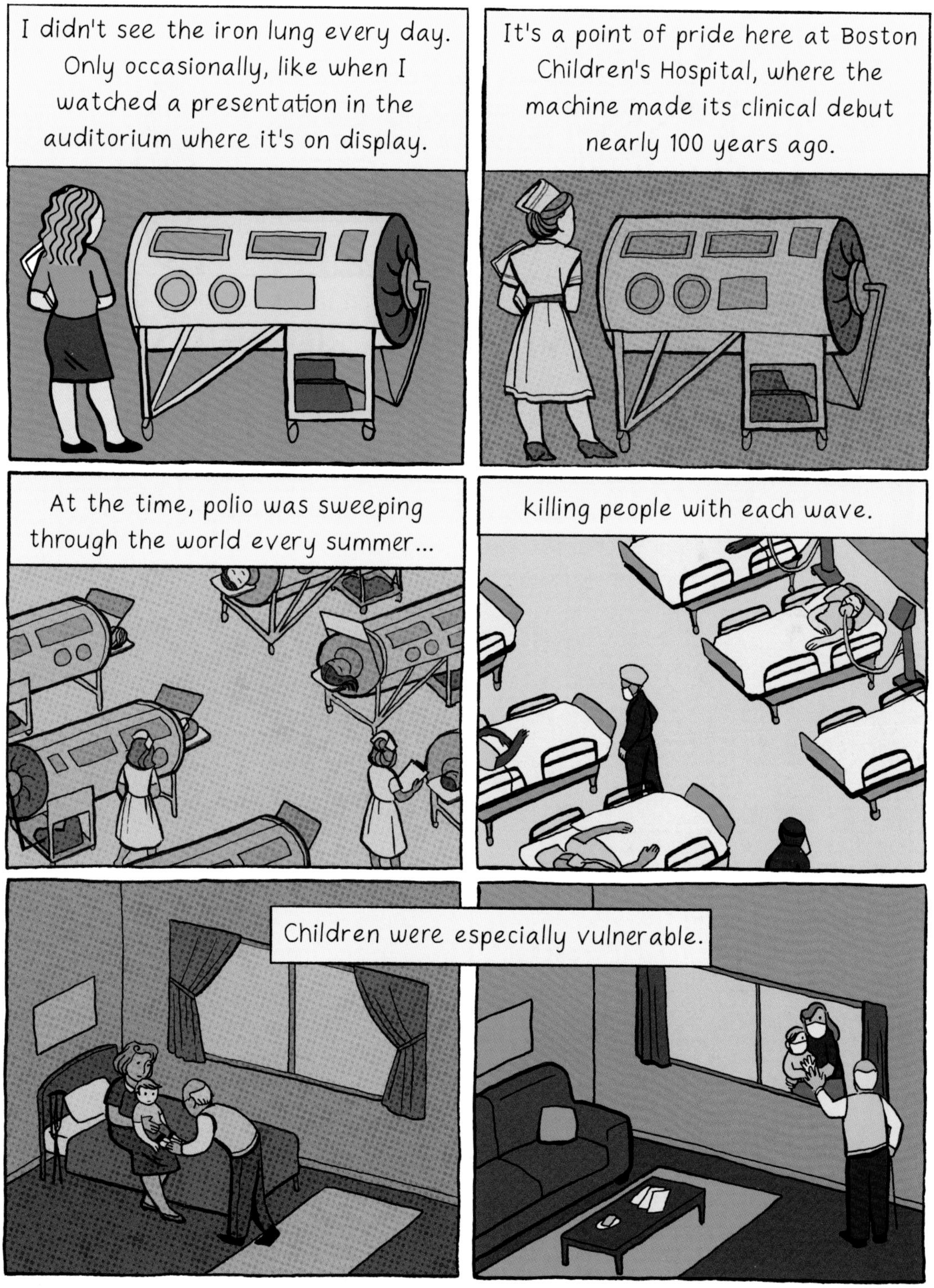
I didn't see the iron lung every day. Only occasionally, like when I watched a presentation in the auditorium where it's on display.
It's a point of pride here at Boston Children's Hospital, where the machine made its clinical debut nearly 100 years ago.
At the time, polio was sweeping through the world every summer...
killing people with each wave.
Children were especially vulnerable.

This machine, ancestor of the modern ventilator, stimulated breathing in paralyzed lungs by outsourcing the work of the diaphragm muscle to a mechanical diaphragm. The changes in air pressure forced air in and out of the lungs.

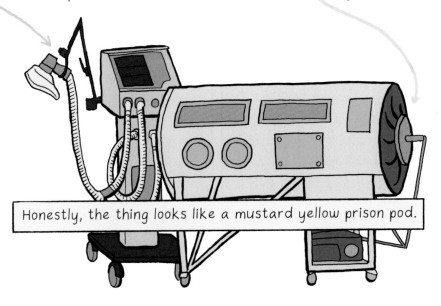

Honestly, the thing looks like a mustard yellow prison pod.

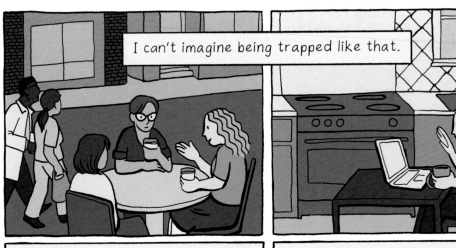

I can't imagine being trapped like that.

It was better than the alternative, though. Patients called it "restful."

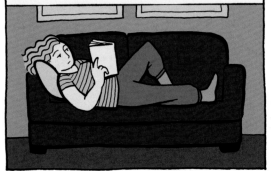

"There wasn't much for you to do in the iron lung," they said.

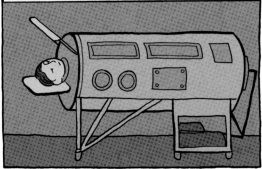

The lung is on display in the John Enders Research Lab...

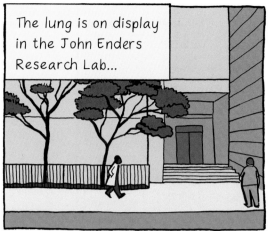

in front of a portrait of the lab's namesake.

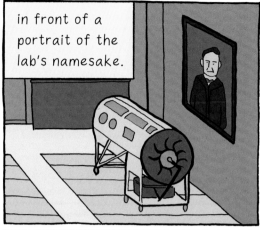

Enders's team managed to cultivate the polio virus using a neat little trick involving a mouse brain.

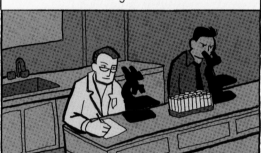

Jonas Salk developed a vaccine 4 years later.

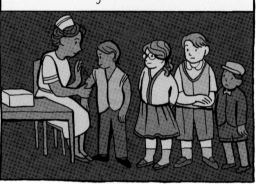

Here in this 150-year-old hospital, you see these artifacts and discoveries stacked on top of each other in the same place.

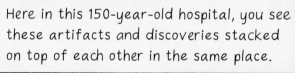

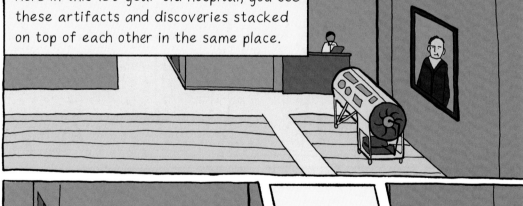

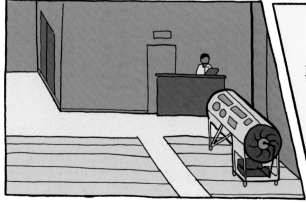

It's easy to forget the gaps in the timeline.

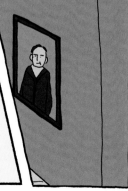

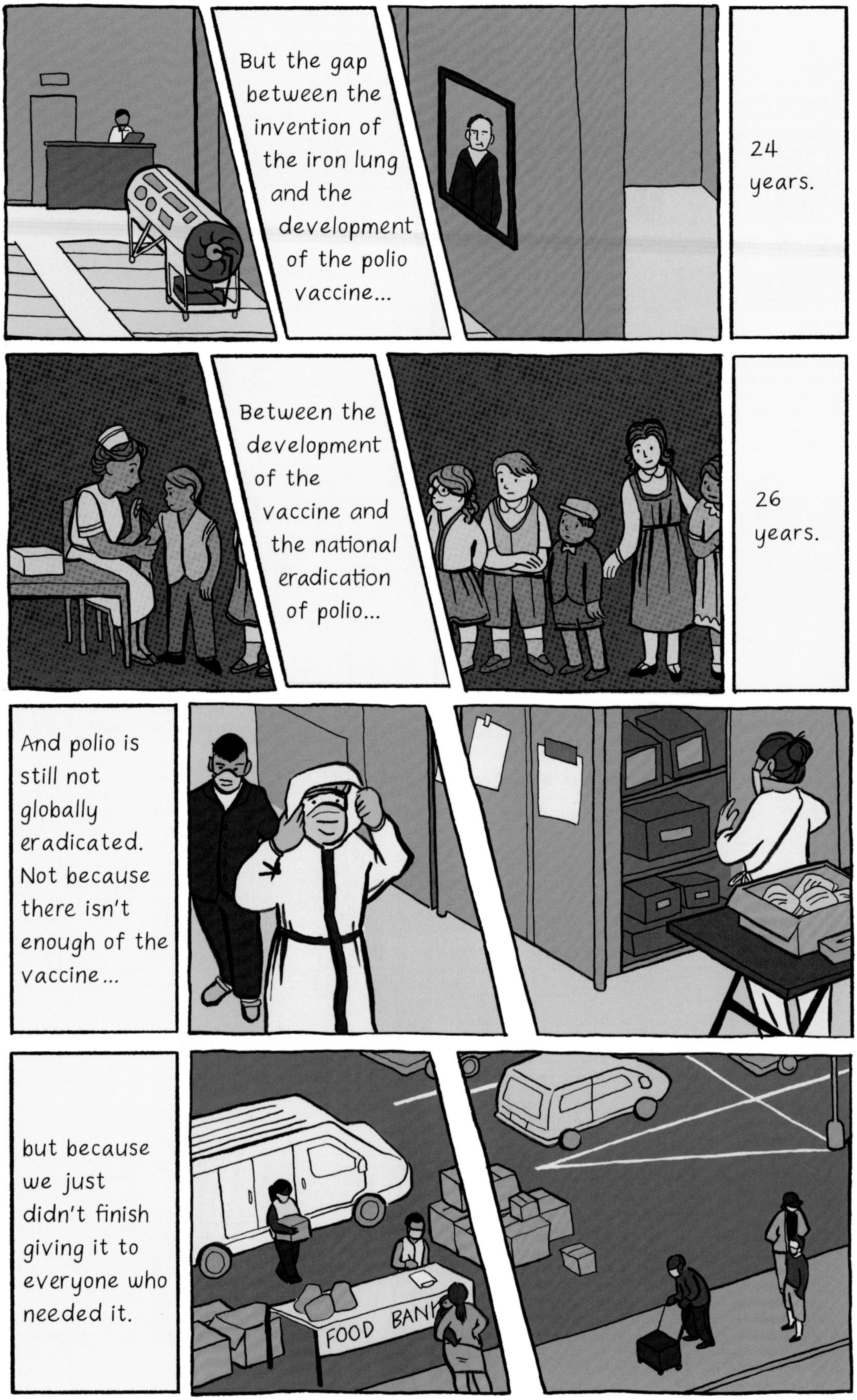
But the gap between the invention of the iron lung and the development of the polio vaccine...
24 years.
Between the development of the vaccine and the national eradication of polio...
26 years.
And polio is still not globally eradicated. Not because there isn't enough of the vaccine...
but because we just didn't finish giving it to everyone who needed it.
FOOD BANK

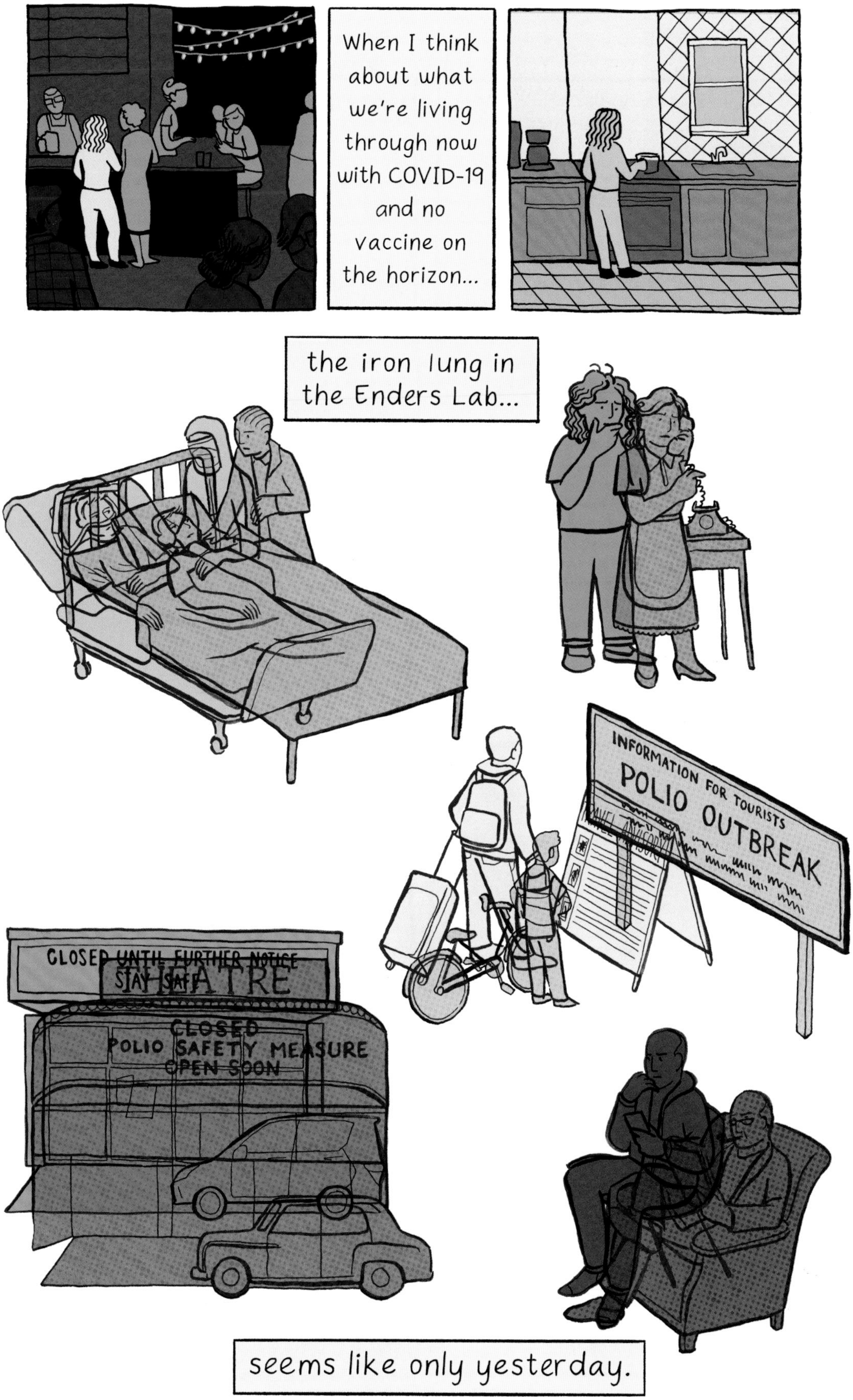
When I think about what we're living through now with COVID-19 and no vaccine on the horizon...
the iron lung in the Enders Lab...
INFORMATION FOR TOURISTS
POLIO OUTBREAK
CLOSED UNTIL FURTHER NOTICE
STAY SAFE
THEATRE
CLOSED
POLIO SAFETY MEASURE
OPEN SOON
seems like only yesterday.

PAST PANDEMICS

BY NED BARNETT

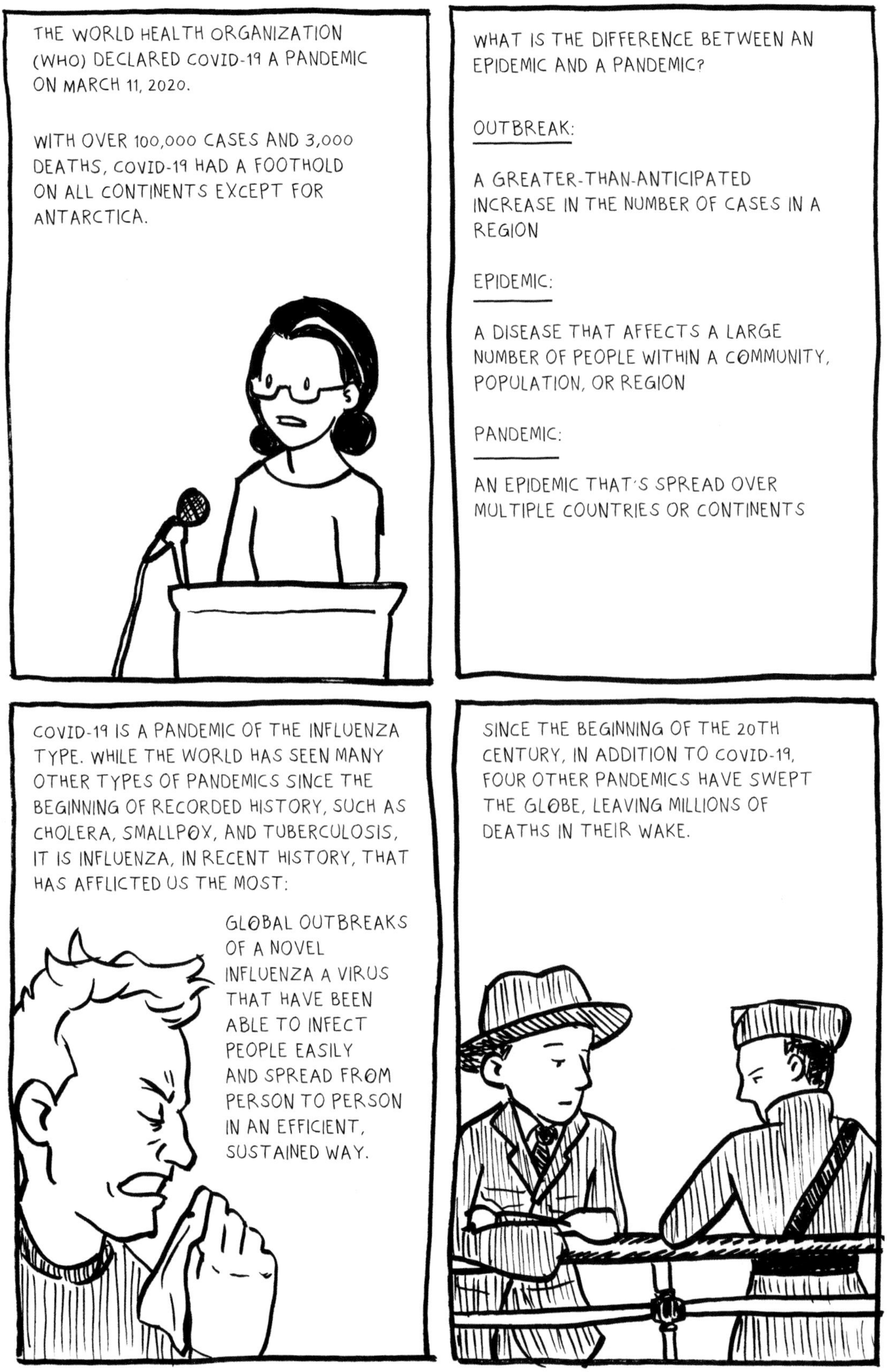
THE WORLD HEALTH ORGANIZATION (WHO) DECLARED COVID-19 A PANDEMIC ON MARCH 11, 2020.
WITH OVER 100,000 CASES AND 3,000 DEATHS, COVID-19 HAD A FOOTHOLD ON ALL CONTINENTS EXCEPT FOR ANTARCTICA.
WHAT IS THE DIFFERENCE BETWEEN AN EPIDEMIC AND A PANDEMIC?
OUTBREAK:
A GREATER-THAN-ANTICIPATED INCREASE IN THE NUMBER OF CASES IN A REGION
EPIDEMIC:
A DISEASE THAT AFFECTS A LARGE NUMBER OF PEOPLE WITHIN A COMMUNITY, POPULATION, OR REGION
PANDEMIC:
AN EPIDEMIC THAT'S SPREAD OVER MULTIPLE COUNTRIES OR CONTINENTS
COVID-19 IS A PANDEMIC OF THE INFLUENZA TYPE. WHILE THE WORLD HAS SEEN MANY OTHER TYPES OF PANDEMICS SINCE THE BEGINNING OF RECORDED HISTORY, SUCH AS CHOLERA, SMALLPOX, AND TUBERCULOSIS, IT IS INFLUENZA, IN RECENT HISTORY, THAT HAS AFFLICTED US THE MOST:
GLOBAL OUTBREAKS OF A NOVEL INFLUENZA A VIRUS THAT HAVE BEEN ABLE TO INFECT PEOPLE EASILY AND SPREAD FROM PERSON TO PERSON IN AN EFFICIENT, SUSTAINED WAY.
SINCE THE BEGINNING OF THE 20TH CENTURY, IN ADDITION TO COVID-19, FOUR OTHER PANDEMICS HAVE SWEPT THE GLOBE, LEAVING MILLIONS OF DEATHS IN THEIR WAKE.

INFLUENZA OF 1918 (H1N1)

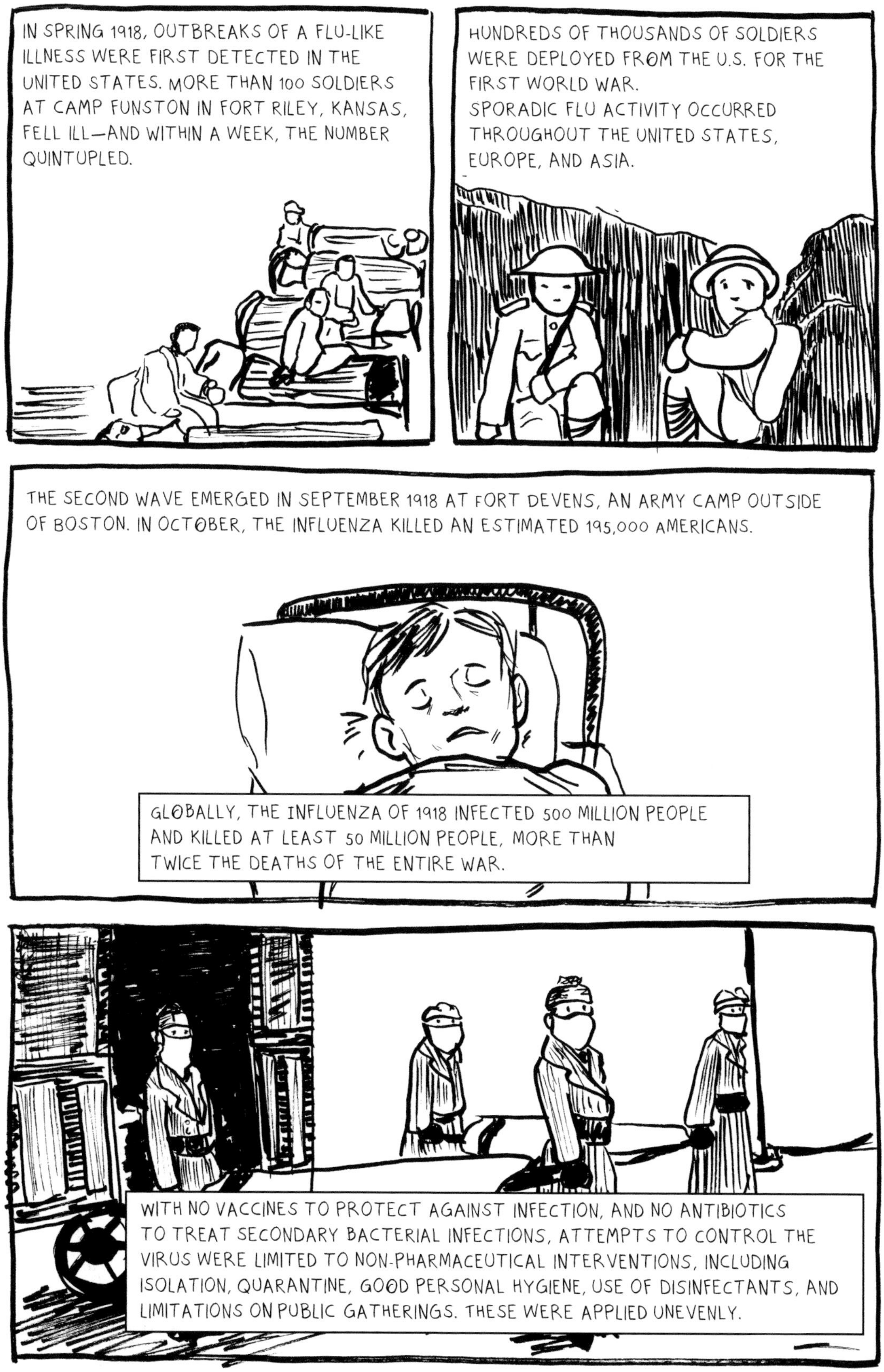
IN SPRING 1918, OUTBREAKS OF A FLU-LIKE ILLNESS WERE FIRST DETECTED IN THE UNITED STATES. MORE THAN 100 SOLDIERS AT CAMP FUNSTON IN FORT RILEY, KANSAS, FELL ILL—AND WITHIN A WEEK, THE NUMBER QUINTUPLED.
HUNDREDS OF THOUSANDS OF SOLDIERS WERE DEPLOYED FROM THE U.S. FOR THE FIRST WORLD WAR.
SPORADIC FLU ACTIVITY OCCURRED THROUGHOUT THE UNITED STATES, EUROPE, AND ASIA.
THE SECOND WAVE EMERGED IN SEPTEMBER 1918 AT FORT DEVENS, AN ARMY CAMP OUTSIDE OF BOSTON. IN OCTOBER, THE INFLUENZA KILLED AN ESTIMATED 195,000 AMERICANS.
GLOBALLY, THE INFLUENZA OF 1918 INFECTED 500 MILLION PEOPLE AND KILLED AT LEAST 50 MILLION PEOPLE, MORE THAN TWICE THE DEATHS OF THE ENTIRE WAR.
WITH NO VACCINES TO PROTECT AGAINST INFECTION, AND NO ANTIBIOTICS TO TREAT SECONDARY BACTERIAL INFECTIONS, ATTEMPTS TO CONTROL THE VIRUS WERE LIMITED TO NON-PHARMACEUTICAL INTERVENTIONS, INCLUDING ISOLATION, QUARANTINE, GOOD PERSONAL HYGIENE, USE OF DISINFECTANTS, AND LIMITATIONS ON PUBLIC GATHERINGS. THESE WERE APPLIED UNEVENLY.

1957-1958 PANDEMIC (H2N2)

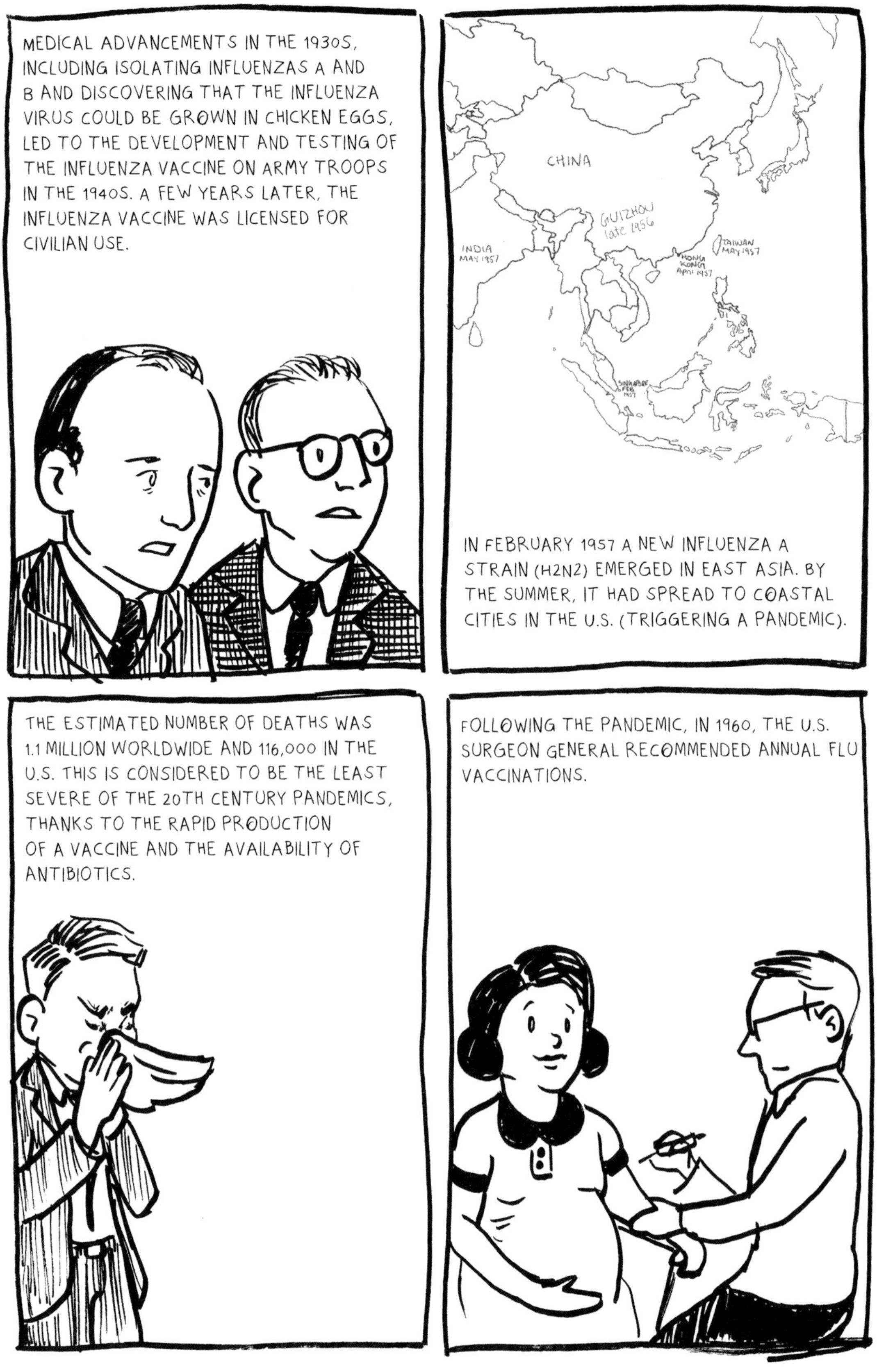
MEDICAL ADVANCEMENTS IN THE 1930S, INCLUDING ISOLATING INFLUENZAS A AND B AND DISCOVERING THAT THE INFLUENZA VIRUS COULD BE GROWN IN CHICKEN EGGS, LED TO THE DEVELOPMENT AND TESTING OF THE INFLUENZA VACCINE ON ARMY TROOPS IN THE 1940S. A FEW YEARS LATER, THE INFLUENZA VACCINE WAS LICENSED FOR CIVILIAN USE.
CHINA
GUIZHOU late 1956
INDIA MAY 1957
TAIWAN MAY 1957
HONG KONG April 1957
IN FEBRUARY 1957 A NEW INFLUENZA A STRAIN (H2N2) EMERGED IN EAST ASIA. BY THE SUMMER, IT HAD SPREAD TO COASTAL CITIES IN THE U.S. (TRIGGERING A PANDEMIC).
THE ESTIMATED NUMBER OF DEATHS WAS 1.1 MILLION WORLDWIDE AND 116,000 IN THE U.S. THIS IS CONSIDERED TO BE THE LEAST SEVERE OF THE 20TH CENTURY PANDEMICS, THANKS TO THE RAPID PRODUCTION OF A VACCINE AND THE AVAILABILITY OF ANTIBIOTICS.
FOLLOWING THE PANDEMIC, IN 1960, THE U.S. SURGEON GENERAL RECOMMENDED ANNUAL FLU VACCINATIONS.

1968 PANDEMIC (H3N2)

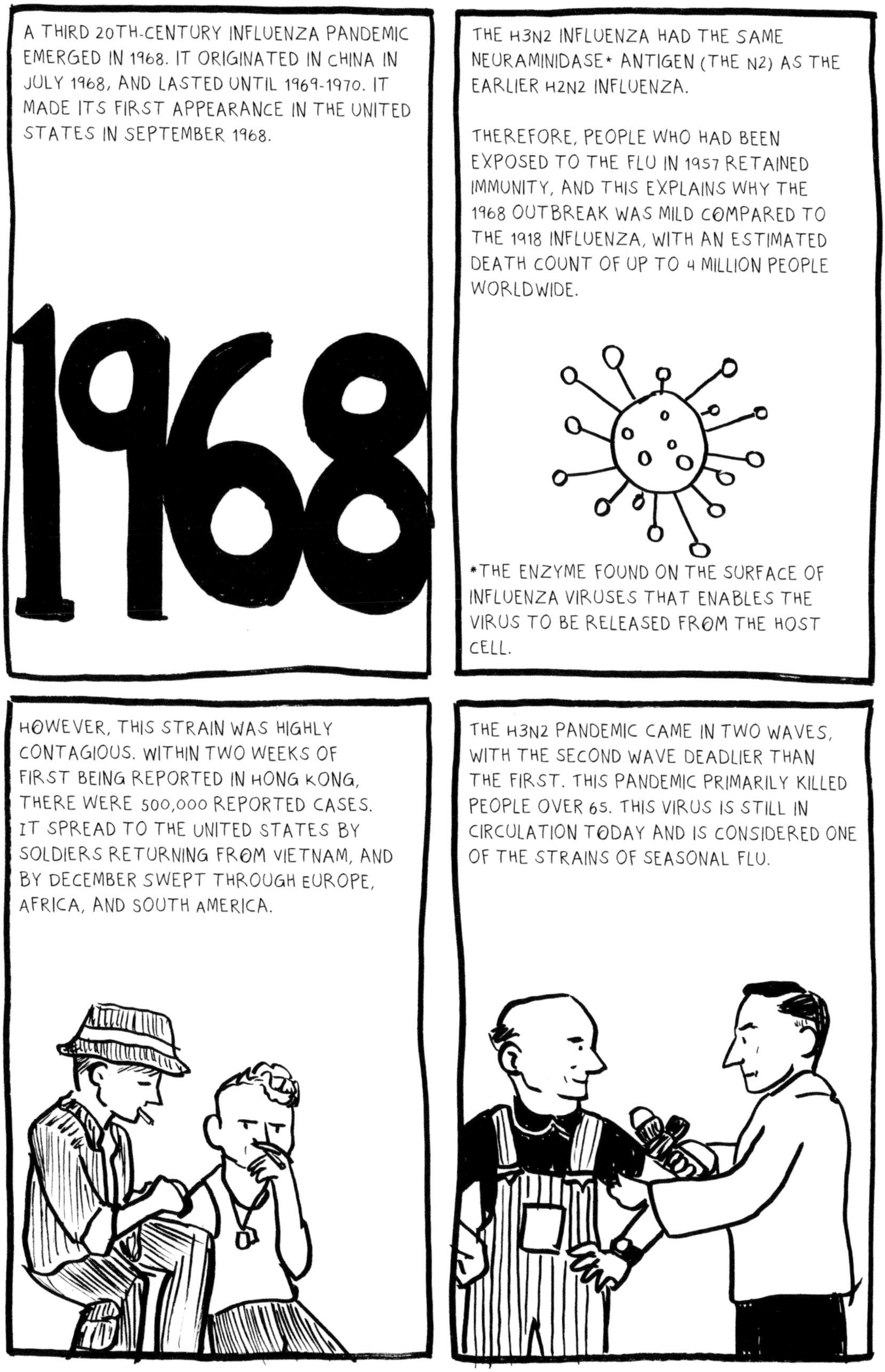

A THIRD 20TH-CENTURY INFLUENZA PANDEMIC EMERGED IN 1968. IT ORIGINATED IN CHINA IN JULY 1968, AND LASTED UNTIL 1969-1970. IT MADE ITS FIRST APPEARANCE IN THE UNITED STATES IN SEPTEMBER 1968.

1968

THE H3N2 INFLUENZA HAD THE SAME NEURAMINIDASE* ANTIGEN (THE N2) AS THE EARLIER H2N2 INFLUENZA.

THEREFORE, PEOPLE WHO HAD BEEN EXPOSED TO THE FLU IN 1957 RETAINED IMMUNITY, AND THIS EXPLAINS WHY THE 1968 OUTBREAK WAS MILD COMPARED TO THE 1918 INFLUENZA, WITH AN ESTIMATED DEATH COUNT OF UP TO 4 MILLION PEOPLE WORLDWIDE.

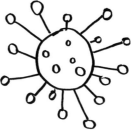

*THE ENZYME FOUND ON THE SURFACE OF INFLUENZA VIRUSES THAT ENABLES THE VIRUS TO BE RELEASED FROM THE HOST CELL.

HOWEVER, THIS STRAIN WAS HIGHLY CONTAGIOUS. WITHIN TWO WEEKS OF FIRST BEING REPORTED IN HONG KONG, THERE WERE 500,000 REPORTED CASES. IT SPREAD TO THE UNITED STATES BY SOLDIERS RETURNING FROM VIETNAM, AND BY DECEMBER SWEPT THROUGH EUROPE, AFRICA, AND SOUTH AMERICA.

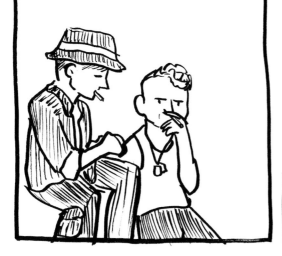

THE H3N2 PANDEMIC CAME IN TWO WAVES, WITH THE SECOND WAVE DEADLIER THAN THE FIRST. THIS PANDEMIC PRIMARILY KILLED PEOPLE OVER 65. THIS VIRUS IS STILL IN CIRCULATION TODAY AND IS CONSIDERED ONE OF THE STRAINS OF SEASONAL FLU.

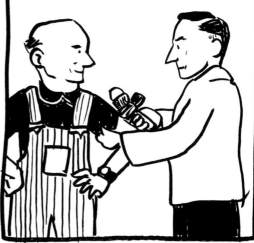

2009 SWINE FLU PANDEMIC (H1N1)

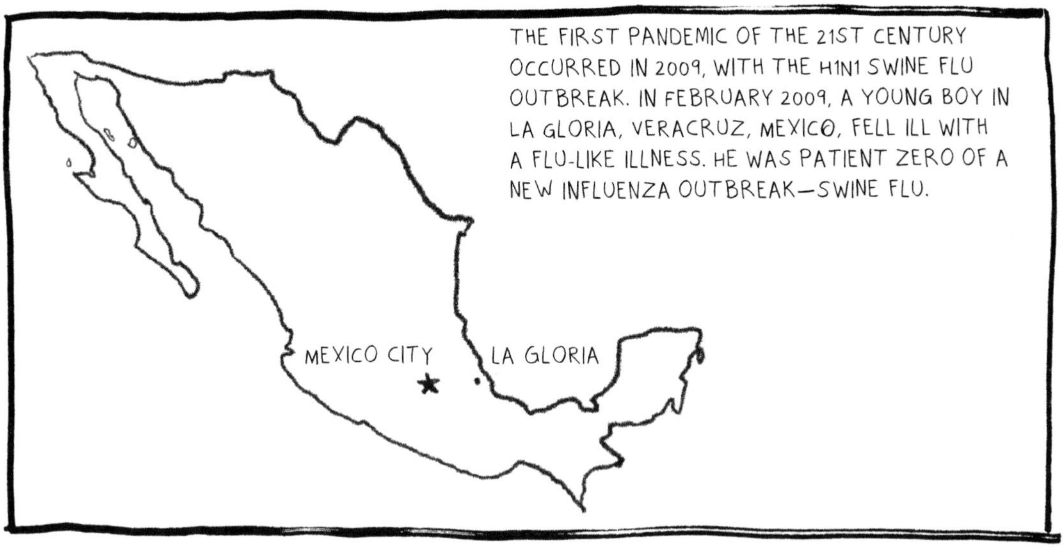
THE FIRST PANDEMIC OF THE 21ST CENTURY OCCURRED IN 2009, WITH THE H1N1 SWINE FLU OUTBREAK. IN FEBRUARY 2009, A YOUNG BOY IN LA GLORIA, VERACRUZ, MEXICO, FELL ILL WITH A FLU-LIKE ILLNESS. HE WAS PATIENT ZERO OF A NEW INFLUENZA OUTBREAK—SWINE FLU.
MEXICO CITY
LA GLORIA

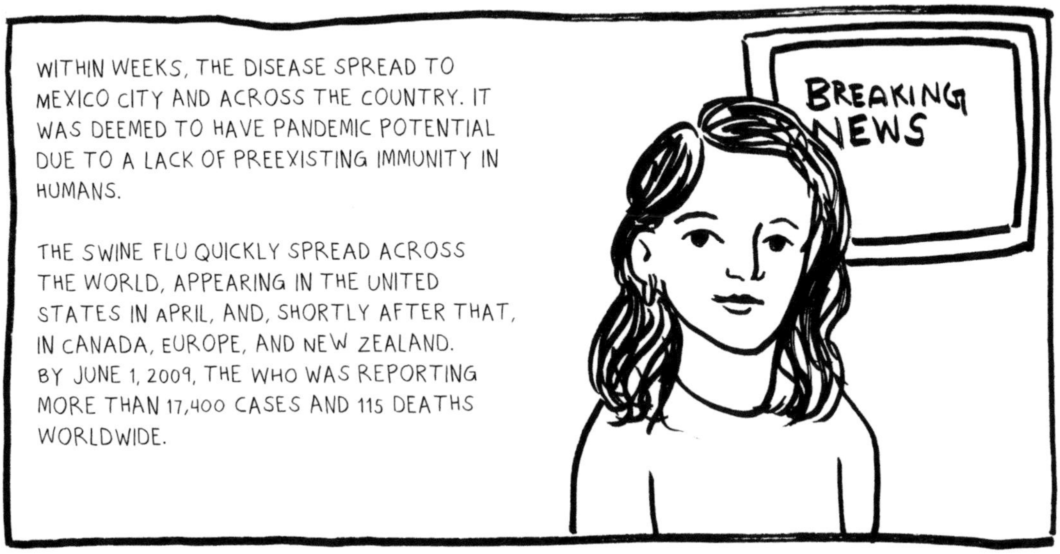
WITHIN WEEKS, THE DISEASE SPREAD TO MEXICO CITY AND ACROSS THE COUNTRY. IT WAS DEEMED TO HAVE PANDEMIC POTENTIAL DUE TO A LACK OF PREEXISTING IMMUNITY IN HUMANS.
THE SWINE FLU QUICKLY SPREAD ACROSS THE WORLD, APPEARING IN THE UNITED STATES IN APRIL, AND, SHORTLY AFTER THAT, IN CANADA, EUROPE, AND NEW ZEALAND. BY JUNE 1, 2009, THE WHO WAS REPORTING MORE THAN 17,400 CASES AND 115 DEATHS WORLDWIDE.
BREAKING NEWS

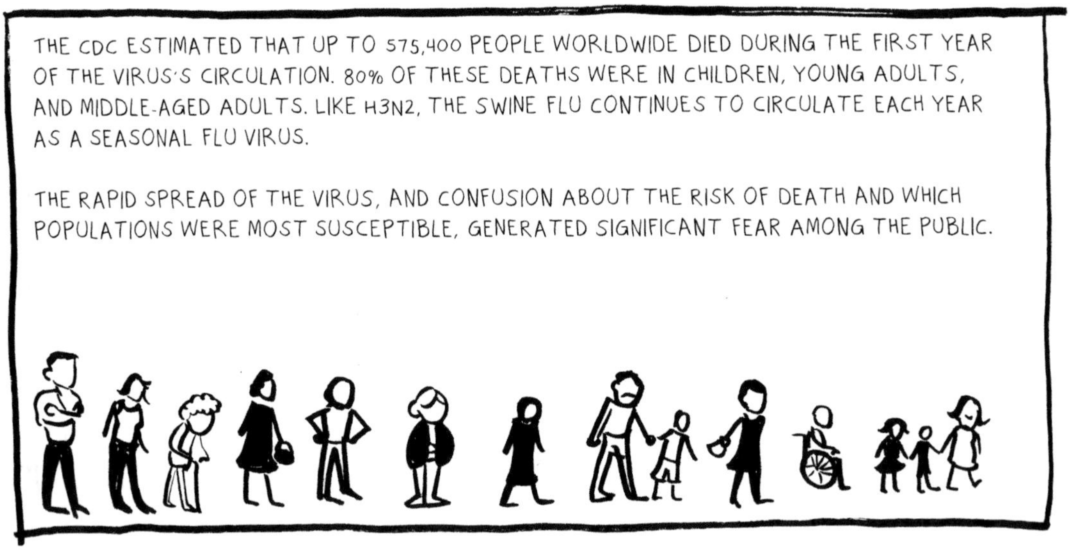
THE CDC ESTIMATED THAT UP TO 575,400 PEOPLE WORLDWIDE DIED DURING THE FIRST YEAR OF THE VIRUS'S CIRCULATION. 80% OF THESE DEATHS WERE IN CHILDREN, YOUNG ADULTS, AND MIDDLE-AGED ADULTS. LIKE H3N2, THE SWINE FLU CONTINUES TO CIRCULATE EACH YEAR AS A SEASONAL FLU VIRUS.
THE RAPID SPREAD OF THE VIRUS, AND CONFUSION ABOUT THE RISK OF DEATH AND WHICH POPULATIONS WERE MOST SUSCEPTIBLE, GENERATED SIGNIFICANT FEAR AMONG THE PUBLIC.

2020 COVID-19

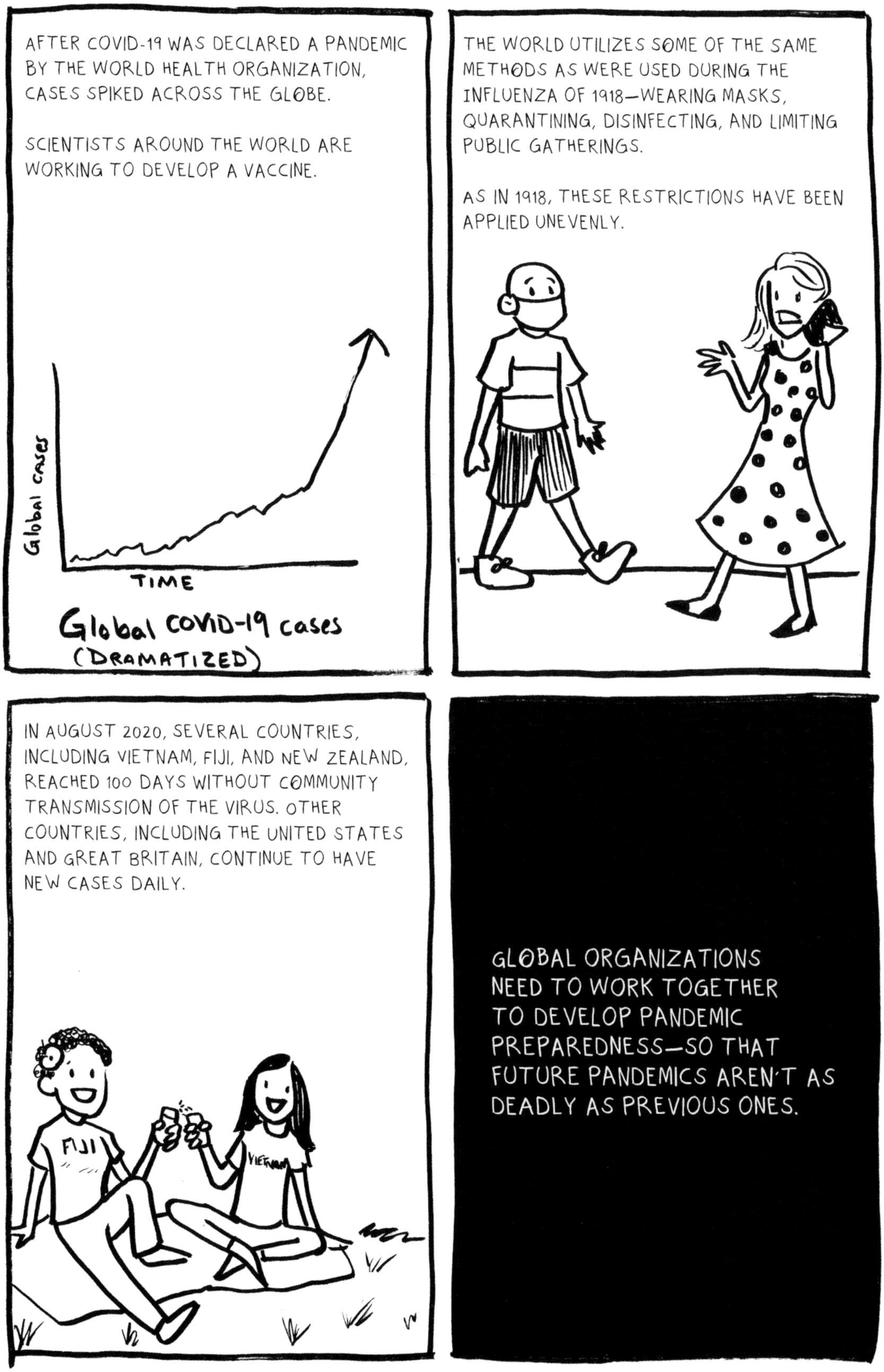
AFTER COVID-19 WAS DECLARED A PANDEMIC BY THE WORLD HEALTH ORGANIZATION, CASES SPIKED ACROSS THE GLOBE.
SCIENTISTS AROUND THE WORLD ARE WORKING TO DEVELOP A VACCINE.
Global cases
TIME
Global COVID-19 cases (DRAMATIZED)
THE WORLD UTILIZES SOME OF THE SAME METHODS AS WERE USED DURING THE INFLUENZA OF 1918—WEARING MASKS, QUARANTINING, DISINFECTING, AND LIMITING PUBLIC GATHERINGS.
AS IN 1918, THESE RESTRICTIONS HAVE BEEN APPLIED UNEVENLY.
IN AUGUST 2020, SEVERAL COUNTRIES, INCLUDING VIETNAM, FIJI, AND NEW ZEALAND, REACHED 100 DAYS WITHOUT COMMUNITY TRANSMISSION OF THE VIRUS. OTHER COUNTRIES, INCLUDING THE UNITED STATES AND GREAT BRITAIN, CONTINUE TO HAVE NEW CASES DAILY.
FIJI
VIETNAM
GLOBAL ORGANIZATIONS NEED TO WORK TOGETHER TO DEVELOP PANDEMIC PREPAREDNESS—SO THAT FUTURE PANDEMICS AREN'T AS DEADLY AS PREVIOUS ONES.

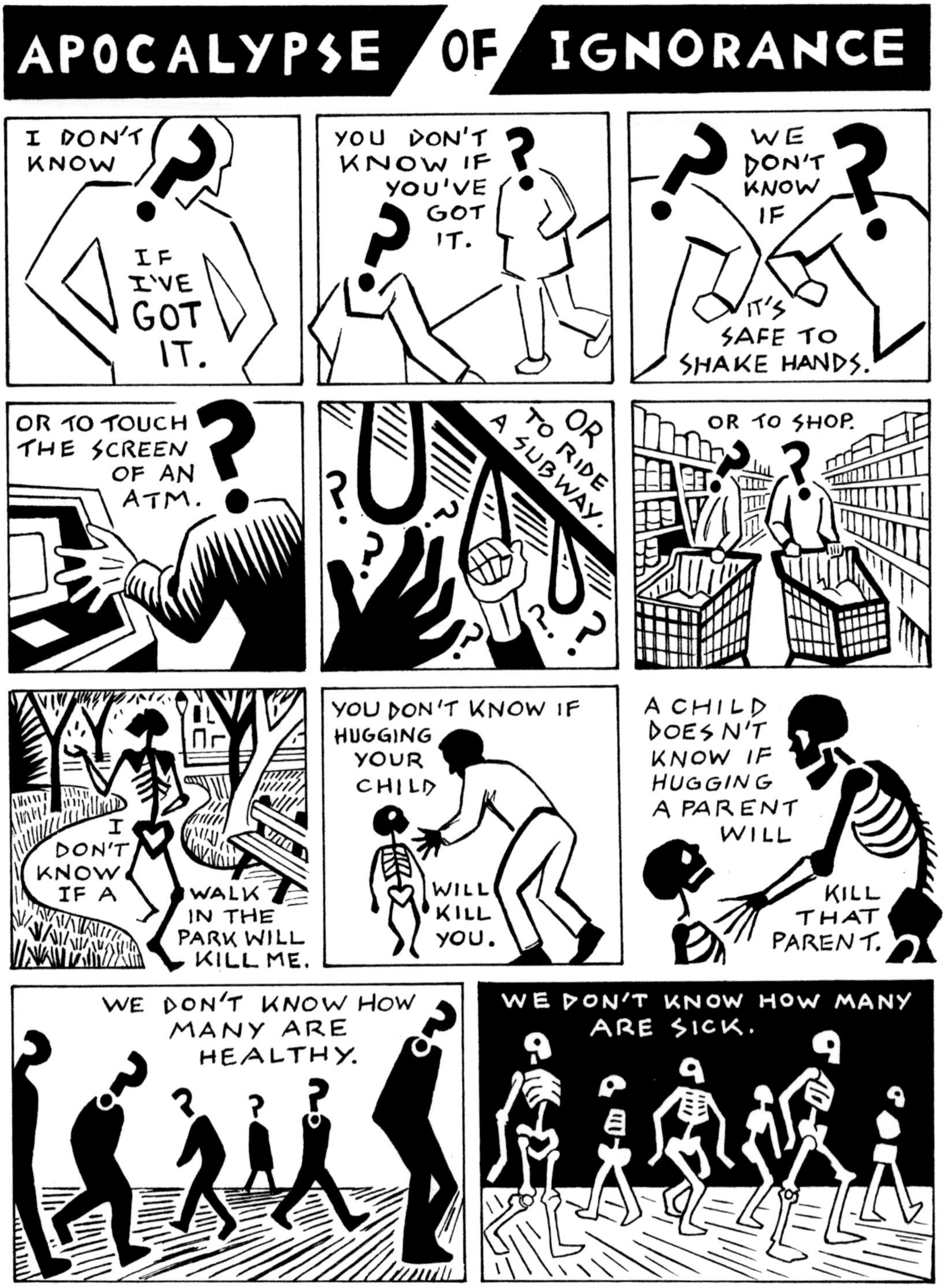
APOCALYPSE OF IGNORANCE
I DON'T KNOW
IF I'VE GOT IT.
YOU DON'T KNOW IF YOU'VE GOT IT.
WE DON'T KNOW IF
IT'S SAFE TO SHAKE HANDS.
OR TO TOUCH THE SCREEN OF AN ATM.
OR TO RIDE A SUBWAY.
OR TO SHOP.
I DON'T KNOW IF A
WALK IN THE PARK WILL KILL ME.
YOU DON'T KNOW IF HUGGING YOUR CHILD
WILL KILL YOU.
A CHILD DOESN'T KNOW IF HUGGING A PARENT WILL
KILL THAT PARENT.
WE DON'T KNOW HOW MANY ARE HEALTHY.
WE DON'T KNOW HOW MANY ARE SICK.

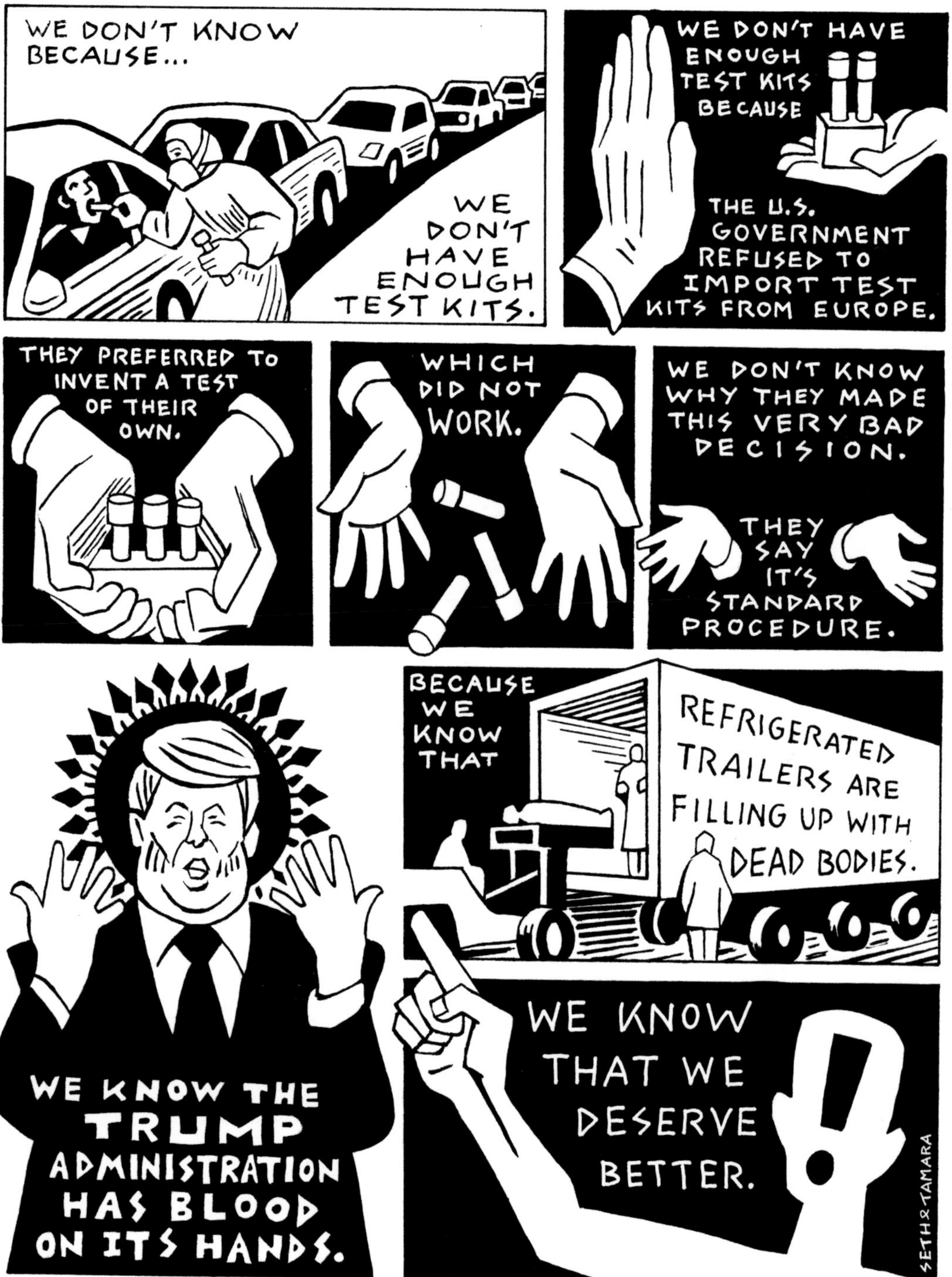
WE DON'T KNOW BECAUSE...
WE DON'T HAVE ENOUGH TEST KITS.
WE DON'T HAVE ENOUGH TEST KITS BECAUSE
THE U.S. GOVERNMENT REFUSED TO IMPORT TEST KITS FROM EUROPE.
THEY PREFERRED TO INVENT A TEST OF THEIR OWN.
WHICH DID NOT WORK.
WE DON'T KNOW WHY THEY MADE THIS VERY BAD DECISION.
THEY SAY IT'S STANDARD PROCEDURE.
WE KNOW THE TRUMP ADMINISTRATION HAS BLOOD ON ITS HANDS.
BECAUSE WE KNOW THAT
REFRIGERATED TRAILERS ARE FILLING UP WITH DEAD BODIES.
WE KNOW THAT WE DESERVE BETTER.
SETH & TAMARA

WRITTEN IN MARCH OF 2020 WHEN WE DID NOT KNOW.

ISOLATION EXERCISES

– LAURA HOLZMAN –

DURING THE STAY-AT-HOME ORDER IN INDIANAPOLIS,
AGAINST A BACKDROP OF FEAR, ILLNESS, AND EMERGENCY,
I FIXATED ON THE GLIMPSES I GOT INTO OTHER PEOPLE'S LIVES.

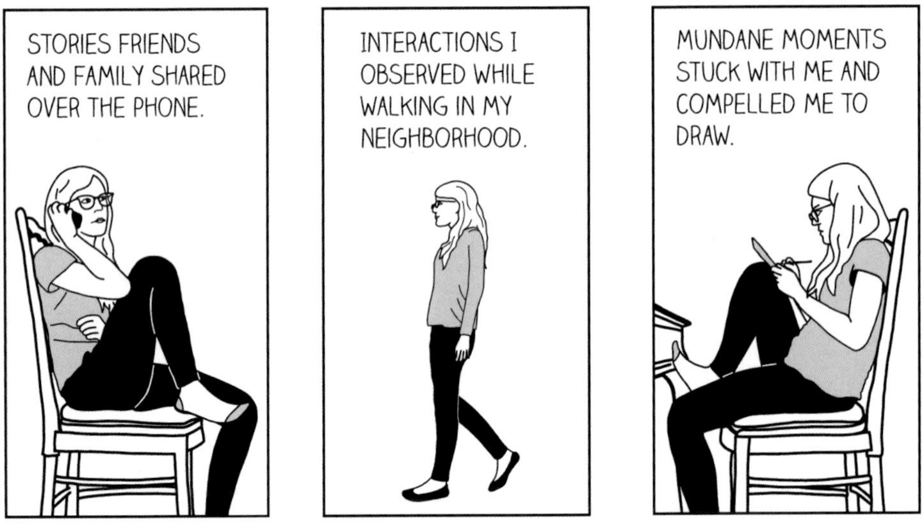
STORIES FRIENDS AND FAMILY SHARED OVER THE PHONE.
INTERACTIONS I OBSERVED WHILE WALKING IN MY NEIGHBORHOOD.
MUNDANE MOMENTS STUCK WITH ME AND COMPELLED ME TO DRAW.

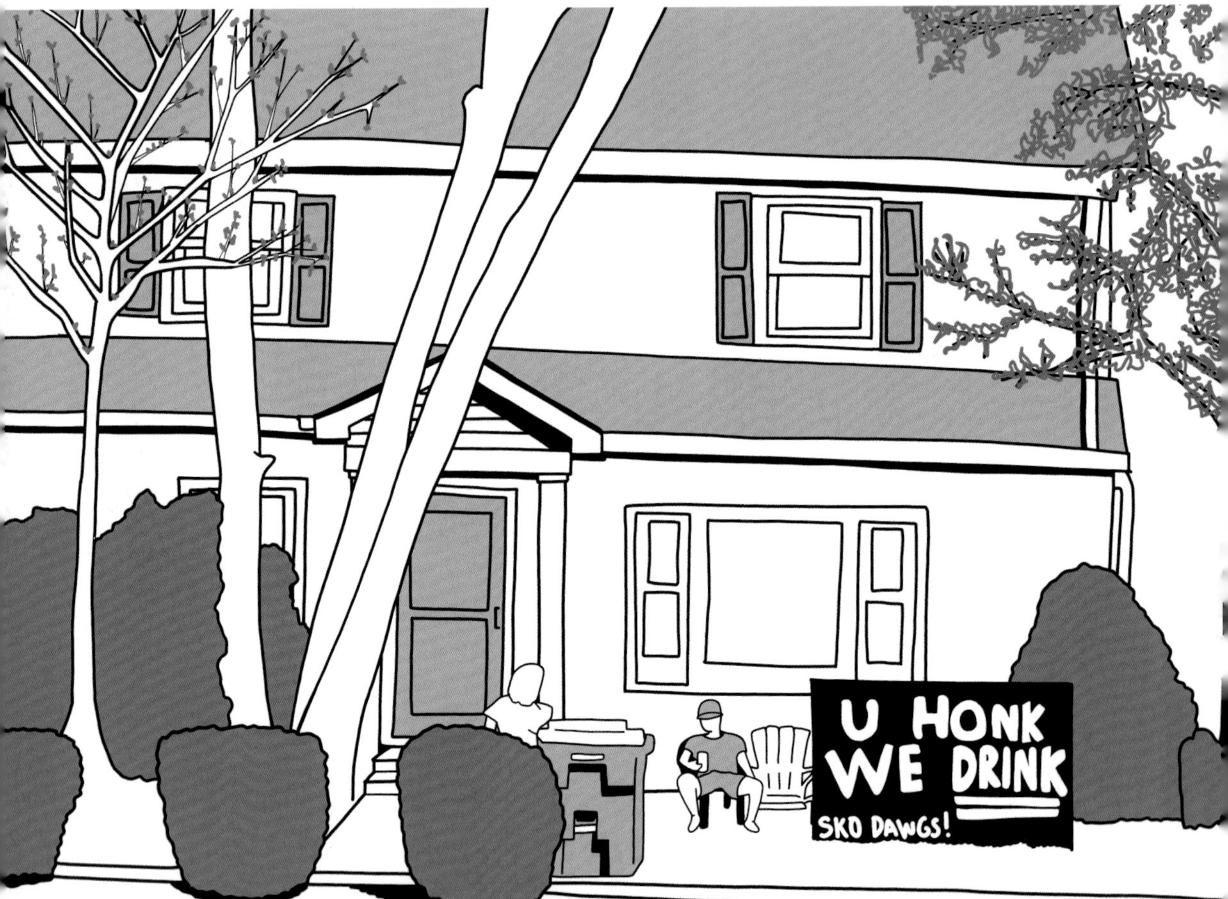
U HONK
WE DRINK
SKO DAWGS!

YOUR DAD SEEMS FINE BUT I'M GOING NUTS.

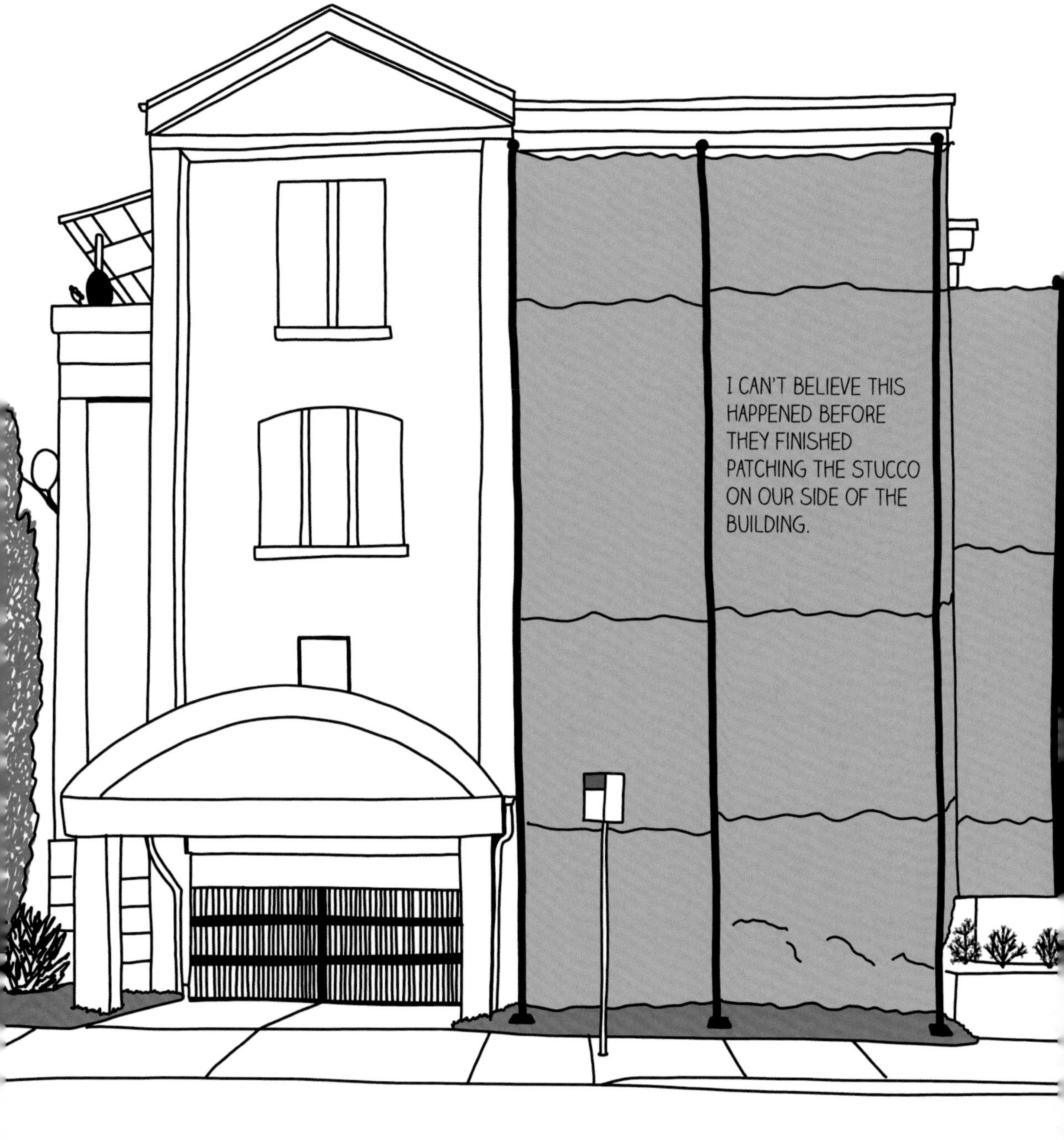
I CAN'T BELIEVE THIS HAPPENED BEFORE THEY FINISHED PATCHING THE STUCCO ON OUR SIDE OF THE BUILDING.

I MIGHT HAVE TO TAKE SOME SCISSORS TO THAT TARP.

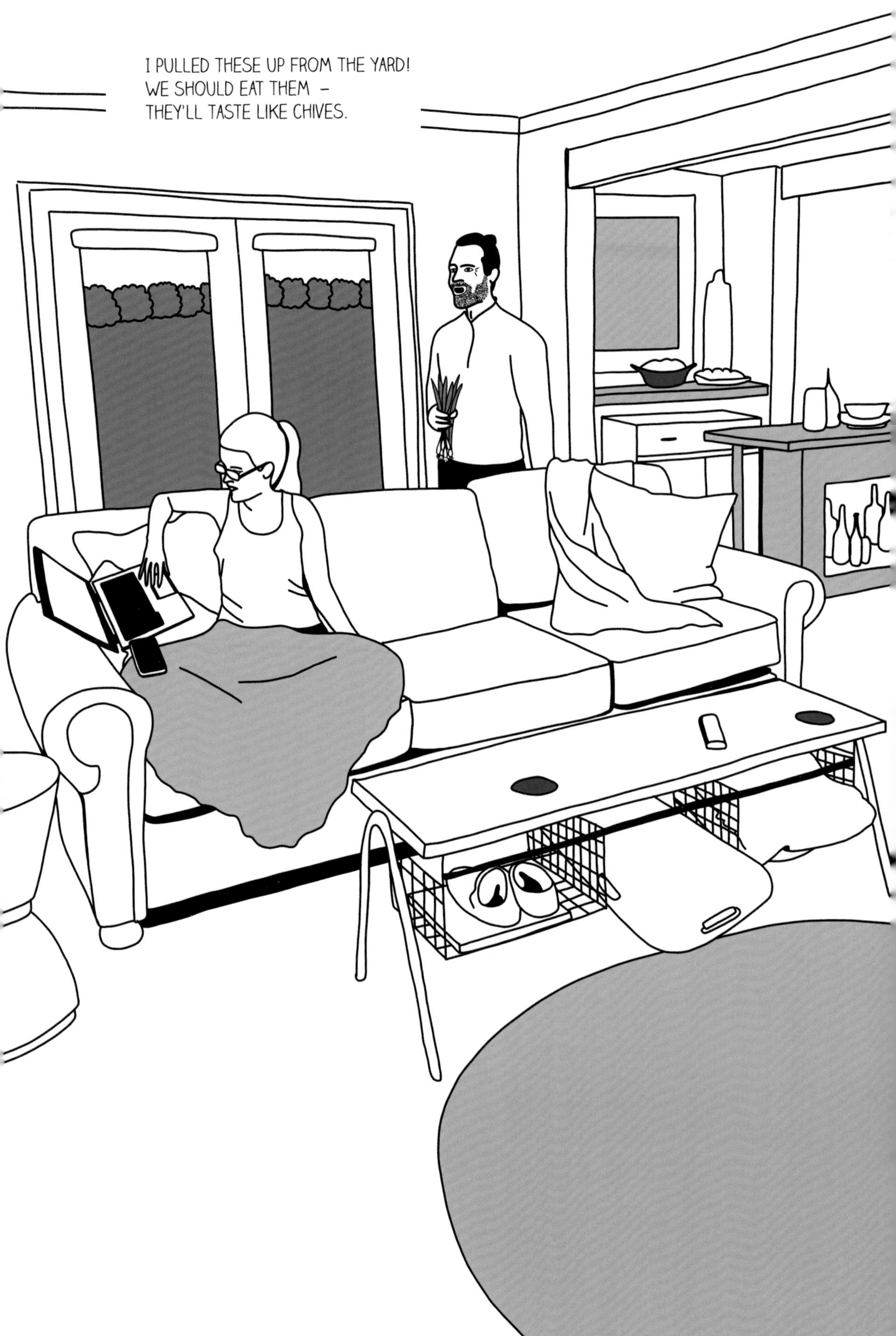
I PULLED THESE UP FROM THE YARD!
WE SHOULD EAT THEM –
THEY'LL TASTE LIKE CHIVES.

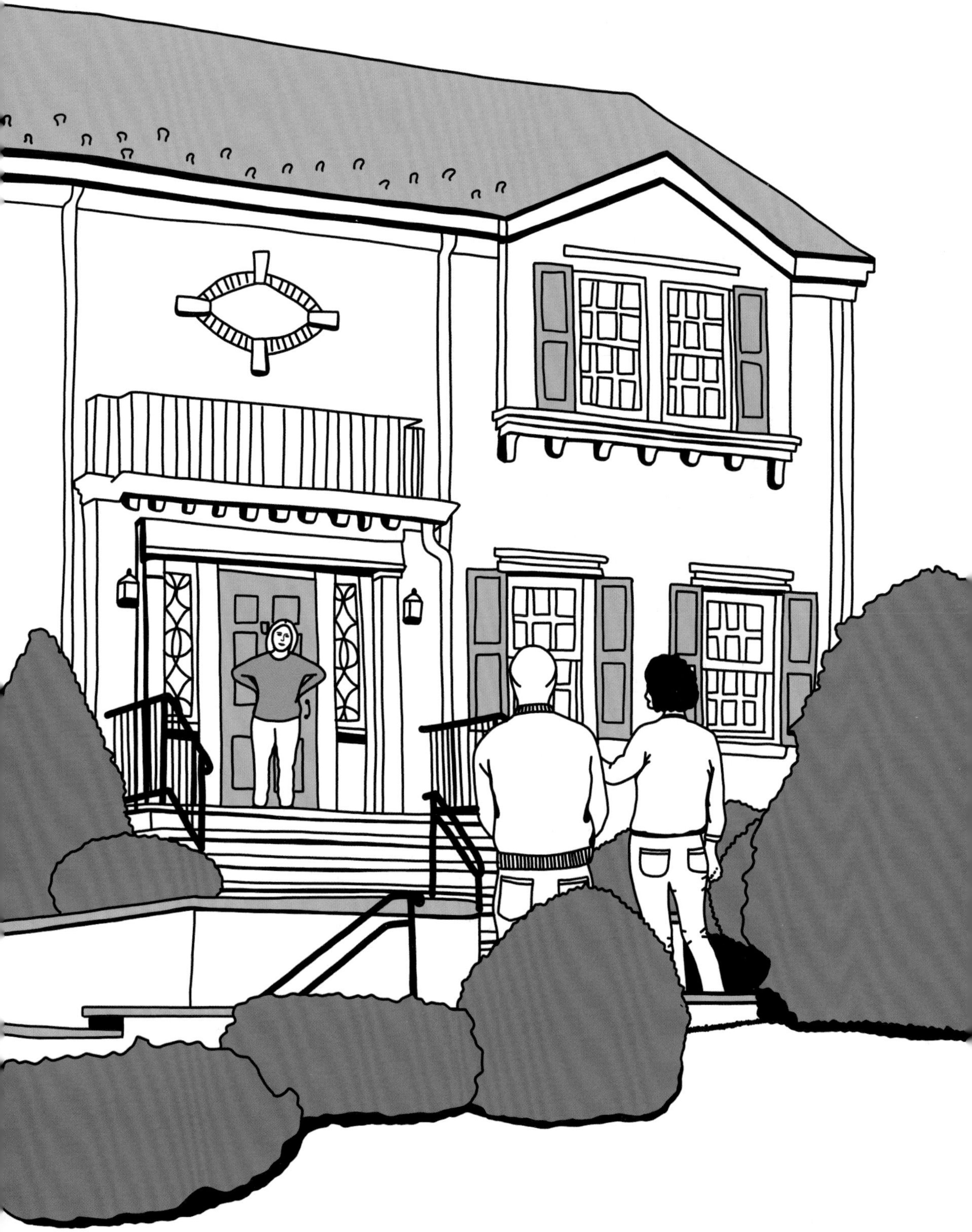

THEY HAD CHICKEN AT THE STORE SO WE GOT YOU SOME.
AND WE THREW IN A FEW HAMANTASCHEN FROM THE FREEZER.

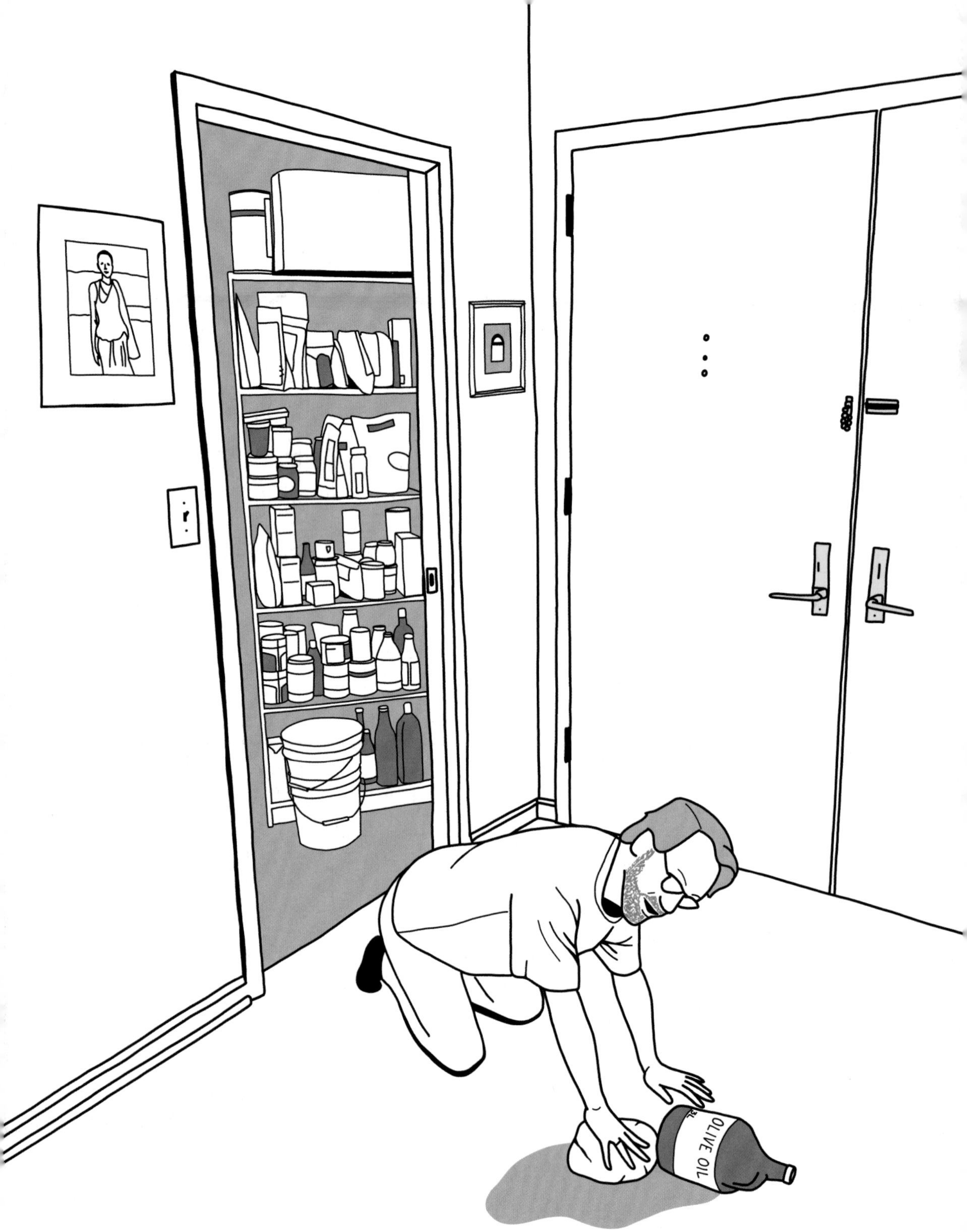
OLIVE OIL
3L

IT'S JUST A CRACK... GRAB A JAR –
IF YOU HURRY WE COULD SALVAGE AT LEAST A LITER.

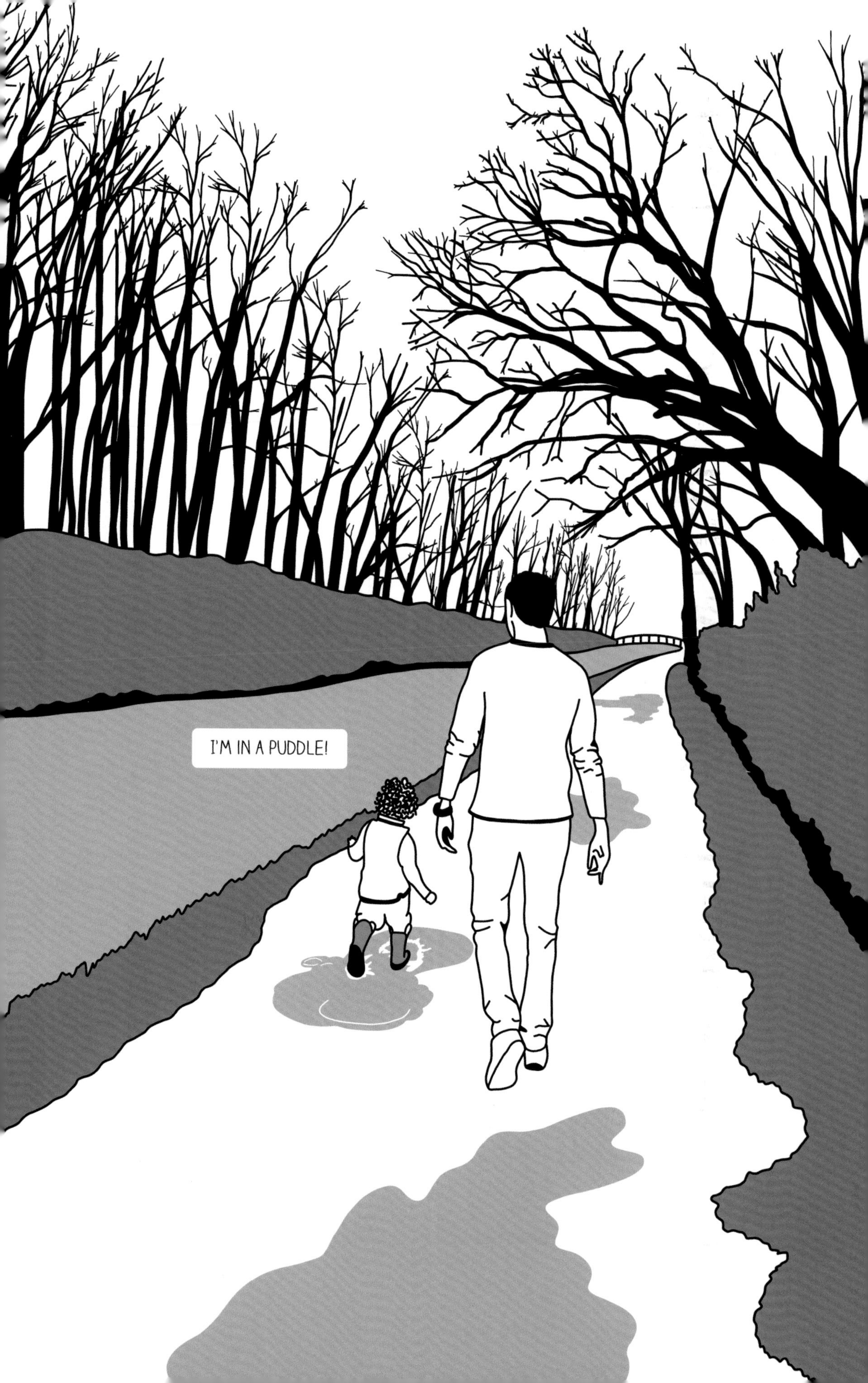
I'M IN A PUDDLE!

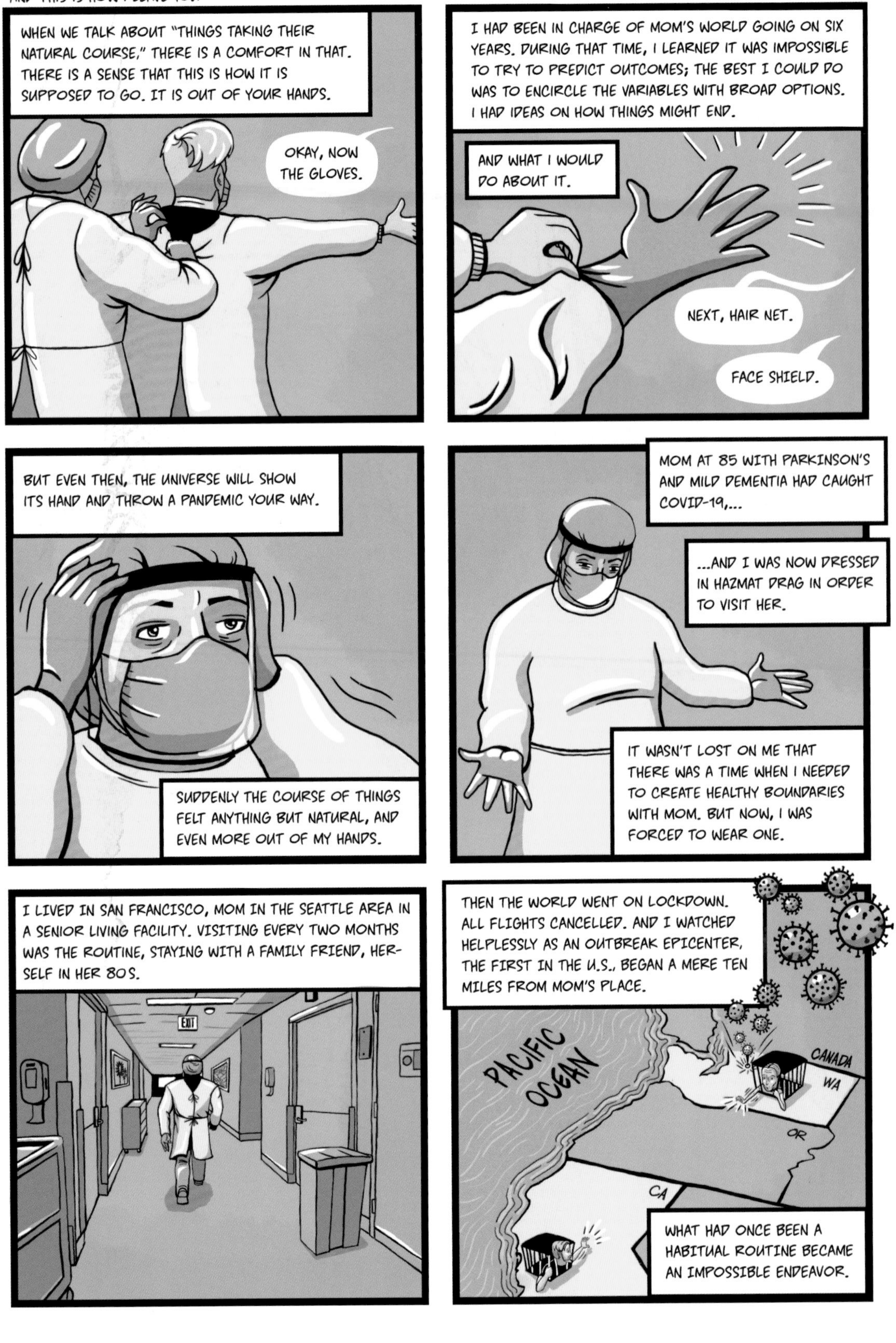
WHEN WE TALK ABOUT "THINGS TAKING THEIR NATURAL COURSE," THERE IS A COMFORT IN THAT. THERE IS A SENSE THAT THIS IS HOW IT IS SUPPOSED TO GO. IT IS OUT OF YOUR HANDS.
OKAY, NOW THE GLOVES.
I HAD BEEN IN CHARGE OF MOM'S WORLD GOING ON SIX YEARS. DURING THAT TIME, I LEARNED IT WAS IMPOSSIBLE TO TRY TO PREDICT OUTCOMES; THE BEST I COULD DO WAS TO ENCIRCLE THE VARIABLES WITH BROAD OPTIONS. I HAD IDEAS ON HOW THINGS MIGHT END.
AND WHAT I WOULD DO ABOUT IT.
NEXT, HAIR NET.
FACE SHIELD.
BUT EVEN THEN, THE UNIVERSE WILL SHOW ITS HAND AND THROW A PANDEMIC YOUR WAY.
SUDDENLY THE COURSE OF THINGS FELT ANYTHING BUT NATURAL, AND EVEN MORE OUT OF MY HANDS.
MOM AT 85 WITH PARKINSON'S AND MILD DEMENTIA HAD CAUGHT COVID-19,...
...AND I WAS NOW DRESSED IN HAZMAT DRAG IN ORDER TO VISIT HER.
IT WASN'T LOST ON ME THAT THERE WAS A TIME WHEN I NEEDED TO CREATE HEALTHY BOUNDARIES WITH MOM. BUT NOW, I WAS FORCED TO WEAR ONE.
I LIVED IN SAN FRANCISCO, MOM IN THE SEATTLE AREA IN A SENIOR LIVING FACILITY. VISITING EVERY TWO MONTHS WAS THE ROUTINE, STAYING WITH A FAMILY FRIEND, HER-SELF IN HER 80S.
EXIT
THEN THE WORLD WENT ON LOCKDOWN. ALL FLIGHTS CANCELLED. AND I WATCHED HELPLESSLY AS AN OUTBREAK EPICENTER, THE FIRST IN THE U.S., BEGAN A MERE TEN MILES FROM MOM'S PLACE.
PACIFIC OCEAN
CANADA
WA
OR
CA
WHAT HAD ONCE BEEN A HABITUAL ROUTINE BECAME AN IMPOSSIBLE ENDEAVOR.

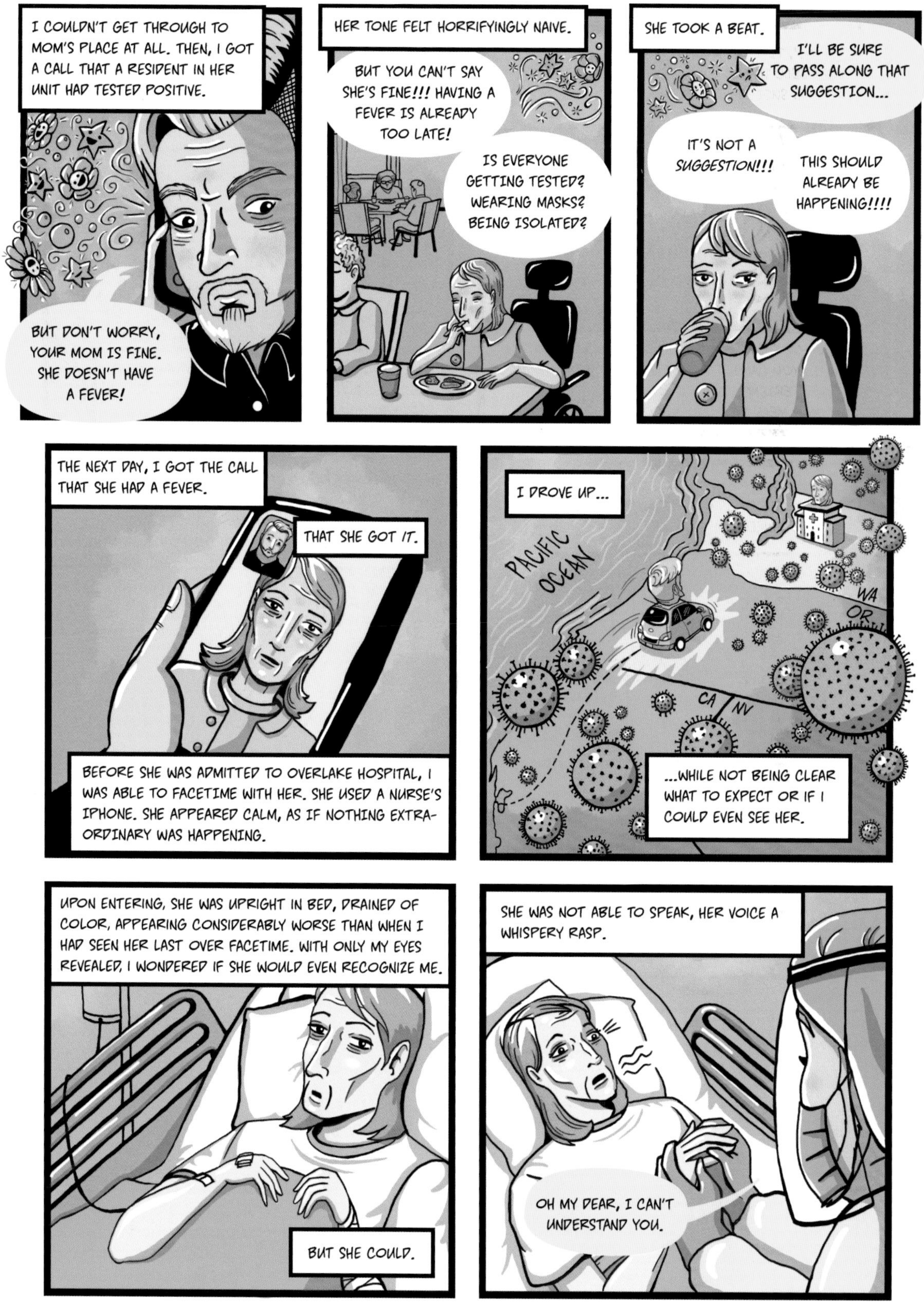
I COULDN'T GET THROUGH TO MOM'S PLACE AT ALL. THEN, I GOT A CALL THAT A RESIDENT IN HER UNIT HAD TESTED POSITIVE.
BUT DON'T WORRY, YOUR MOM IS FINE. SHE DOESN'T HAVE A FEVER!
HER TONE FELT HORRIFYINGLY NAIVE.
BUT YOU CAN'T SAY SHE'S FINE!!! HAVING A FEVER IS ALREADY TOO LATE!
IS EVERYONE GETTING TESTED? WEARING MASKS? BEING ISOLATED?
SHE TOOK A BEAT.
I'LL BE SURE TO PASS ALONG THAT SUGGESTION...
IT'S NOT A SUGGESTION!!!
THIS SHOULD ALREADY BE HAPPENING!!!!
THE NEXT DAY, I GOT THE CALL THAT SHE HAD A FEVER.
THAT SHE GOT IT.
BEFORE SHE WAS ADMITTED TO OVERLAKE HOSPITAL, I WAS ABLE TO FACETIME WITH HER. SHE USED A NURSE'S IPHONE. SHE APPEARED CALM, AS IF NOTHING EXTRA-ORDINARY WAS HAPPENING.
I DROVE UP...
PACIFIC OCEAN
WA
OR
CA
NV
...WHILE NOT BEING CLEAR WHAT TO EXPECT OR IF I COULD EVEN SEE HER.
UPON ENTERING, SHE WAS UPRIGHT IN BED, DRAINED OF COLOR, APPEARING CONSIDERABLY WORSE THAN WHEN I HAD SEEN HER LAST OVER FACETIME. WITH ONLY MY EYES REVEALED, I WONDERED IF SHE WOULD EVEN RECOGNIZE ME.
BUT SHE COULD.
SHE WAS NOT ABLE TO SPEAK, HER VOICE A WHISPERY RASP.
OH MY DEAR, I CAN'T UNDERSTAND YOU.

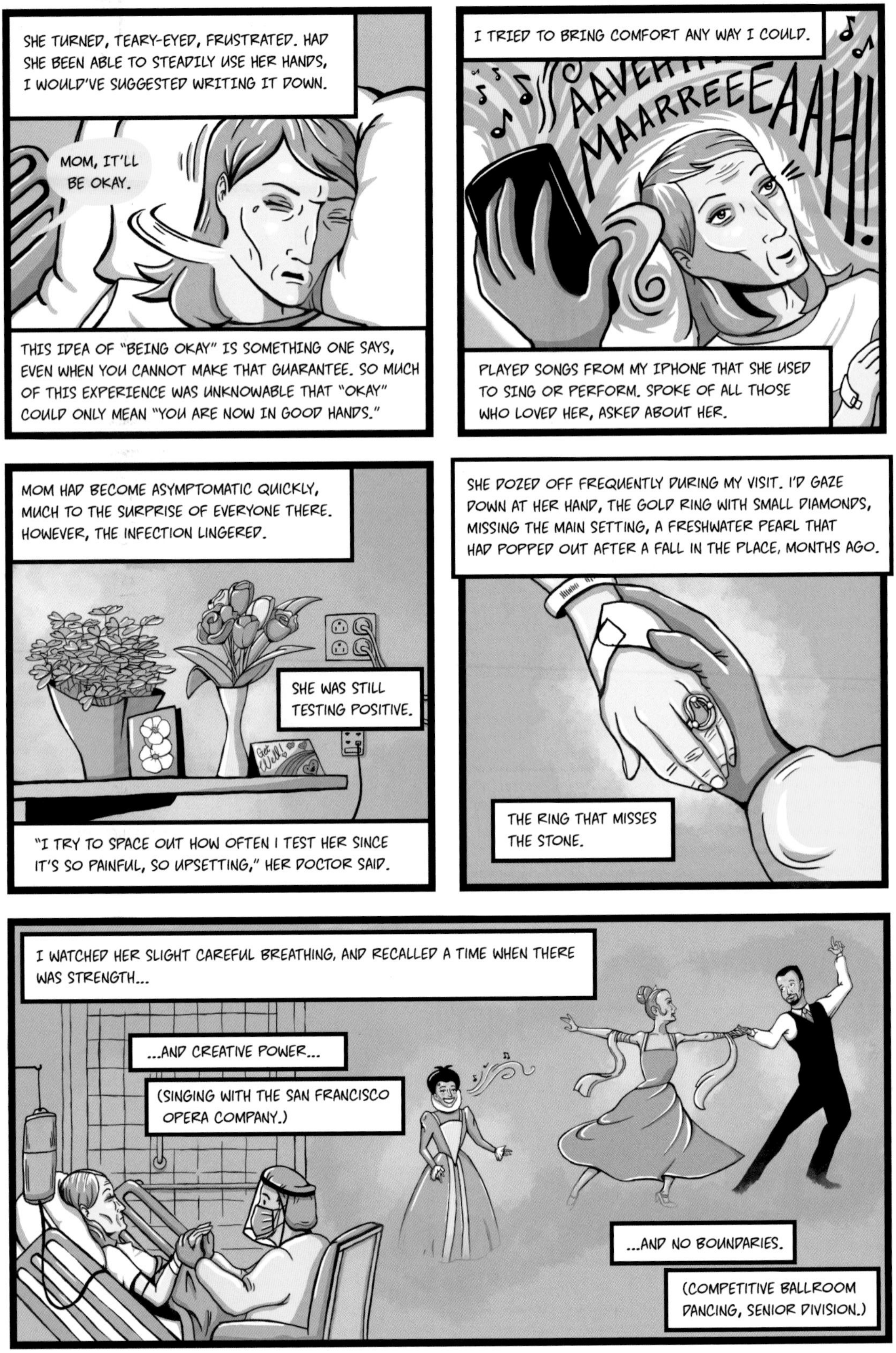
SHE TURNED, TEARY-EYED, FRUSTRATED. HAD SHE BEEN ABLE TO STEADILY USE HER HANDS, I WOULD'VE SUGGESTED WRITING IT DOWN.
MOM, IT'LL BE OKAY.
THIS IDEA OF "BEING OKAY" IS SOMETHING ONE SAYS, EVEN WHEN YOU CANNOT MAKE THAT GUARANTEE. SO MUCH OF THIS EXPERIENCE WAS UNKNOWABLE THAT "OKAY" COULD ONLY MEAN "YOU ARE NOW IN GOOD HANDS."
I TRIED TO BRING COMFORT ANY WAY I COULD.
MAARREEEAAH!!
PLAYED SONGS FROM MY IPHONE THAT SHE USED TO SING OR PERFORM. SPOKE OF ALL THOSE WHO LOVED HER, ASKED ABOUT HER.
MOM HAD BECOME ASYMPTOMATIC QUICKLY, MUCH TO THE SURPRISE OF EVERYONE THERE. HOWEVER, THE INFECTION LINGERED.
SHE WAS STILL TESTING POSITIVE.
Get Well!
"I TRY TO SPACE OUT HOW OFTEN I TEST HER SINCE IT'S SO PAINFUL, SO UPSETTING," HER DOCTOR SAID.
SHE DOZED OFF FREQUENTLY DURING MY VISIT. I'D GAZE DOWN AT HER HAND, THE GOLD RING WITH SMALL DIAMONDS, MISSING THE MAIN SETTING, A FRESHWATER PEARL THAT HAD POPPED OUT AFTER A FALL IN THE PLACE, MONTHS AGO.
THE RING THAT MISSES THE STONE.
I WATCHED HER SLIGHT CAREFUL BREATHING, AND RECALLED A TIME WHEN THERE WAS STRENGTH...
...AND CREATIVE POWER...
(SINGING WITH THE SAN FRANCISCO OPERA COMPANY.)
...AND NO BOUNDARIES.
(COMPETITIVE BALLROOM DANCING, SENIOR DIVISION.)

THE PALLIATIVE CARE NURSES WHO HAD MANAGED TO CHAMPION THIS VISIT AGAINST ALL ODDS SAID I WOULD HAVE ONE HOUR TO VISIT.

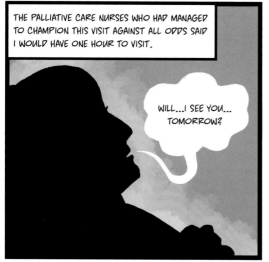

WILL...I SEE YOU... TOMORROW?

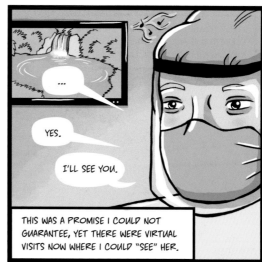

...

YES.

I'LL SEE YOU.

THIS WAS A PROMISE I COULD NOT GUARANTEE, YET THERE WERE VIRTUAL VISITS NOW WHERE I COULD "SEE" HER.

MY EXIT FROM THE COVID WARD WAS JUST AS PRECISE WITH PROTOCOL FOR THE DISROBING.

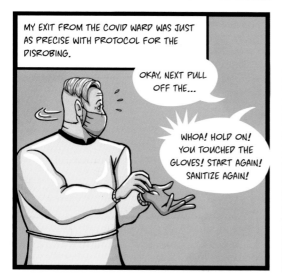

OKAY, NEXT PULL OFF THE...

WHOA! HOLD ON! YOU TOUCHED THE GLOVES! START AGAIN! SANITIZE AGAIN!

FELT STRANGE TO LEAVE MY MOTHER BEHIND IN A HERMETICALLY SEALED COCOON...

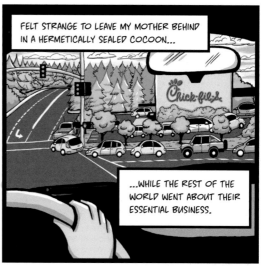

...WHILE THE REST OF THE WORLD WENT ABOUT THEIR ESSENTIAL BUSINESS.

AFTERWARDS, I WAS PHYSICALLY KNOCKED OUT. TOOK A LONG SHOWER AND NAPPED FOR OVER TWO HOURS.

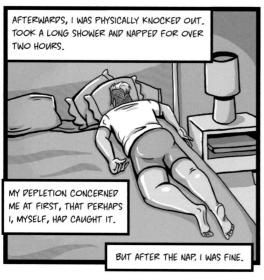

MY DEPLETION CONCERNED ME AT FIRST, THAT PERHAPS I, MYSELF, HAD CAUGHT IT.

BUT AFTER THE NAP, I WAS FINE.

I'D GET UPDATES FROM DOCTORS DAILY, AND HOSPICE WAS PLANNING TO BE ON HAND AFTER SHE WAS DISCHARGED.

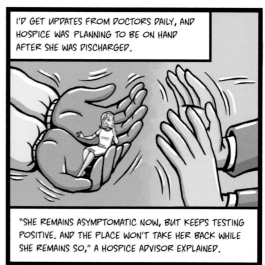

"SHE REMAINS ASYMPTOMATIC NOW, BUT KEEPS TESTING POSITIVE. AND THE PLACE WON'T TAKE HER BACK WHILE SHE REMAINS SO," A HOSPICE ADVISOR EXPLAINED.

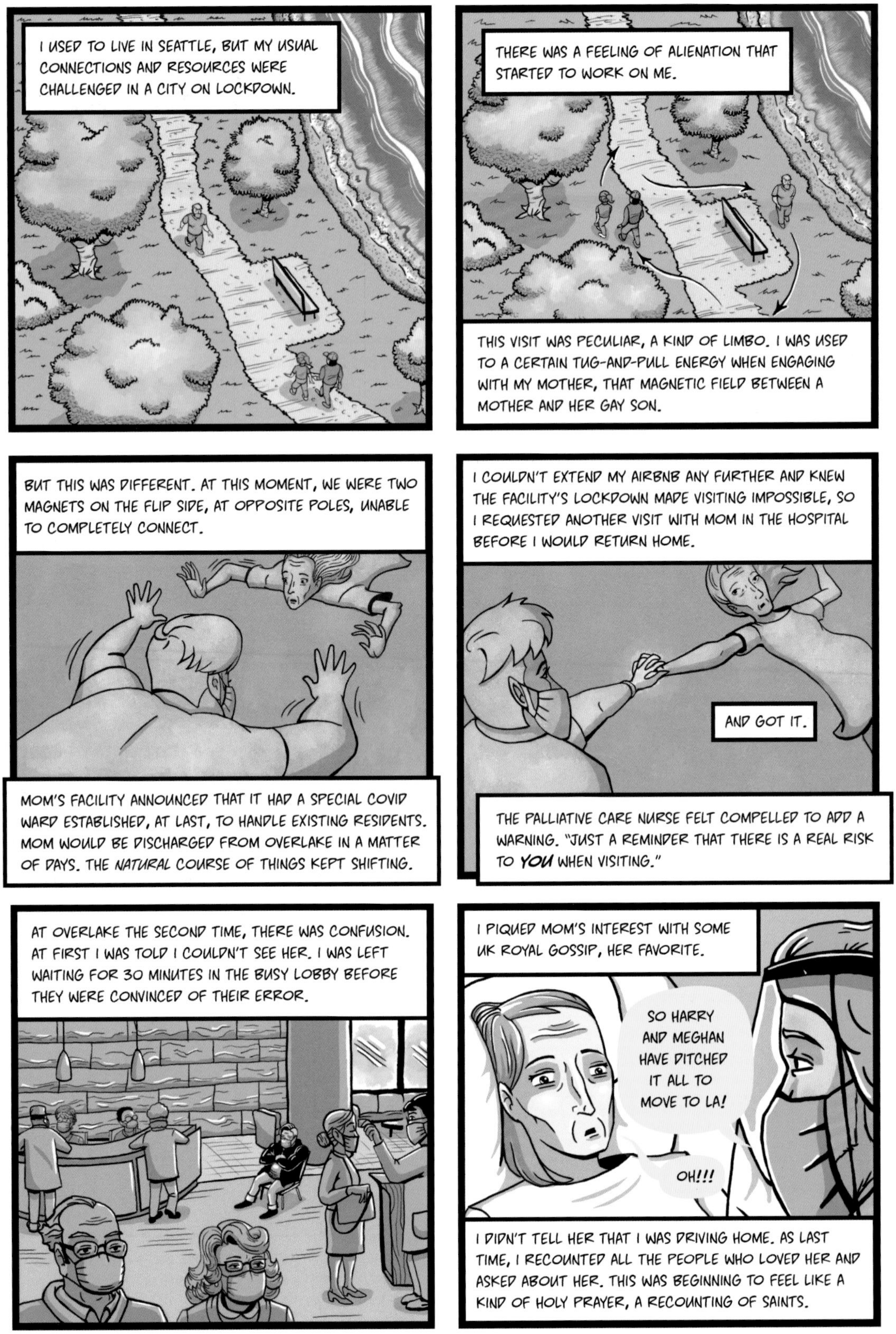
I USED TO LIVE IN SEATTLE, BUT MY USUAL CONNECTIONS AND RESOURCES WERE CHALLENGED IN A CITY ON LOCKDOWN.
THERE WAS A FEELING OF ALIENATION THAT STARTED TO WORK ON ME.
THIS VISIT WAS PECULIAR, A KIND OF LIMBO. I WAS USED TO A CERTAIN TUG-AND-PULL ENERGY WHEN ENGAGING WITH MY MOTHER, THAT MAGNETIC FIELD BETWEEN A MOTHER AND HER GAY SON.
BUT THIS WAS DIFFERENT. AT THIS MOMENT, WE WERE TWO MAGNETS ON THE FLIP SIDE, AT OPPOSITE POLES, UNABLE TO COMPLETELY CONNECT.
MOM'S FACILITY ANNOUNCED THAT IT HAD A SPECIAL COVID WARD ESTABLISHED, AT LAST, TO HANDLE EXISTING RESIDENTS. MOM WOULD BE DISCHARGED FROM OVERLAKE IN A MATTER OF DAYS. THE *NATURAL* COURSE OF THINGS KEPT SHIFTING.
I COULDN'T EXTEND MY AIRBNB ANY FURTHER AND KNEW THE FACILITY'S LOCKDOWN MADE VISITING IMPOSSIBLE, SO I REQUESTED ANOTHER VISIT WITH MOM IN THE HOSPITAL BEFORE I WOULD RETURN HOME.
AND GOT IT.
THE PALLIATIVE CARE NURSE FELT COMPELLED TO ADD A WARNING. "JUST A REMINDER THAT THERE IS A REAL RISK TO ***YOU*** WHEN VISITING."
AT OVERLAKE THE SECOND TIME, THERE WAS CONFUSION. AT FIRST I WAS TOLD I COULDN'T SEE HER. I WAS LEFT WAITING FOR 30 MINUTES IN THE BUSY LOBBY BEFORE THEY WERE CONVINCED OF THEIR ERROR.
I PIQUED MOM'S INTEREST WITH SOME UK ROYAL GOSSIP, HER FAVORITE.
SO HARRY AND MEGHAN HAVE DITCHED IT ALL TO MOVE TO LA!
OH!!!
I DIDN'T TELL HER THAT I WAS DRIVING HOME. AS LAST TIME, I RECOUNTED ALL THE PEOPLE WHO LOVED HER AND ASKED ABOUT HER. THIS WAS BEGINNING TO FEEL LIKE A KIND OF HOLY PRAYER, A RECOUNTING OF SAINTS.

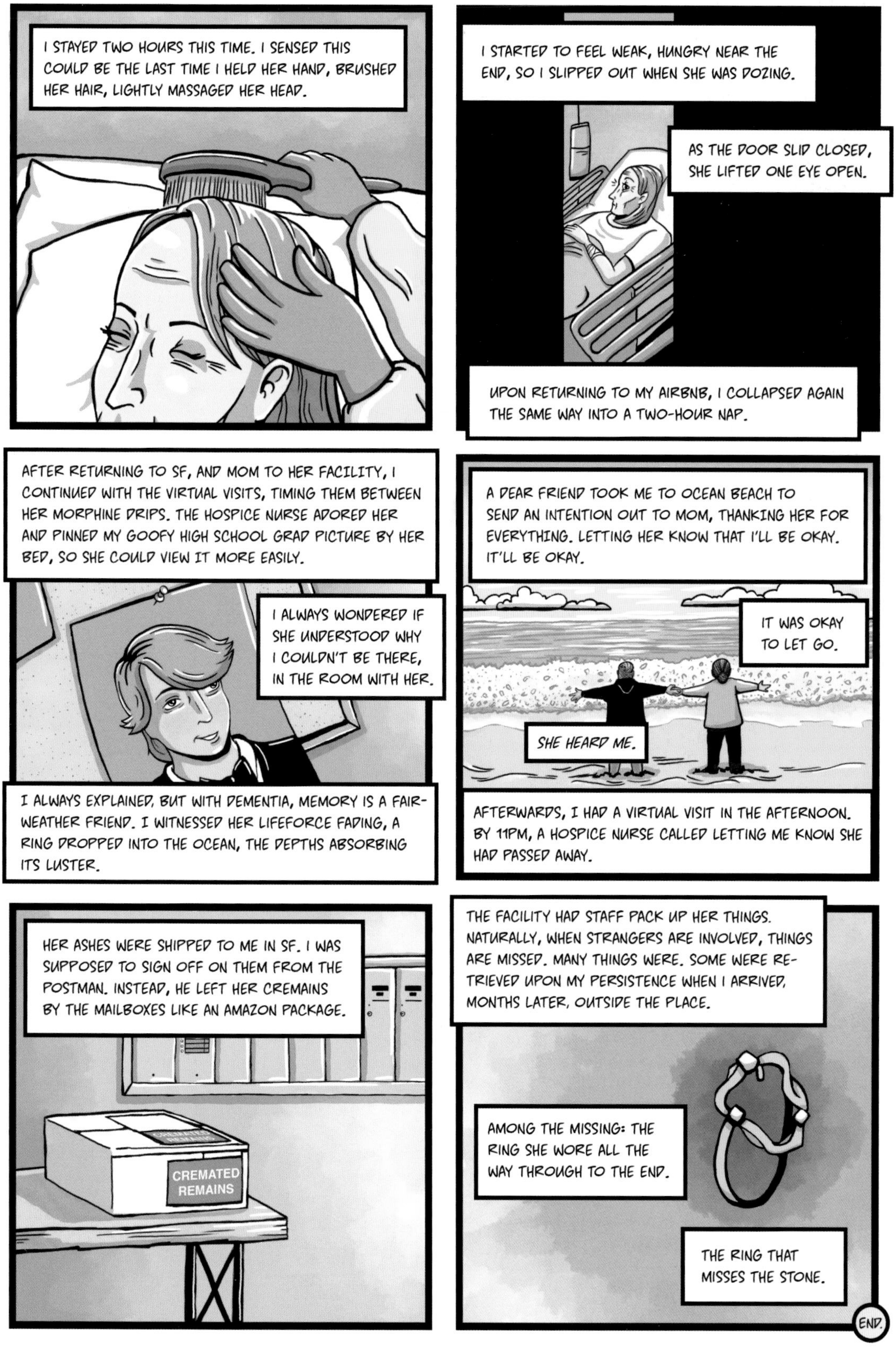
I STAYED TWO HOURS THIS TIME. I SENSED THIS COULD BE THE LAST TIME I HELD HER HAND, BRUSHED HER HAIR, LIGHTLY MASSAGED HER HEAD.
I STARTED TO FEEL WEAK, HUNGRY NEAR THE END, SO I SLIPPED OUT WHEN SHE WAS DOZING.
AS THE DOOR SLID CLOSED, SHE LIFTED ONE EYE OPEN.
UPON RETURNING TO MY AIRBNB, I COLLAPSED AGAIN THE SAME WAY INTO A TWO-HOUR NAP.
AFTER RETURNING TO SF, AND MOM TO HER FACILITY, I CONTINUED WITH THE VIRTUAL VISITS, TIMING THEM BETWEEN HER MORPHINE DRIPS. THE HOSPICE NURSE ADORED HER AND PINNED MY GOOFY HIGH SCHOOL GRAD PICTURE BY HER BED, SO SHE COULD VIEW IT MORE EASILY.
I ALWAYS WONDERED IF SHE UNDERSTOOD WHY I COULDN'T BE THERE, IN THE ROOM WITH HER.
I ALWAYS EXPLAINED, BUT WITH DEMENTIA, MEMORY IS A FAIR-WEATHER FRIEND. I WITNESSED HER LIFEFORCE FADING, A RING DROPPED INTO THE OCEAN, THE DEPTHS ABSORBING ITS LUSTER.
A DEAR FRIEND TOOK ME TO OCEAN BEACH TO SEND AN INTENTION OUT TO MOM, THANKING HER FOR EVERYTHING. LETTING HER KNOW THAT I'LL BE OKAY. IT'LL BE OKAY.
IT WAS OKAY TO LET GO.
SHE HEARD ME.
AFTERWARDS, I HAD A VIRTUAL VISIT IN THE AFTERNOON. BY 11PM, A HOSPICE NURSE CALLED LETTING ME KNOW SHE HAD PASSED AWAY.
HER ASHES WERE SHIPPED TO ME IN SF. I WAS SUPPOSED TO SIGN OFF ON THEM FROM THE POSTMAN. INSTEAD, HE LEFT HER CREMAINS BY THE MAILBOXES LIKE AN AMAZON PACKAGE.
CREMATED REMAINS
THE FACILITY HAD STAFF PACK UP HER THINGS. NATURALLY, WHEN STRANGERS ARE INVOLVED, THINGS ARE MISSED. MANY THINGS WERE. SOME WERE RE-TRIEVED UPON MY PERSISTENCE WHEN I ARRIVED, MONTHS LATER, OUTSIDE THE PLACE.
AMONG THE MISSING: THE RING SHE WORE ALL THE WAY THROUGH TO THE END.
THE RING THAT MISSES THE STONE.
END.

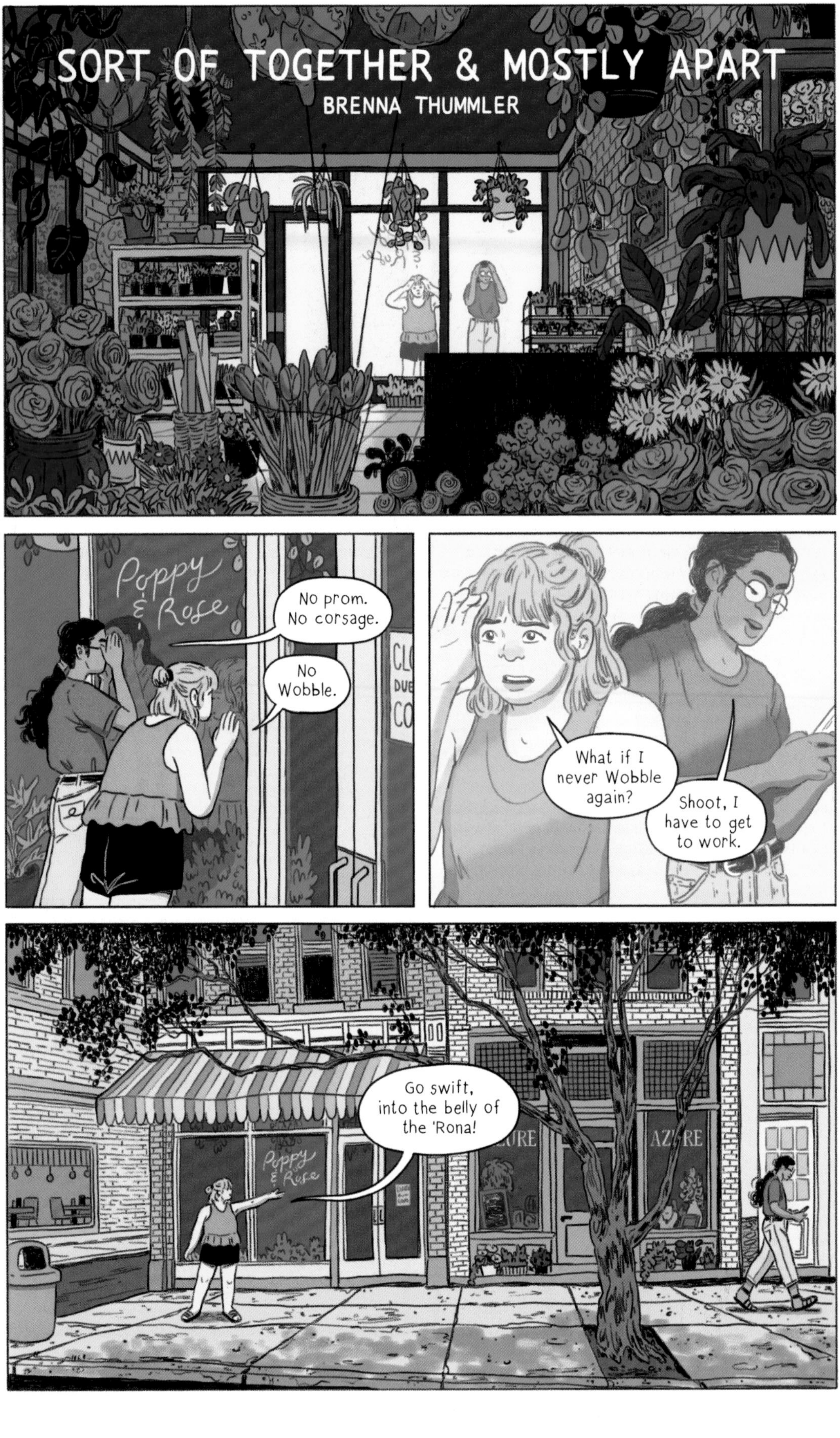
SORT OF TOGETHER & MOSTLY APART
BRENNA THUMMLER
Poppy & Rose
No prom. No corsage.
No Wobble.
What if I never Wobble again?
Shoot, I have to get to work.
Go swift, into the belly of the 'Rona!

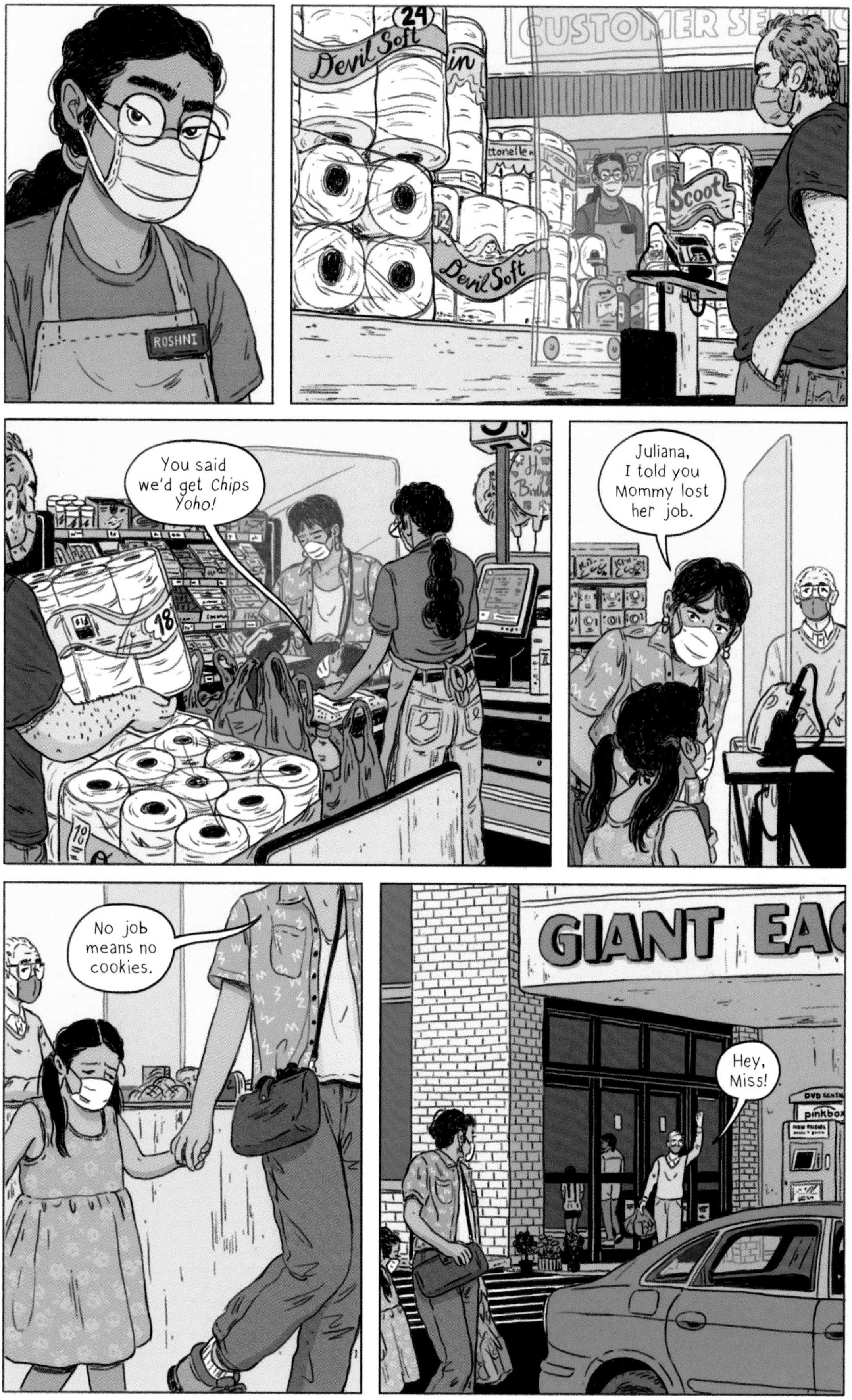
ROSHNI
24
Devil Soft
CUSTOMER SE
Scoot
Devil Soft
You said we'd get Chips Yoho!
Juliana, I told you Mommy lost her job.
No job means no cookies.
GIANT EAG
Hey, Miss!
pinkbox

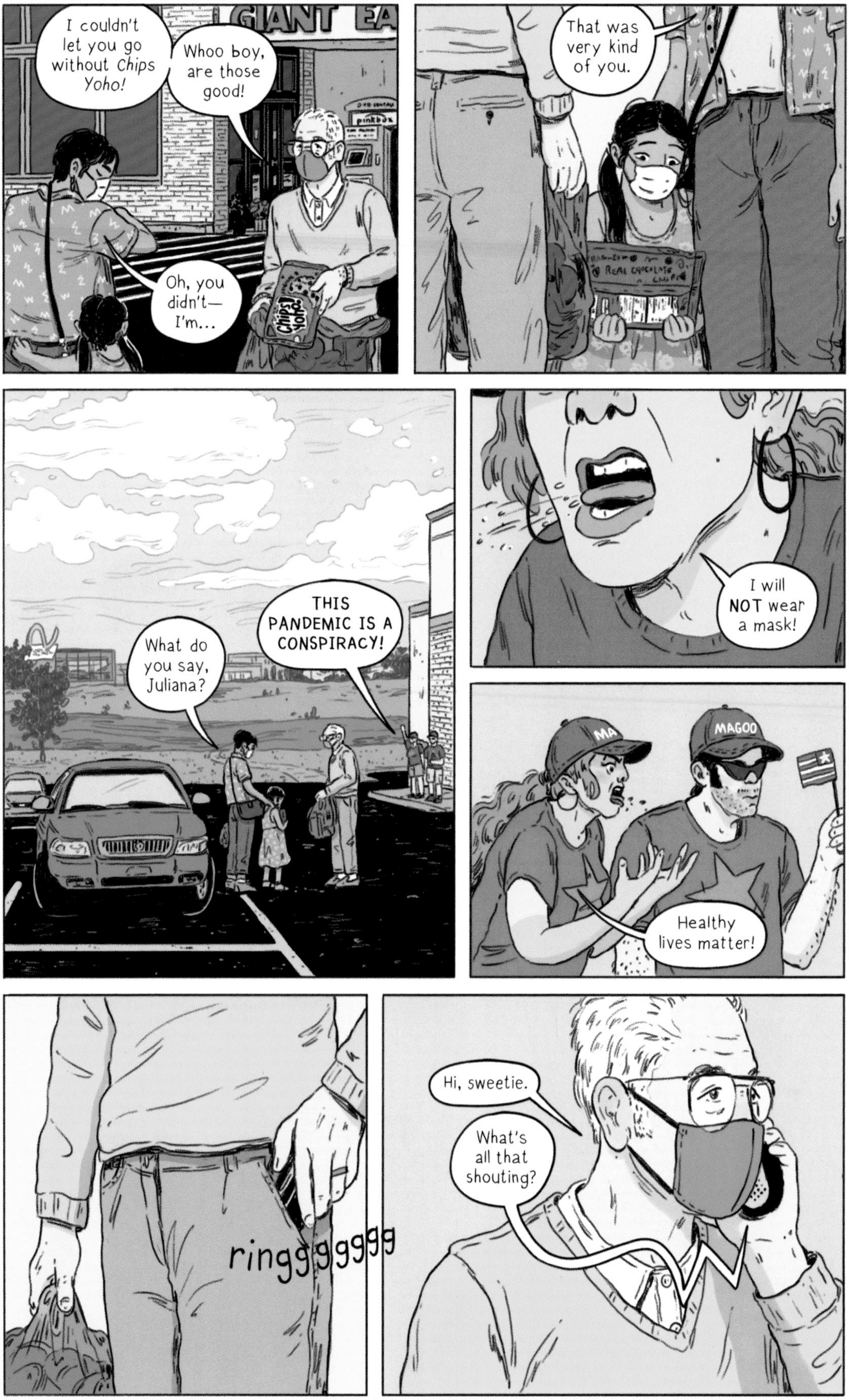
GIANT EA
I couldn't let you go without Chips Yoho!
Whoo boy, are those good!
Oh, you didn't— I'm...
Chips! Yoho
That was very kind of you.
REAL CHOCOLATE
What do you say, Juliana?
THIS PANDEMIC IS A CONSPIRACY!
I will NOT wear a mask!
MA
MAGOO
Healthy lives matter!
ringggggg
Hi, sweetie.
What's all that shouting?

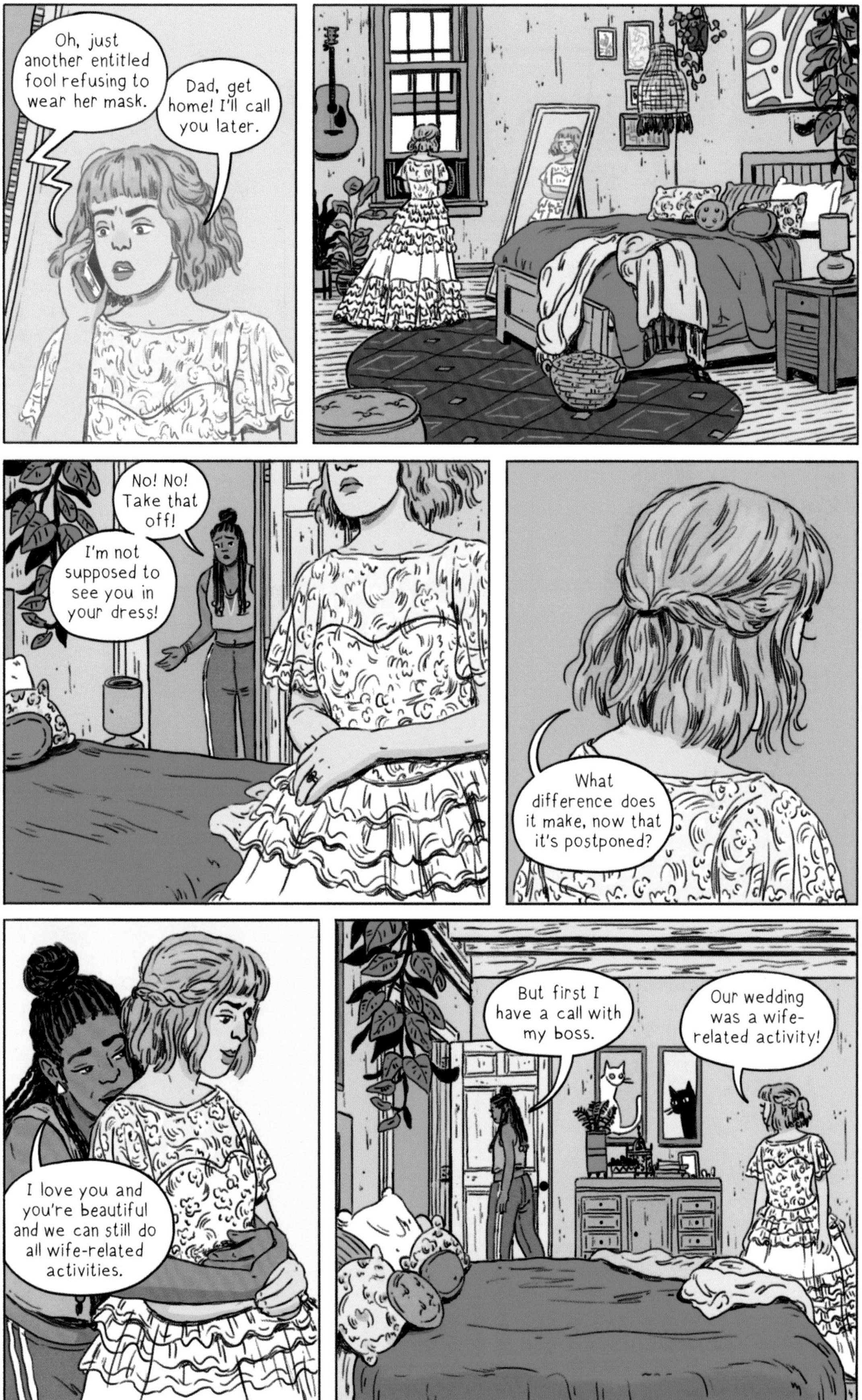

Oh, just another entitled fool refusing to wear her mask.
Dad, get home! I'll call you later.
No! No! Take that off!
I'm not supposed to see you in your dress!
What difference does it make, now that it's postponed?
I love you and you're beautiful and we can still do all wife-related activities.
But first I have a call with my boss.
Our wedding was a wife-related activity!

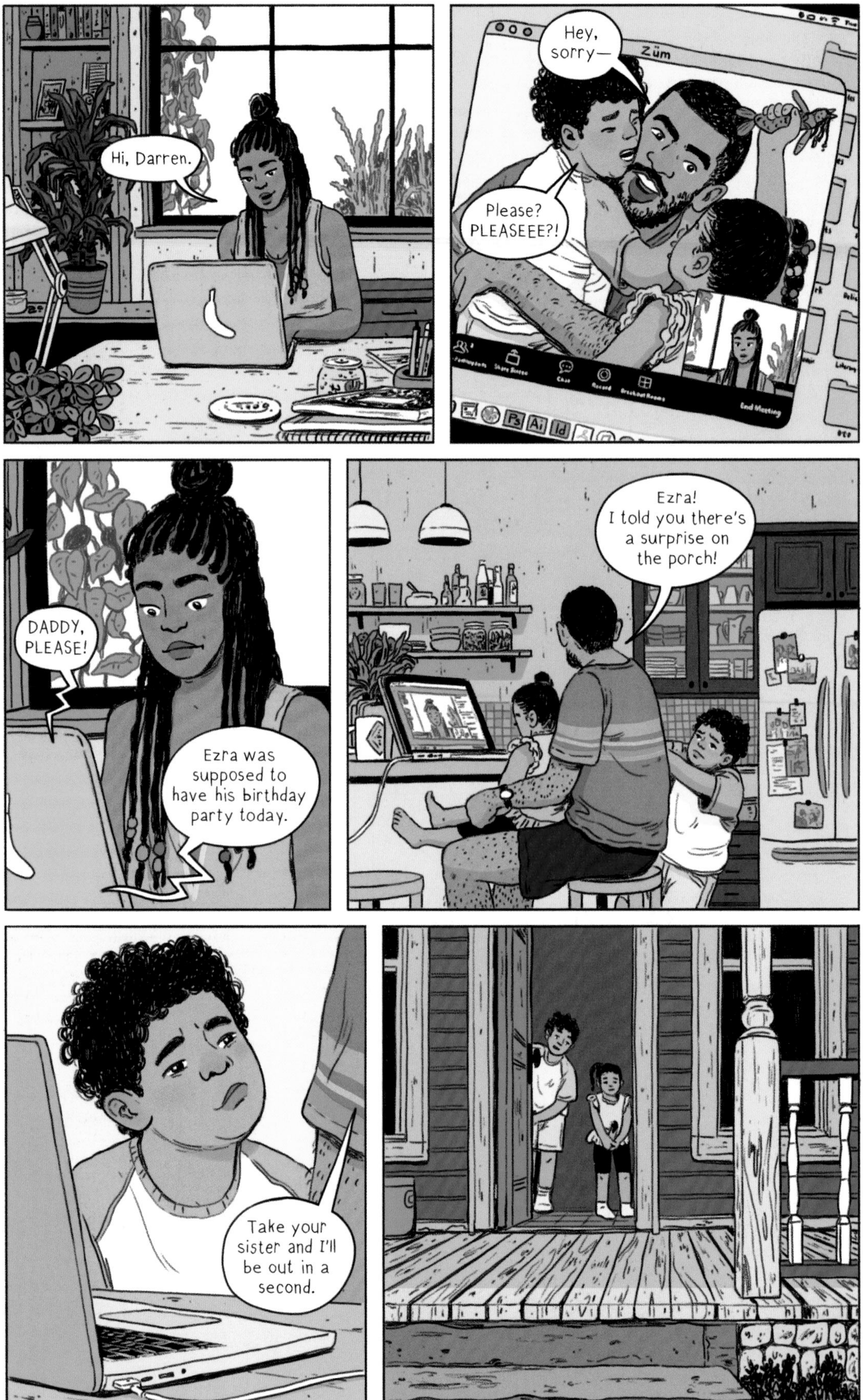
Hi, Darren.
Hey, sorry—
Zūm
Please? PLEASEEE?!
DADDY, PLEASE!
Ezra was supposed to have his birthday party today.
Ezra! I told you there's a surprise on the porch!
Take your sister and I'll be out in a second.

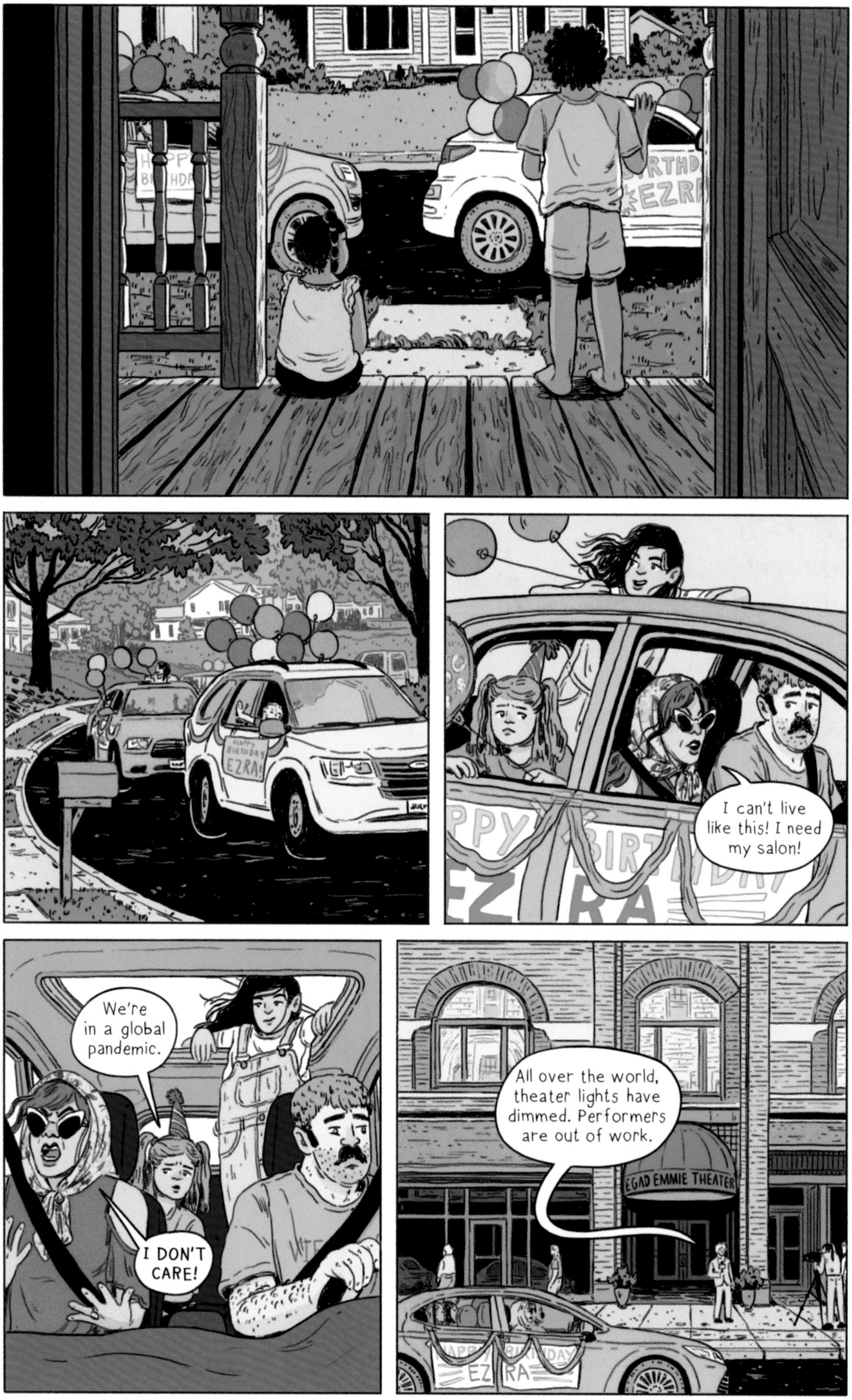

HAPPY BIRTHDAY
BIRTHDAY EZRA
HAPPY BIRTHDAY EZRA!
I can't live like this! I need my salon!
We're in a global pandemic.
I DON'T CARE!
All over the world, theater lights have dimmed. Performers are out of work.
EGAD EMMIE THEATER
HAPPY BIRTHDAY EZRA

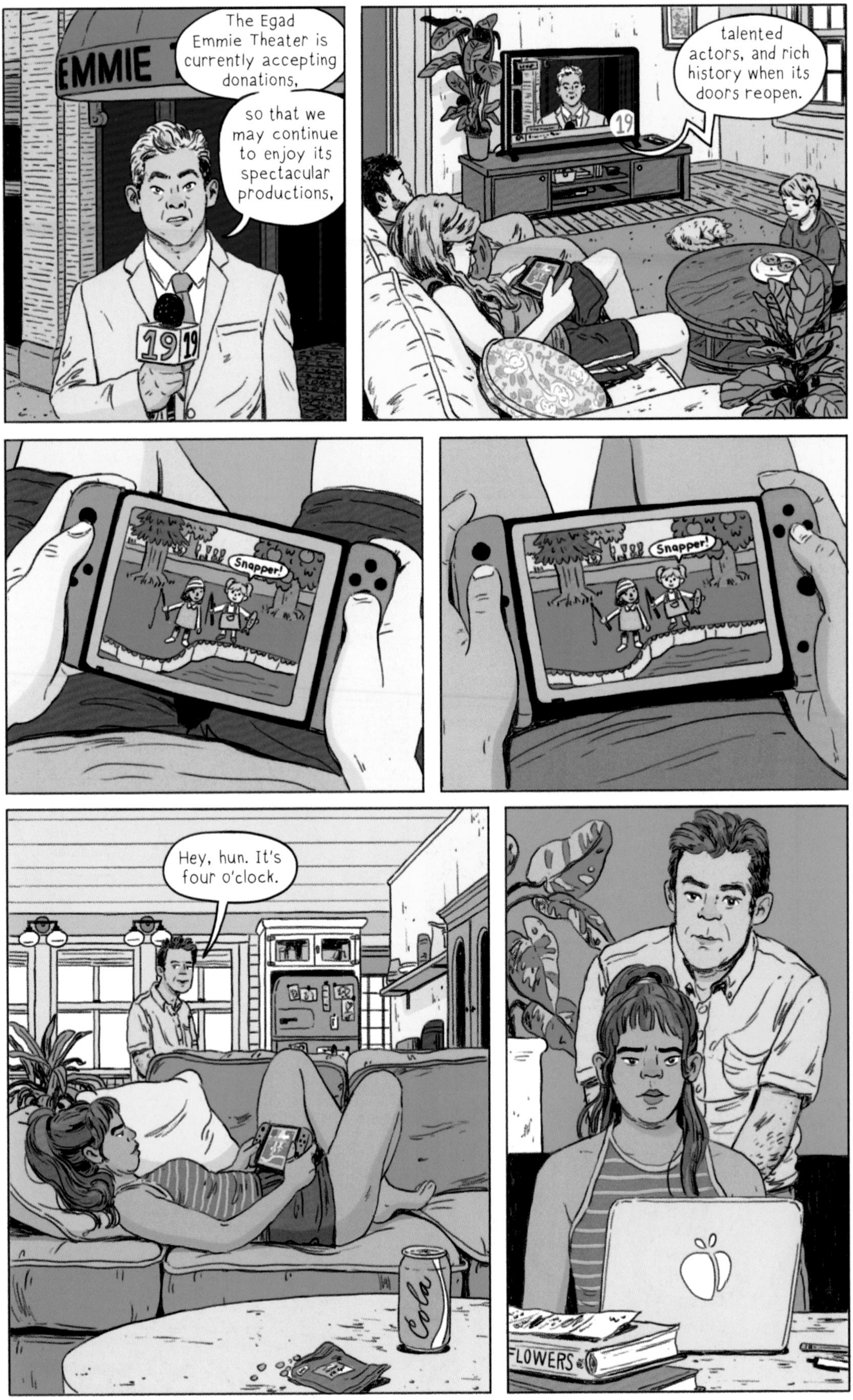
EMMIE
The Egad Emmie Theater is currently accepting donations,
so that we may continue to enjoy its spectacular productions,
19
talented actors, and rich history when its doors reopen.
Snapper!
Snapper!
Hey, hun. It's four o'clock.
Cola
FLOWERS

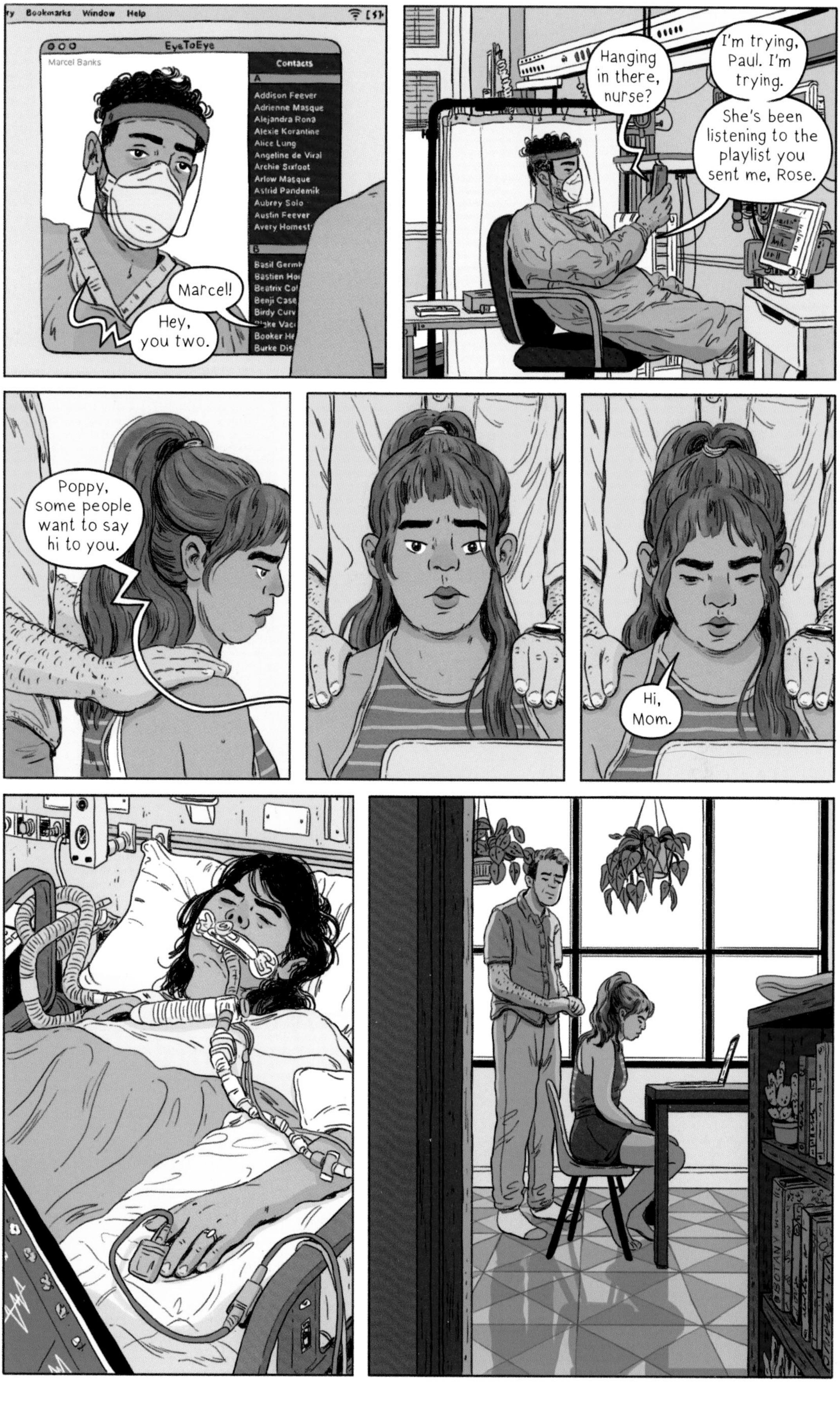

Bookmarks Window Help
EyeToEye
Marcel Banks
Contacts
A
Addison Feever
Adrienne Masque
Alejandra Rona
Alexie Korantine
Alice Lung
Angeline de Viral
Archie Sixfoot
Arlow Masque
Astrid Pandemik
Aubrey Solo
Austin Feever
B
Marcel!
Hey, you two.
Hanging in there, nurse?
I'm trying, Paul. I'm trying.
She's been listening to the playlist you sent me, Rose.
Poppy, some people want to say hi to you.
Hi, Mom.
BOTANY

Hi, Dad. It's Rivi.
Oh Riv'... I just...
mmmph....
mmm....
zzzzzzz.....
Dad?! Do you feel okay? You sound very tired.
...DESPERATELY ....tired....
Get some rest. I just called to hear your voice and send love. I'll call again soon. Bye.

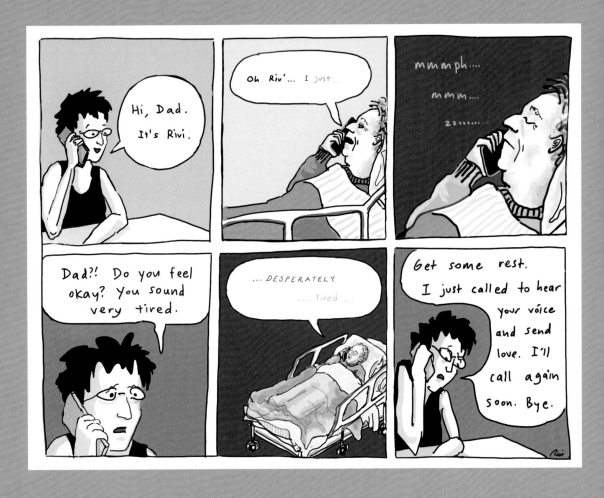

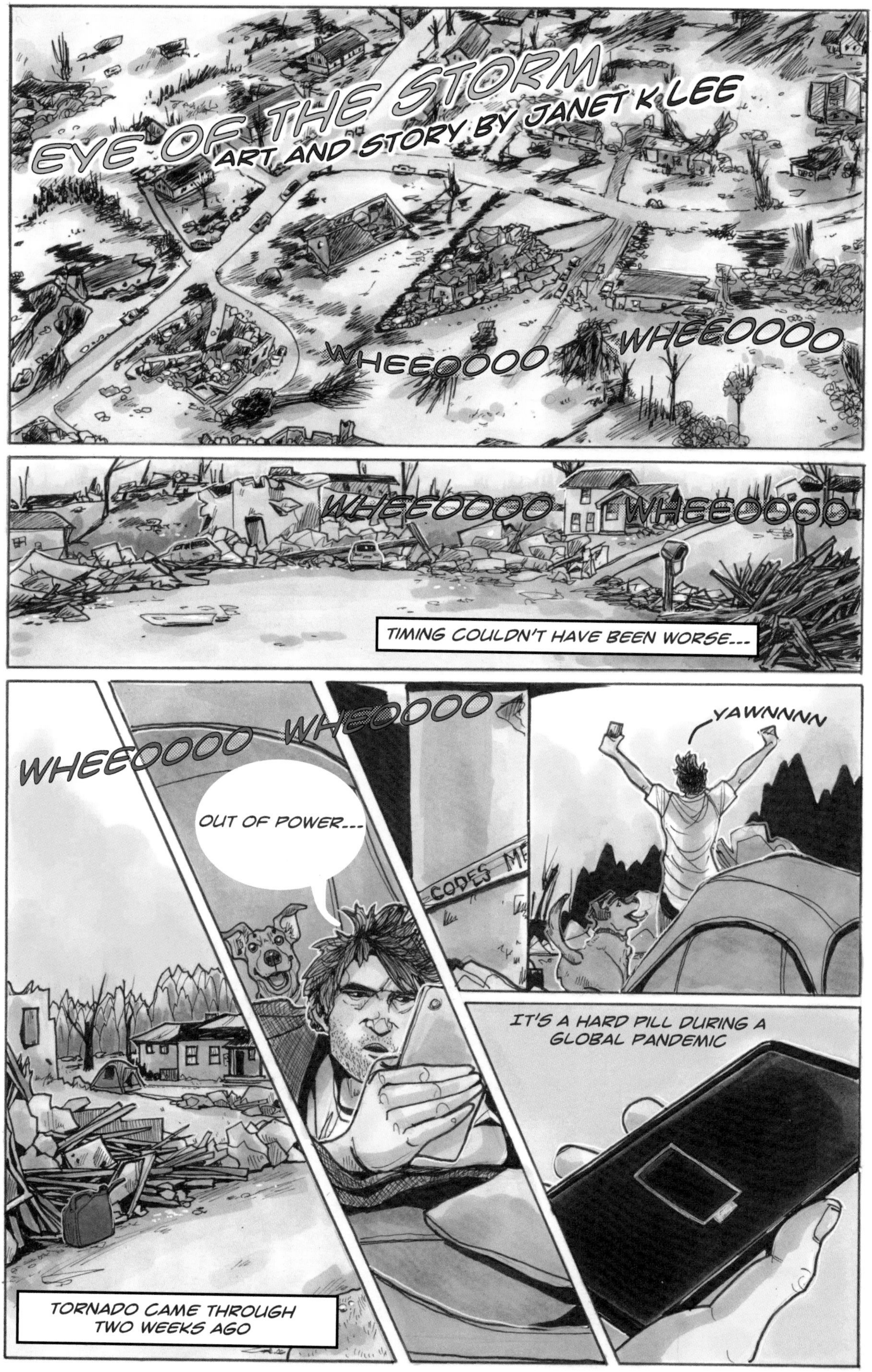
EYE OF THE STORM
ART AND STORY BY JANET K LEE
WHEEOOOO WHEEOOOO
WHEEOOOO WHEEOOOO
TIMING COULDN'T HAVE BEEN WORSE...
WHEEOOOO WHEOOOO
OUT OF POWER...
CODES ME
YAWNNNN
IT'S A HARD PILL DURING A GLOBAL PANDEMIC
TORNADO CAME THROUGH TWO WEEKS AGO

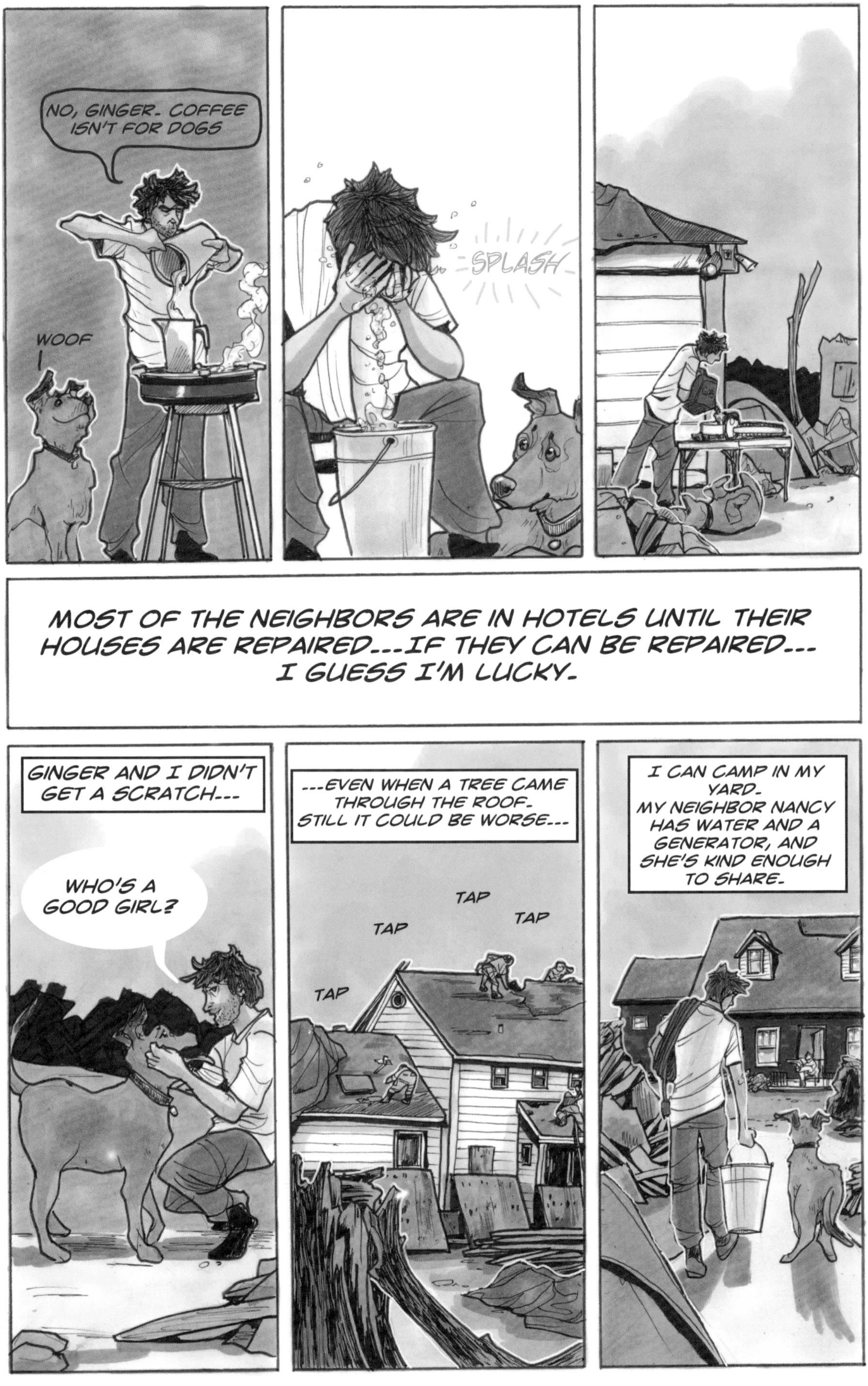
NO, GINGER. COFFEE ISN'T FOR DOGS
WOOF
SPLASH
MOST OF THE NEIGHBORS ARE IN HOTELS UNTIL THEIR HOUSES ARE REPAIRED...IF THEY CAN BE REPAIRED... I GUESS I'M LUCKY.
GINGER AND I DIDN'T GET A SCRATCH...
WHO'S A GOOD GIRL?
...EVEN WHEN A TREE CAME THROUGH THE ROOF. STILL IT COULD BE WORSE...
TAP
TAP
TAP
TAP
I CAN CAMP IN MY YARD. MY NEIGHBOR NANCY HAS WATER AND A GENERATOR, AND SHE'S KIND ENOUGH TO SHARE.

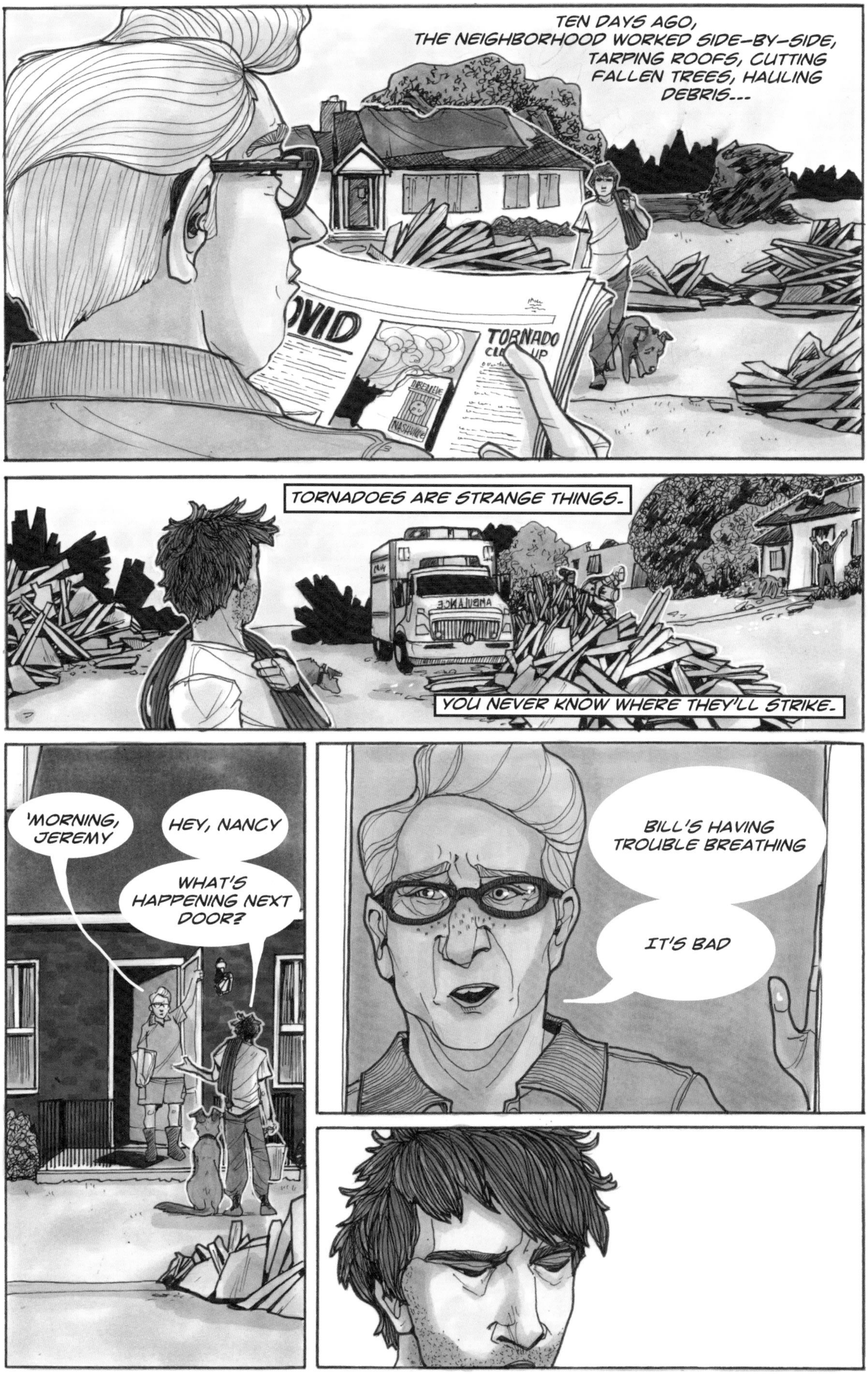
TEN DAYS AGO, THE NEIGHBORHOOD WORKED SIDE-BY-SIDE, TARPING ROOFS, CUTTING FALLEN TREES, HAULING DEBRIS...
COVID
TORNADO
TORNADOES ARE STRANGE THINGS.
AMBULANCE
YOU NEVER KNOW WHERE THEY'LL STRIKE.
'MORNING, JEREMY
HEY, NANCY
WHAT'S HAPPENING NEXT DOOR?
BILL'S HAVING TROUBLE BREATHING
IT'S BAD

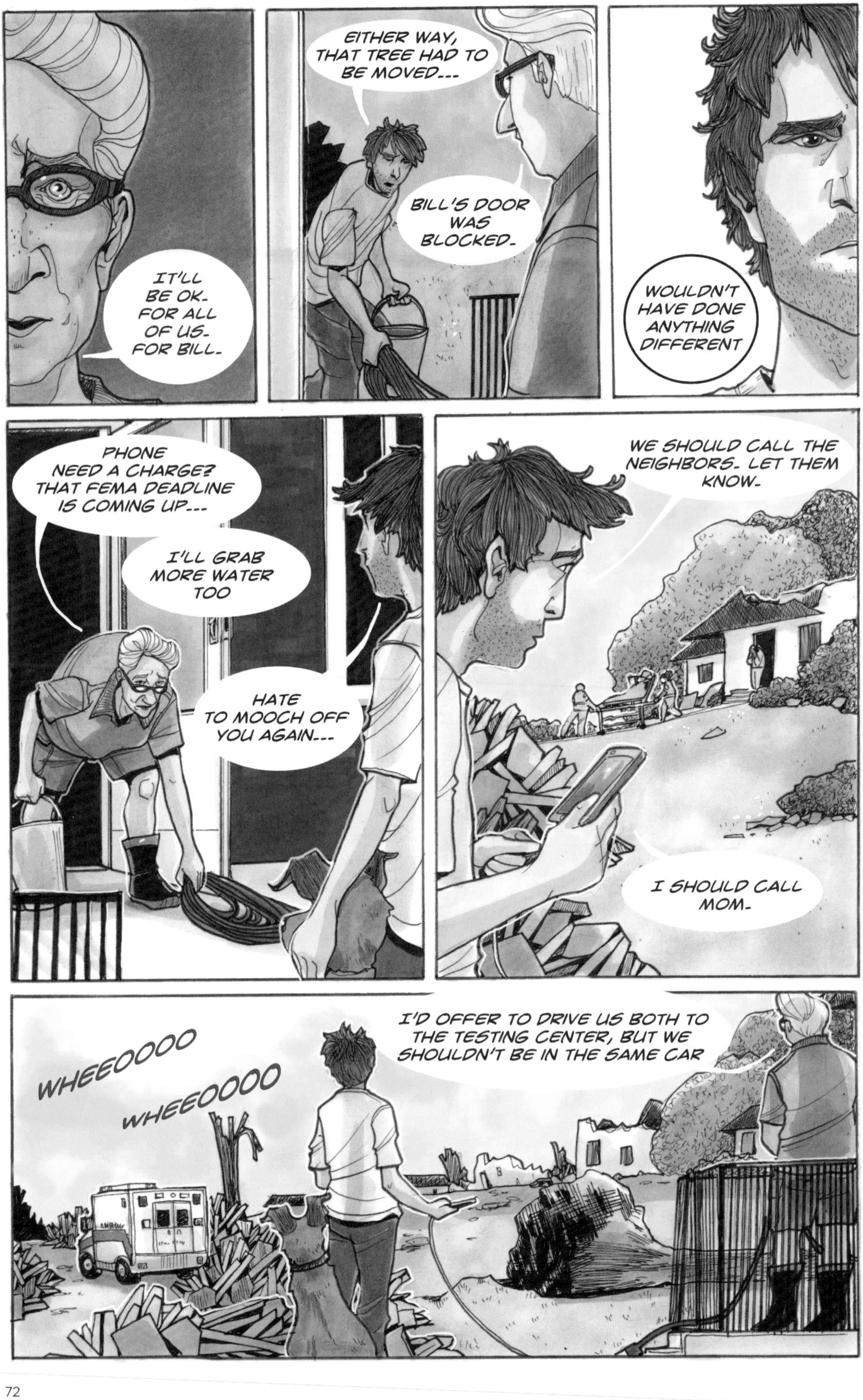
IT'LL BE OK. FOR ALL OF US. FOR BILL.
EITHER WAY, THAT TREE HAD TO BE MOVED...
BILL'S DOOR WAS BLOCKED.
WOULDN'T HAVE DONE ANYTHING DIFFERENT
PHONE NEED A CHARGE? THAT FEMA DEADLINE IS COMING UP...
I'LL GRAB MORE WATER TOO
HATE TO MOOCH OFF YOU AGAIN...
WE SHOULD CALL THE NEIGHBORS. LET THEM KNOW.
I SHOULD CALL MOM.
WHEEOOOO
WHEEOOOO
I'D OFFER TO DRIVE US BOTH TO THE TESTING CENTER, BUT WE SHOULDN'T BE IN THE SAME CAR

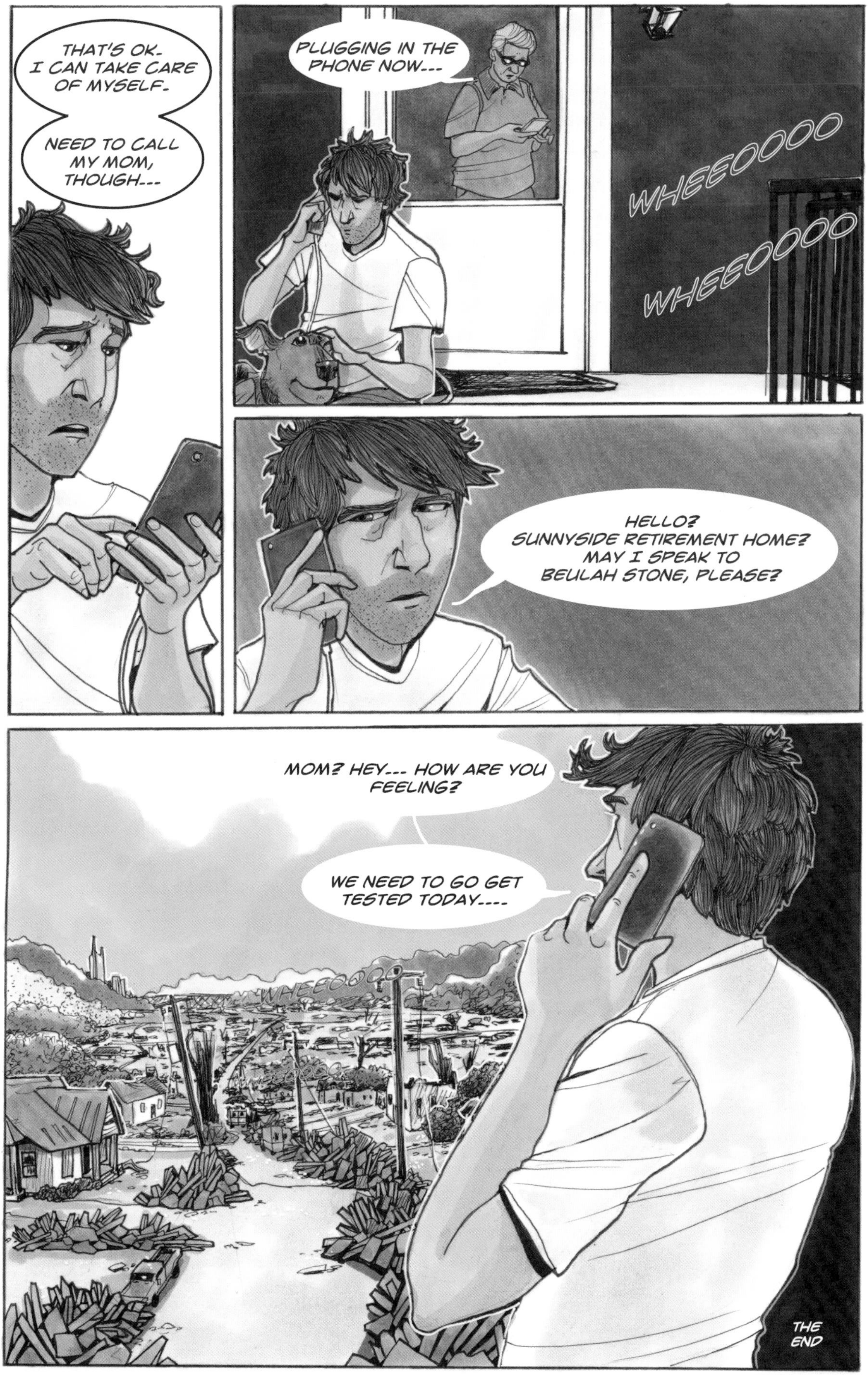
THAT'S OK. I CAN TAKE CARE OF MYSELF.
NEED TO CALL MY MOM, THOUGH...
PLUGGING IN THE PHONE NOW...
WHEEOOOO
WHEEOOOO
HELLO? SUNNYSIDE RETIREMENT HOME? MAY I SPEAK TO BEULAH STONE, PLEASE?
MOM? HEY... HOW ARE YOU FEELING?
WE NEED TO GO GET TESTED TODAY....
THE END

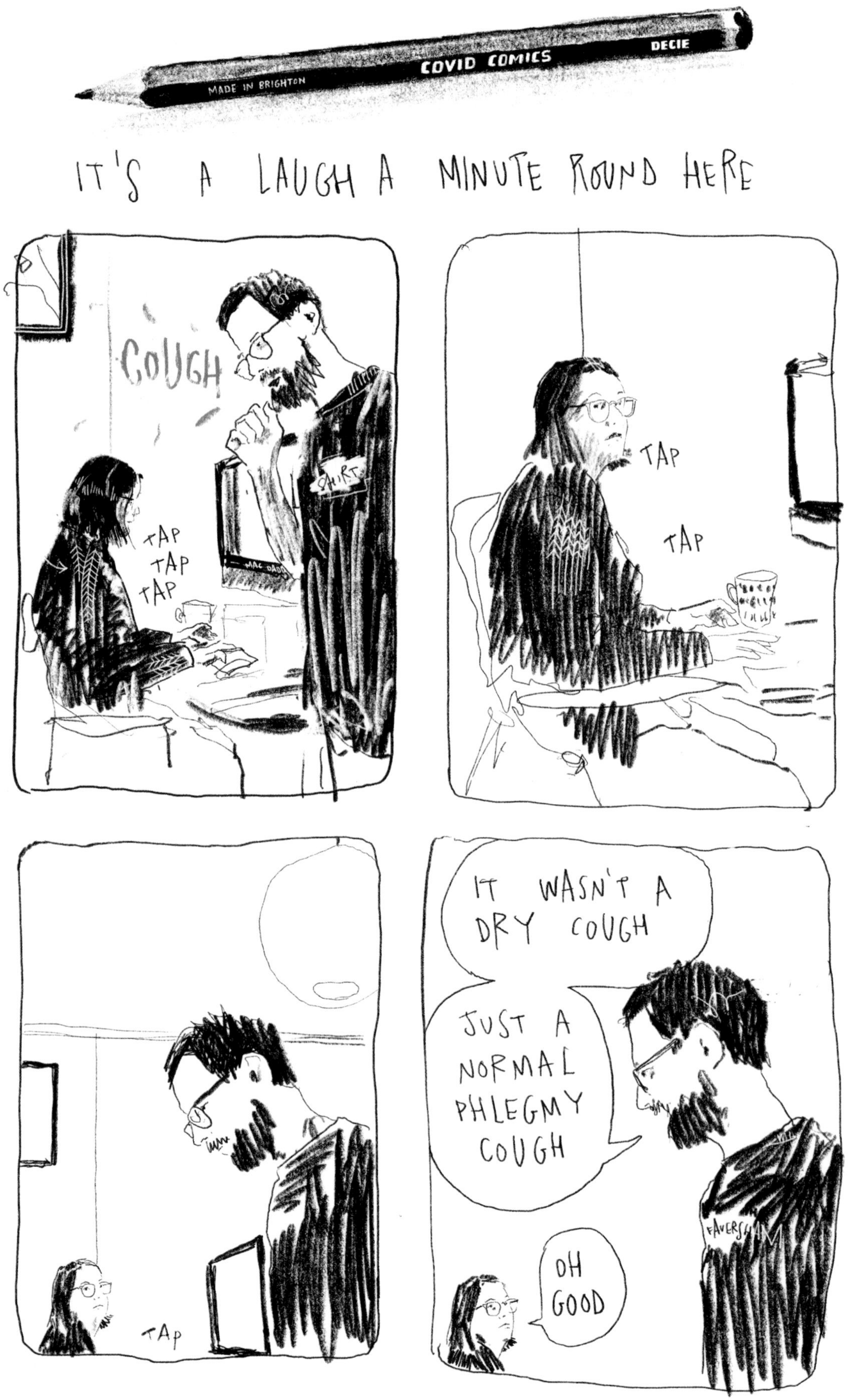
MADE IN BRIGHTON
COVID COMICS
DECIE
IT'S A LAUGH A MINUTE ROUND HERE
COUGH
TAP TAP TAP
TAP
TAP
TAP
IT WASN'T A DRY COUGH
JUST A NORMAL PHLEGMY COUGH
OH GOOD

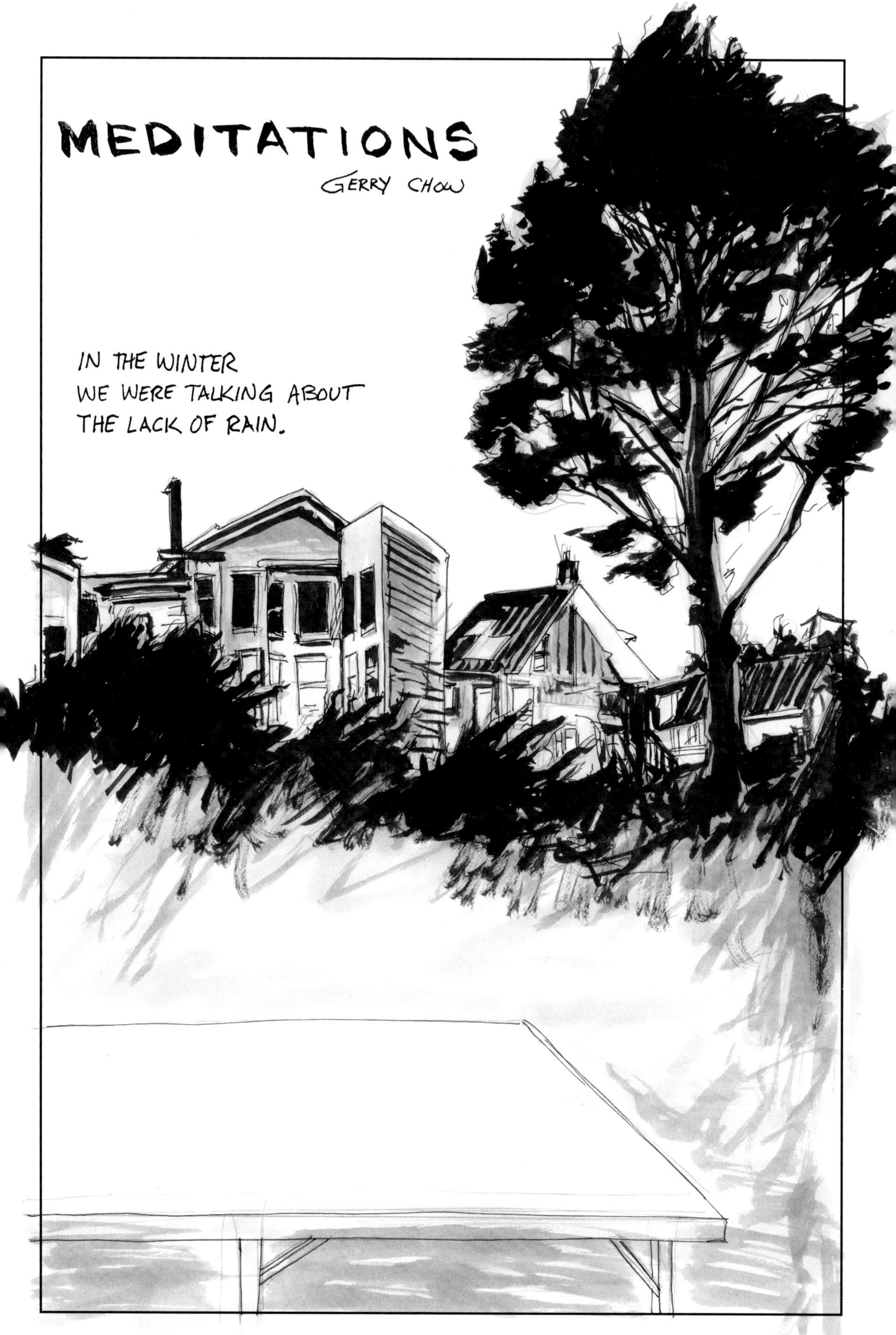
MEDITATIONS
GERRY CHOW
IN THE WINTER
WE WERE TALKING ABOUT
THE LACK OF RAIN.

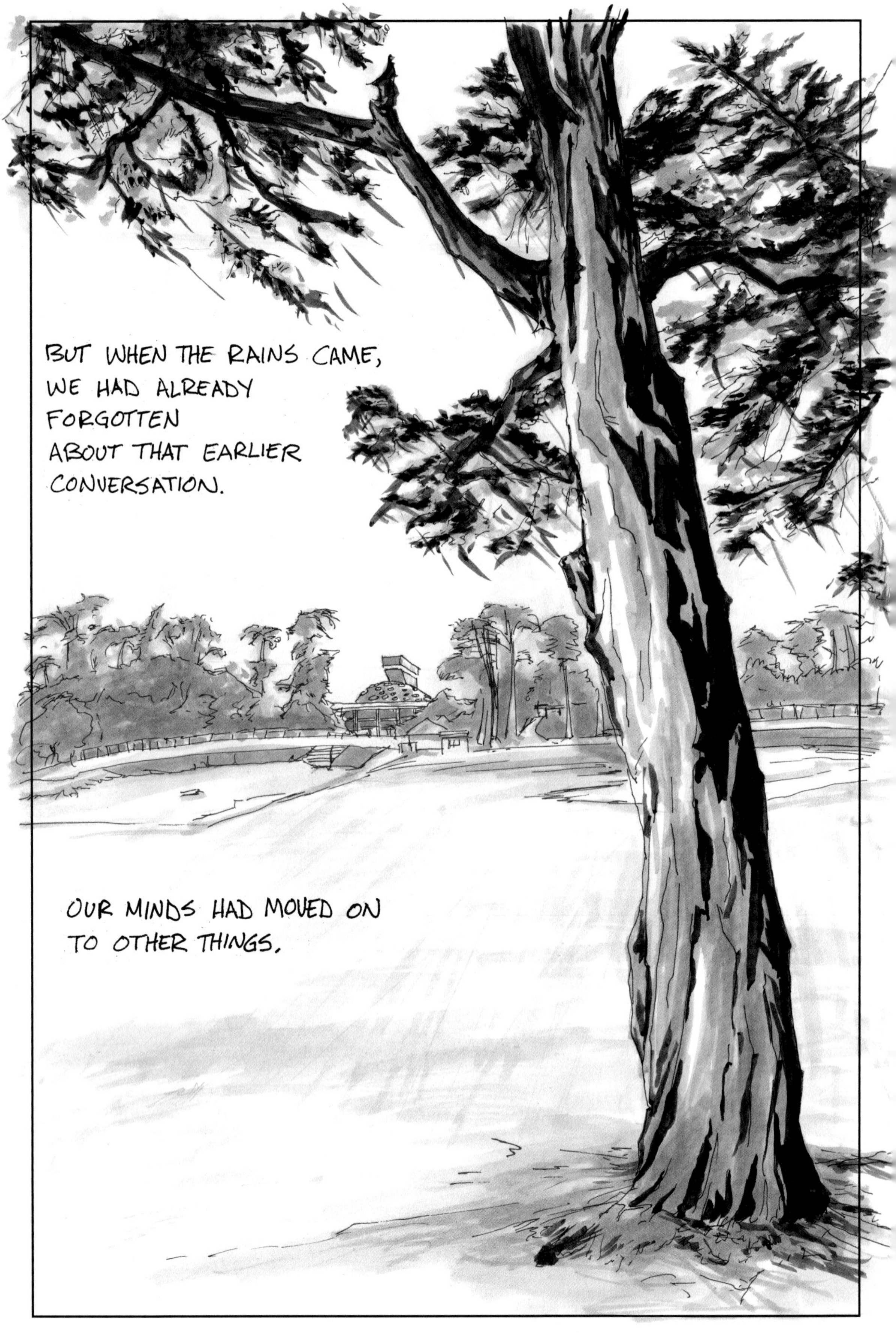
BUT WHEN THE RAINS CAME, WE HAD ALREADY FORGOTTEN ABOUT THAT EARLIER CONVERSATION.
OUR MINDS HAD MOVED ON TO OTHER THINGS.

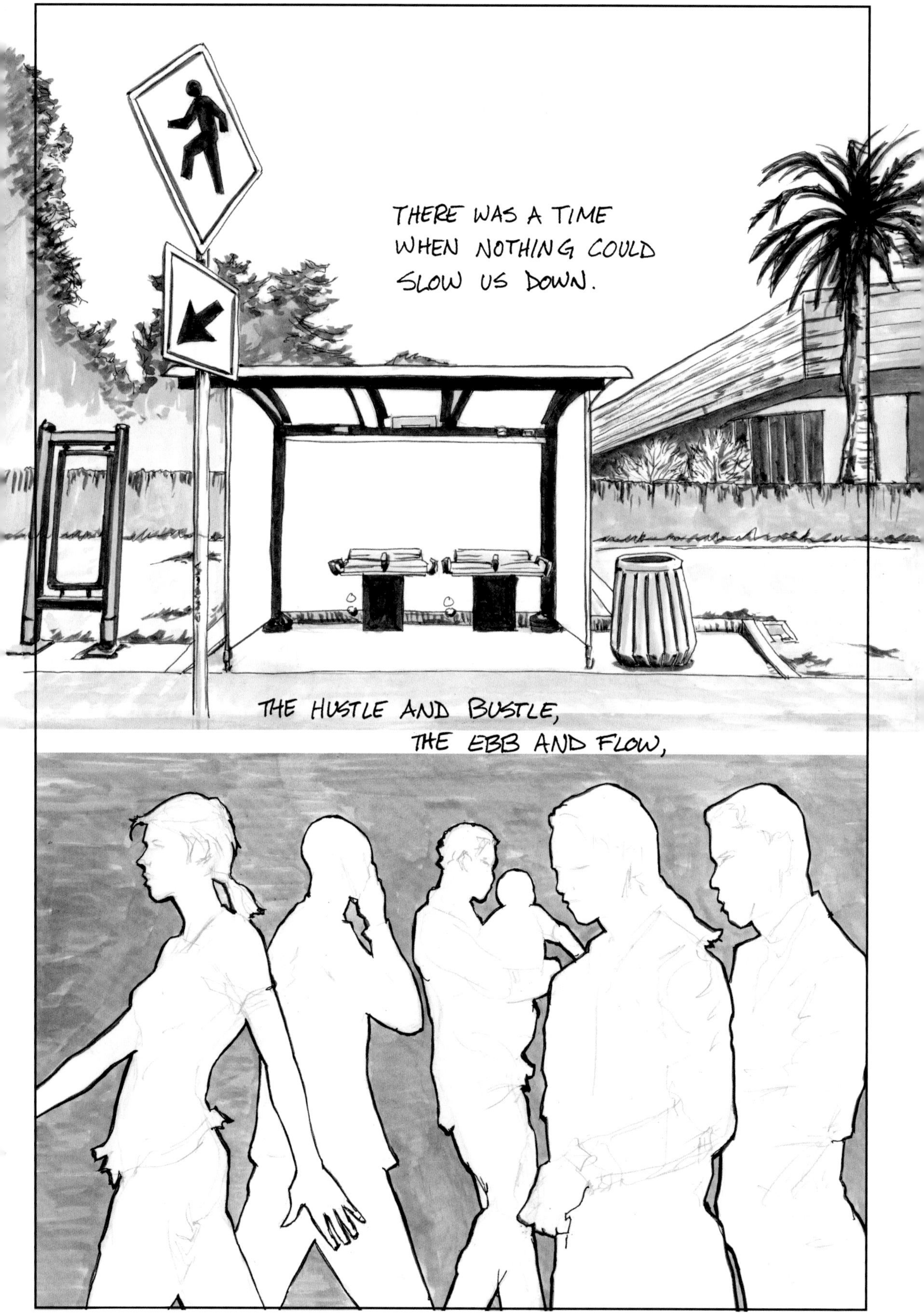
THERE WAS A TIME
WHEN NOTHING COULD
SLOW US DOWN.
THE HUSTLE AND BUSTLE,
THE EBB AND FLOW,

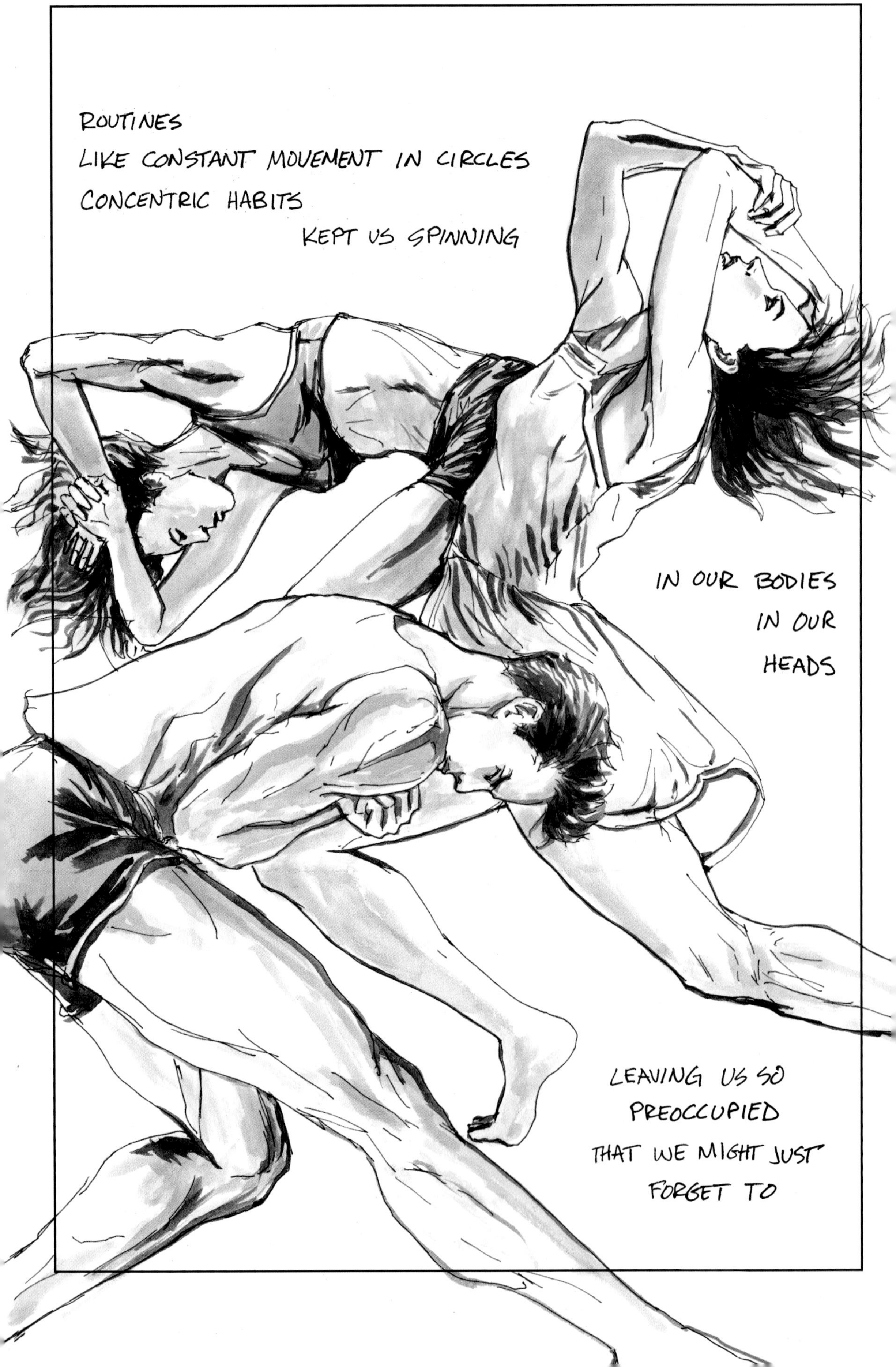
ROUTINES
LIKE CONSTANT MOVEMENT IN CIRCLES
CONCENTRIC HABITS
KEPT US SPINNING
IN OUR BODIES
IN OUR
HEADS
LEAVING US SO
PREOCCUPIED
THAT WE MIGHT JUST
FORGET TO

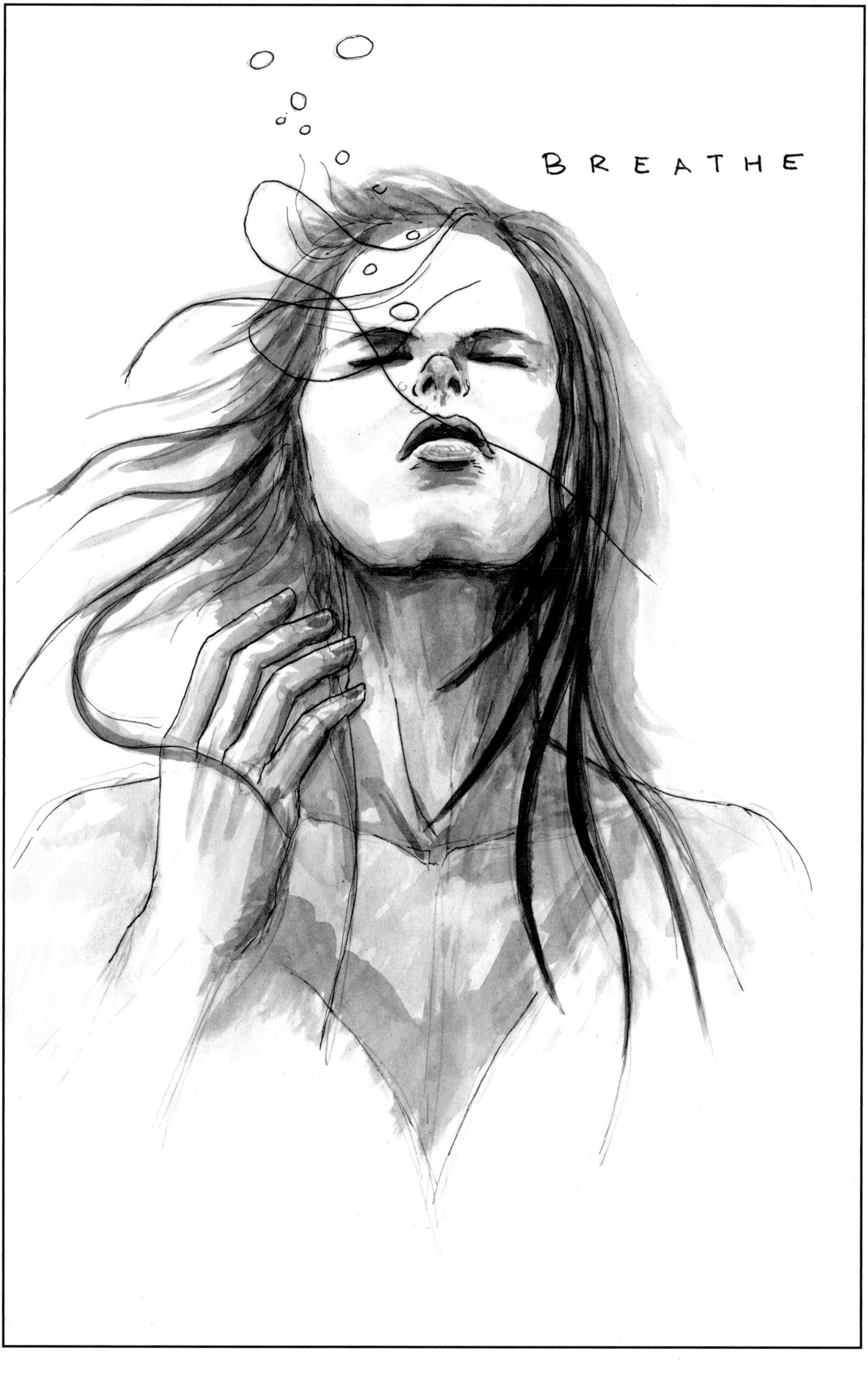
BREATHE

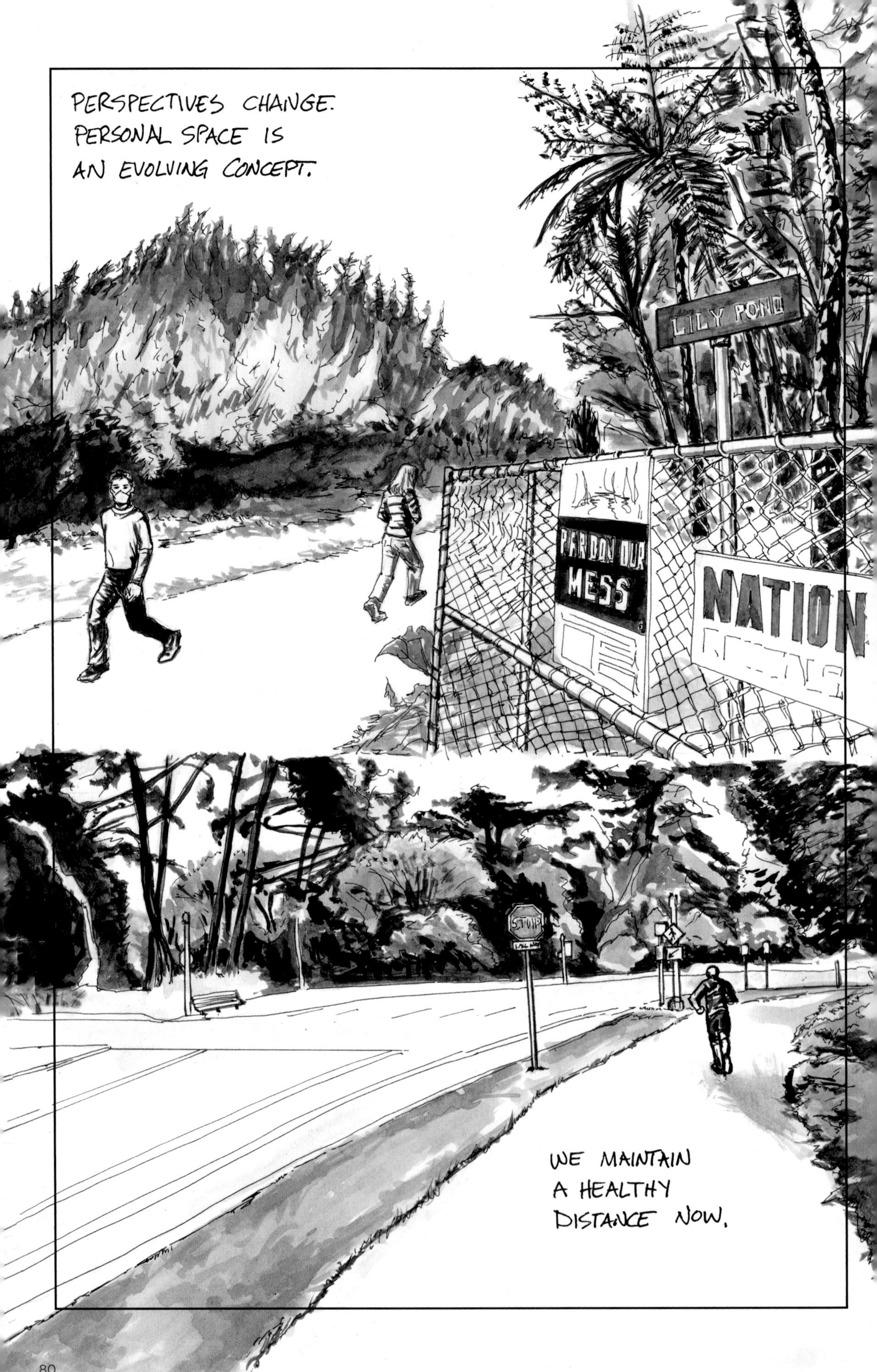
PERSPECTIVES CHANGE.
PERSONAL SPACE IS
AN EVOLVING CONCEPT.
LILY POND
PARDON OUR
MESS
NATION
WE MAINTAIN
A HEALTHY
DISTANCE NOW.

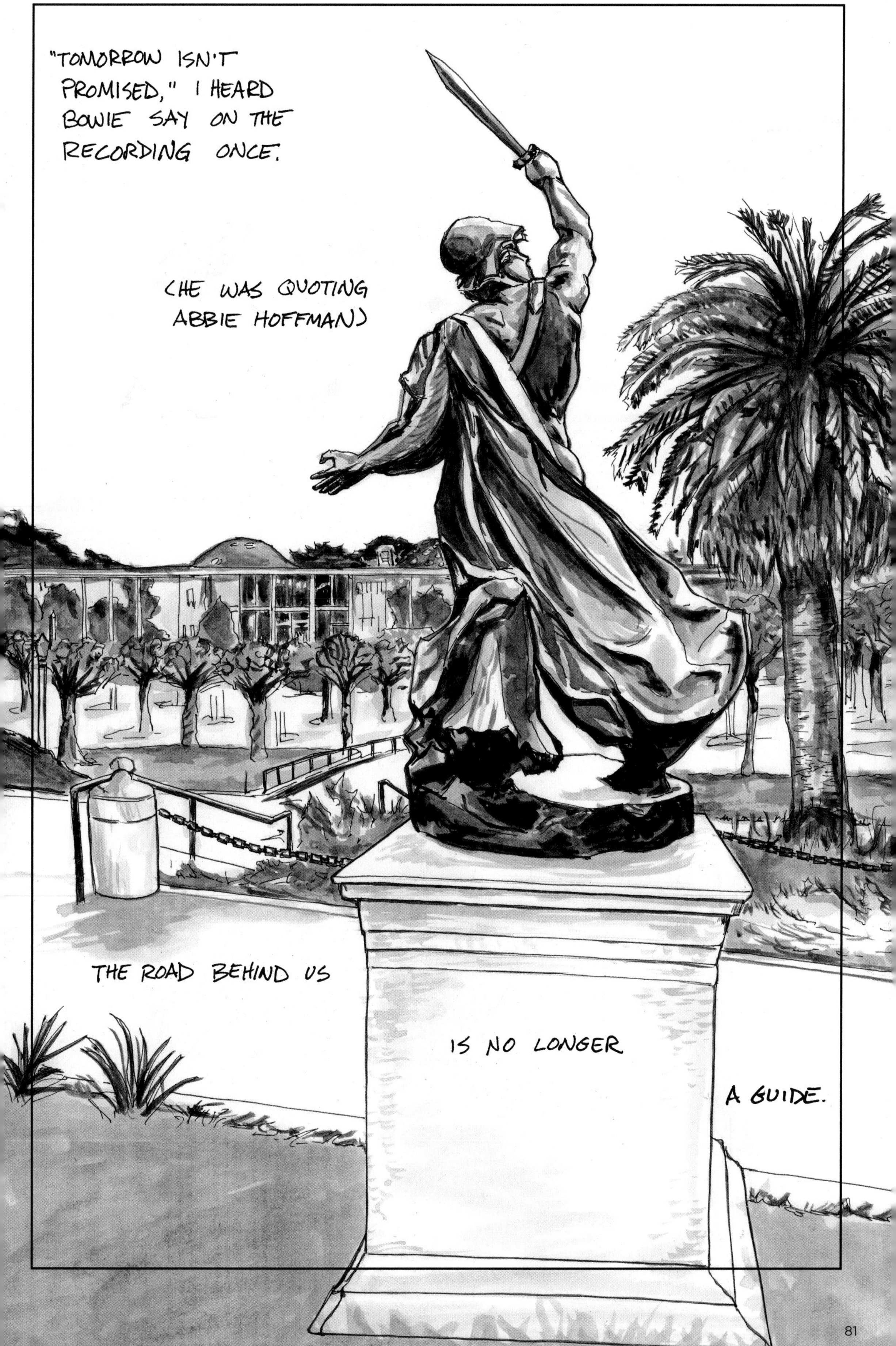
"TOMORROW ISN'T PROMISED," I HEARD BOWIE SAY ON THE RECORDING ONCE.
(HE WAS QUOTING ABBIE HOFFMAN)
THE ROAD BEHIND US
IS NO LONGER
A GUIDE.

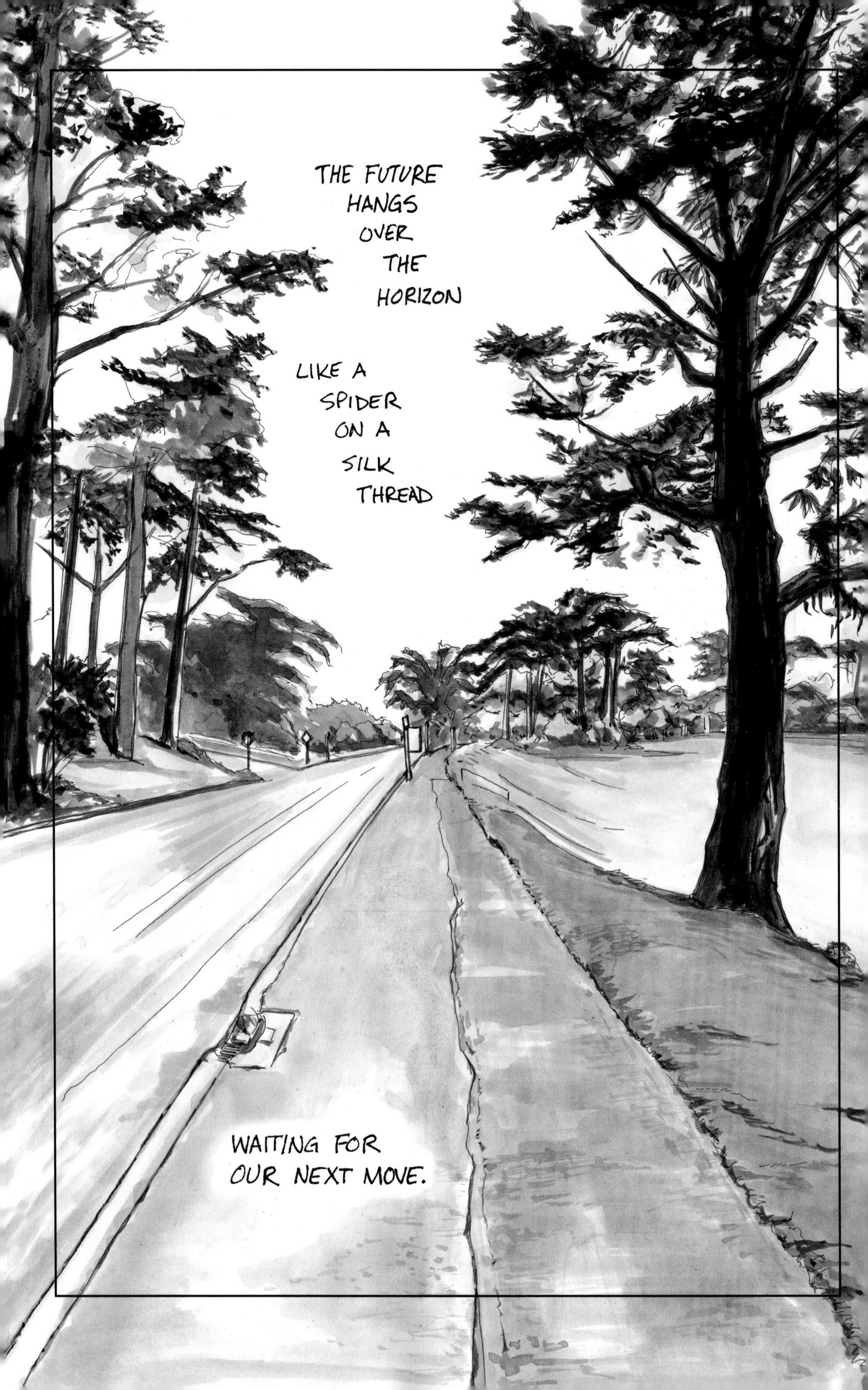
THE FUTURE HANGS OVER THE HORIZON
LIKE A SPIDER ON A SILK THREAD
WAITING FOR OUR NEXT MOVE.

GRIEF CHANGES

Shelley Wall

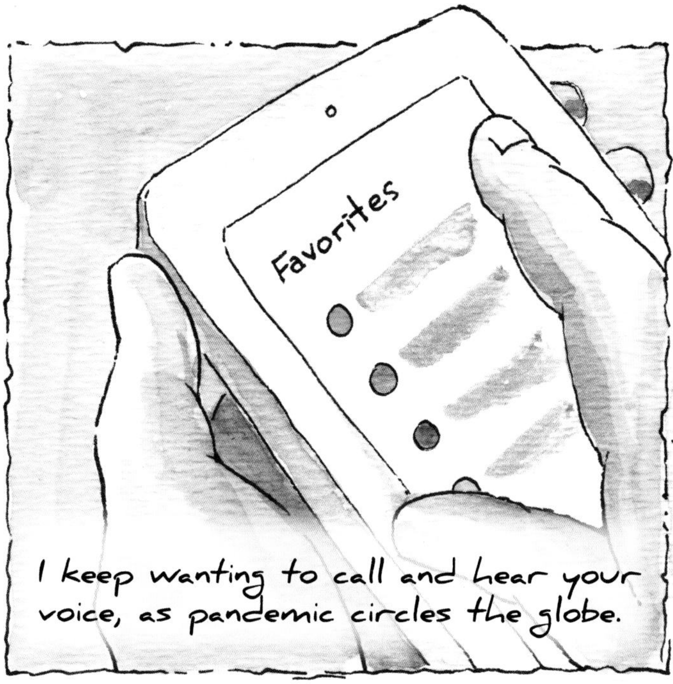
Favorites
I keep wanting to call and hear your voice, as pandemic circles the globe.

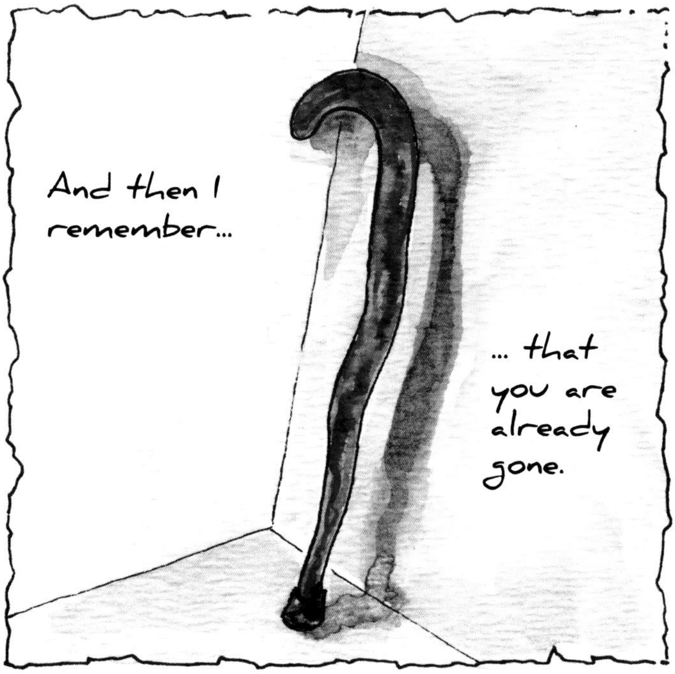
And then I remember...
... that you are already gone.

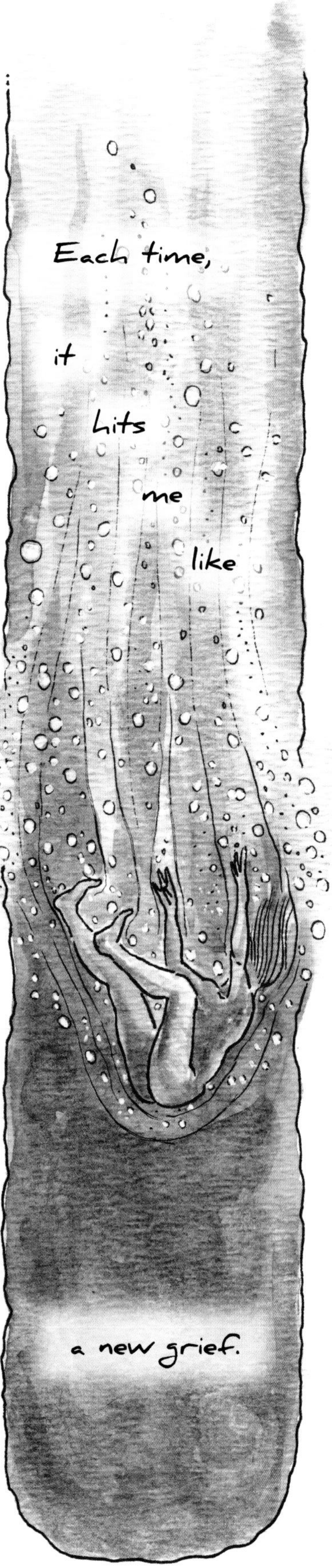
Each time,
it
hits
me
like
a new grief.

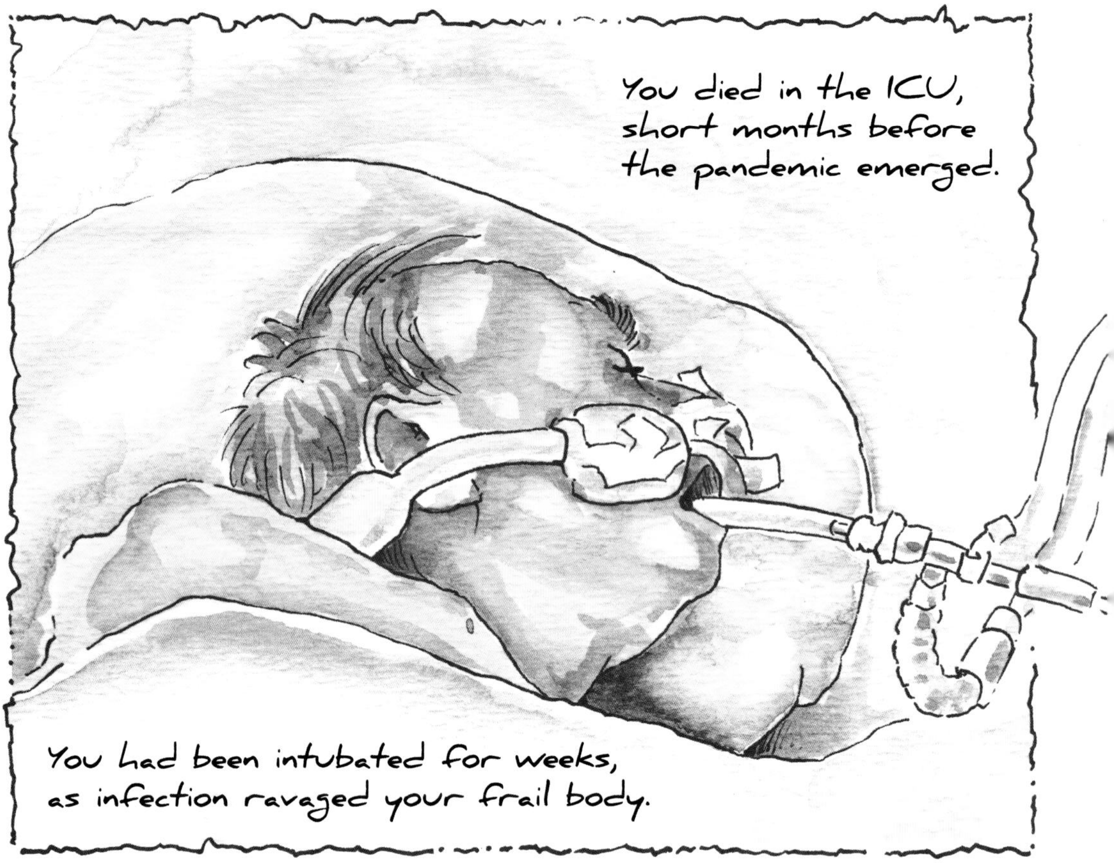
You died in the ICU, short months before the pandemic emerged.
You had been intubated for weeks, as infection ravaged your frail body.

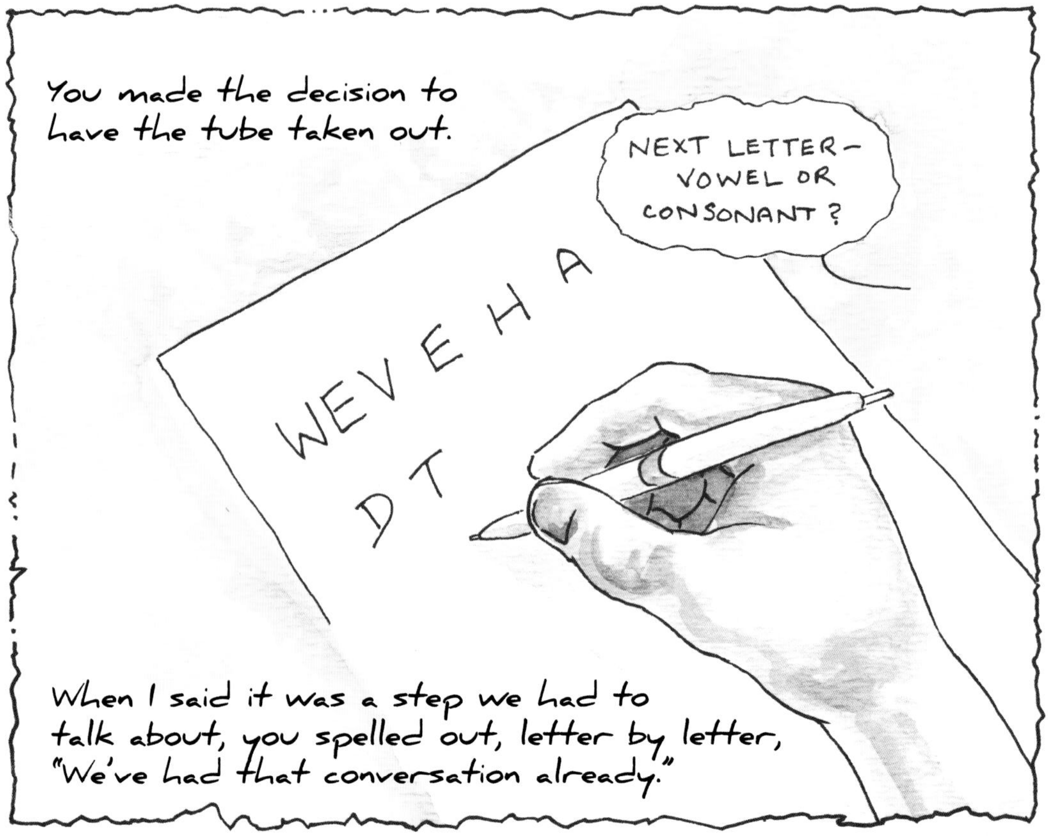
You made the decision to have the tube taken out.
NEXT LETTER - VOWEL OR CONSONANT ?
WEVE HA
DT
When I said it was a step we had to talk about, you spelled out, letter by letter, "We've had that conversation already."

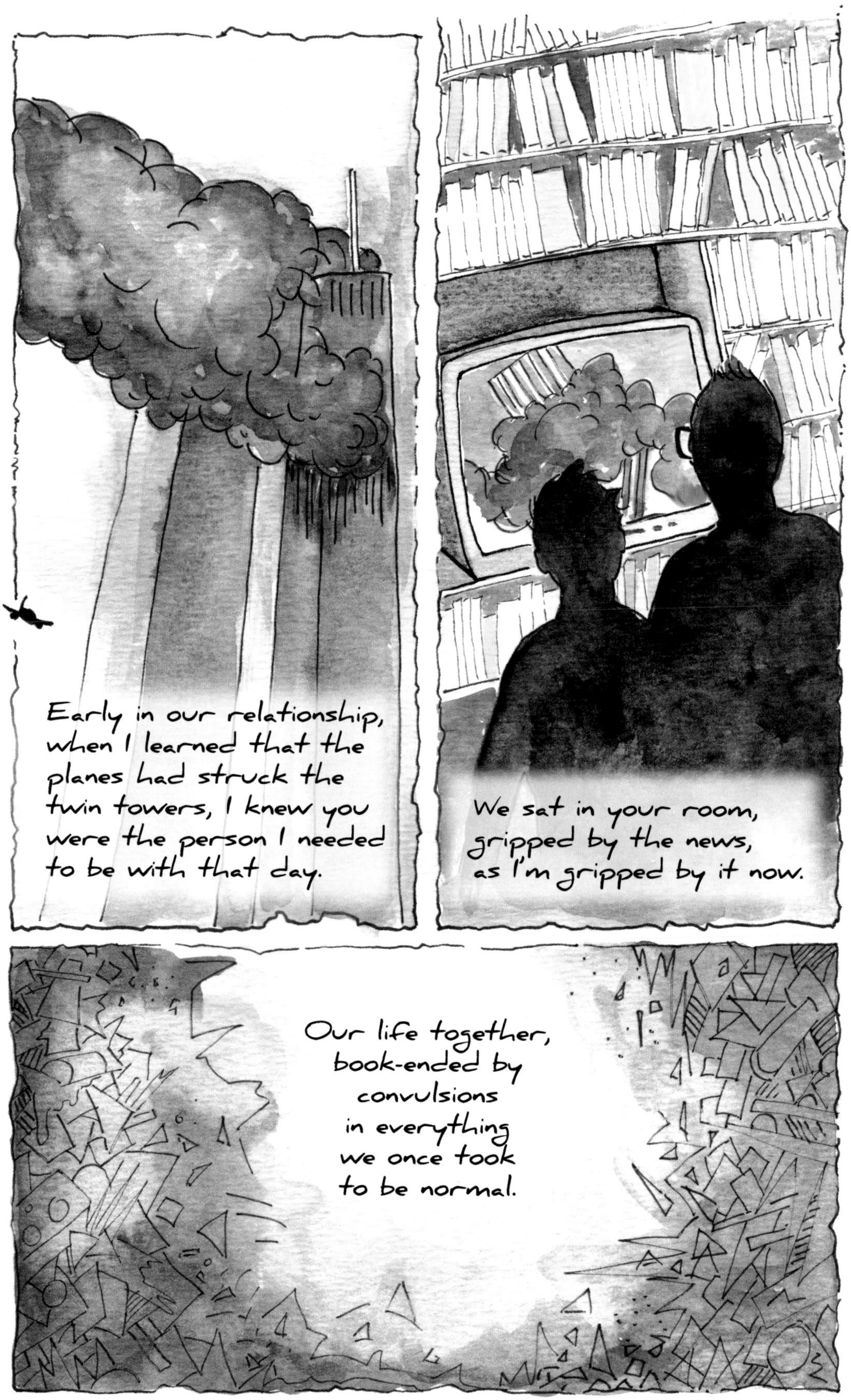
Early in our relationship, when I learned that the planes had struck the twin towers, I knew you were the person I needed to be with that day.
We sat in your room, gripped by the news, as I'm gripped by it now.
Our life together, book-ended by convulsions in everything we once took to be normal.

The fabric of nightmare late last year...

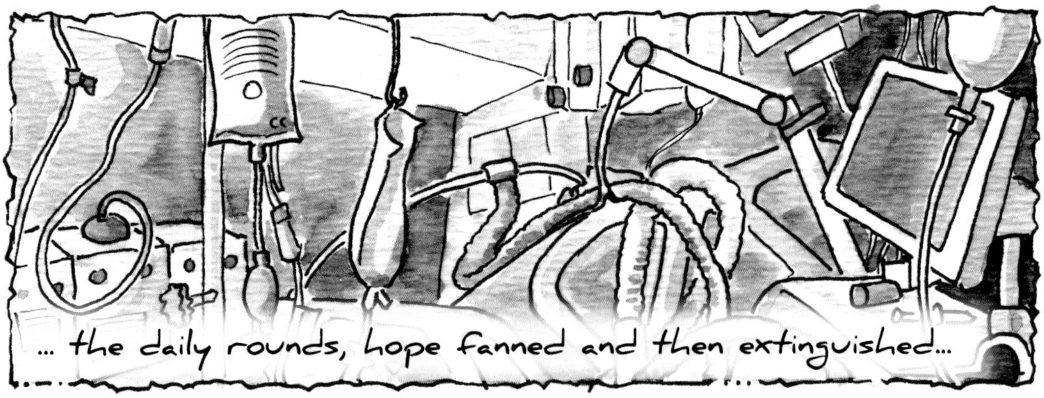
... the daily rounds, hope fanned and then extinguished...

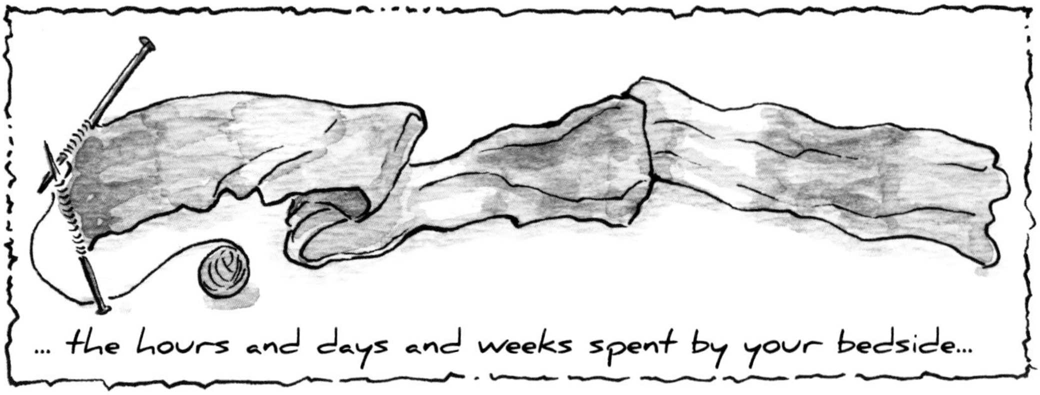
... the hours and days and weeks spent by your bedside...

... holding your hand as you took your last breath...

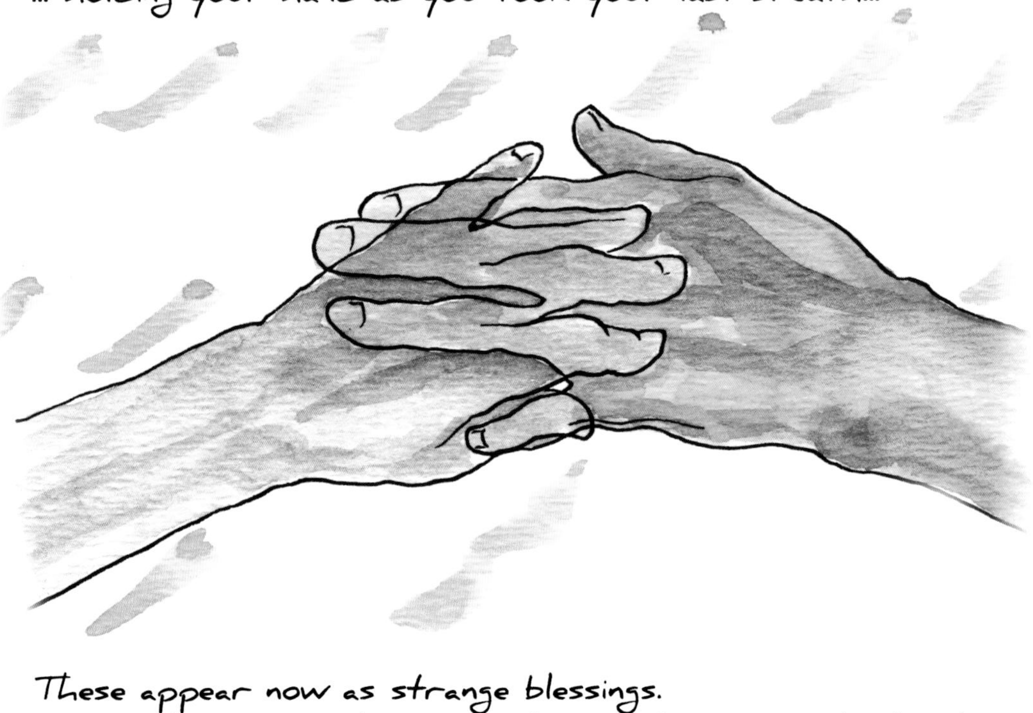

These appear now as strange blessings.
I was able to be with you. In this pandemic, people die alone.

Grief changes when individual, inconceivable loss is overwhelmed by this global wave of catastrophe, fresh on its heels.

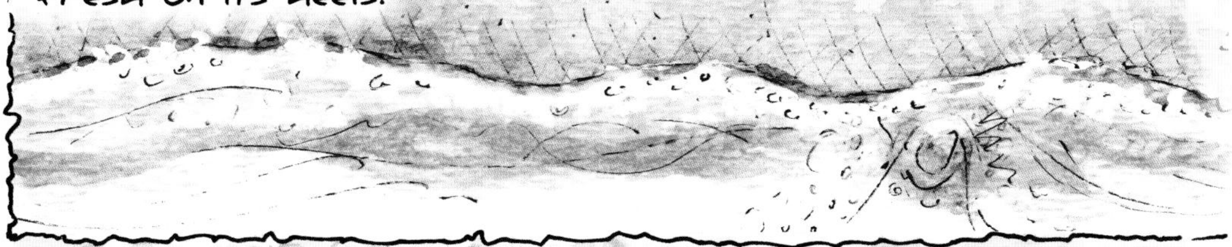

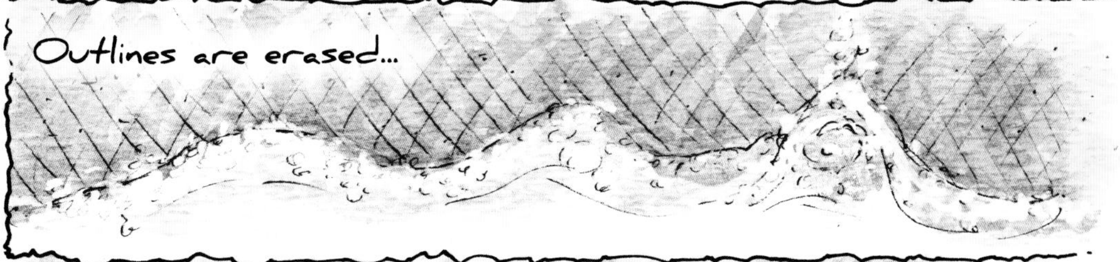
Outlines are erased...

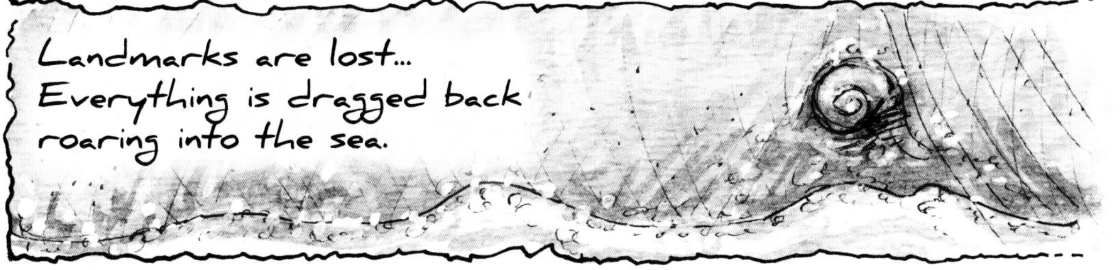
Landmarks are lost...
Everything is dragged back roaring into the sea.

I cling to fragments to stay afloat...

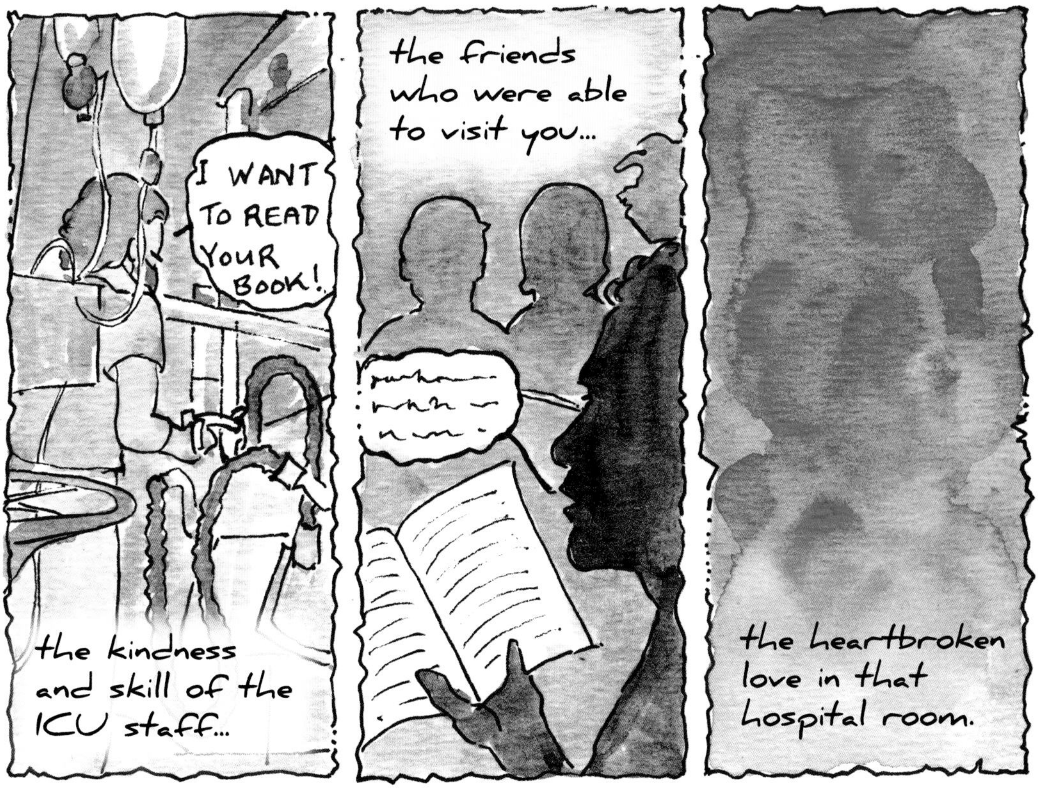
I WANT TO READ YOUR BOOK!
the kindness and skill of the ICU staff...
the friends who were able to visit you...
the heartbroken love in that hospital room.

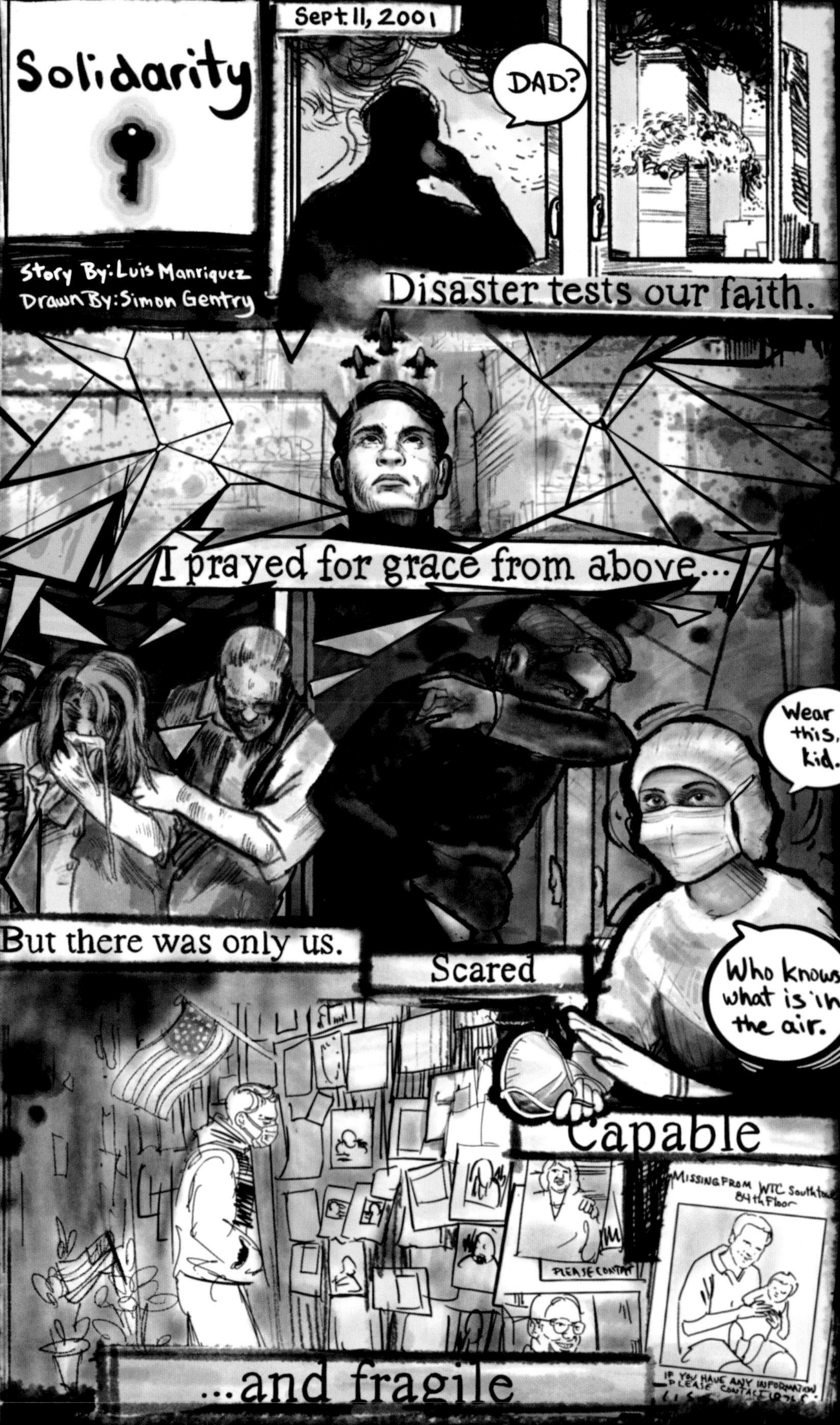
Solidarity
Story By: Luis Manriquez
Drawn By: Simon Gentry
Sept. 11, 2001
DAD?
Disaster tests our faith.
I prayed for grace from above...
Wear this, kid.
But there was only us.
Scared
Who knows what is in the air.
Capable
MISSING FROM WTC South tower 84th Floor
IF YOU HAVE ANY INFORMATION PLEASE CONTACT
PLEASE CONTACT
...and fragile

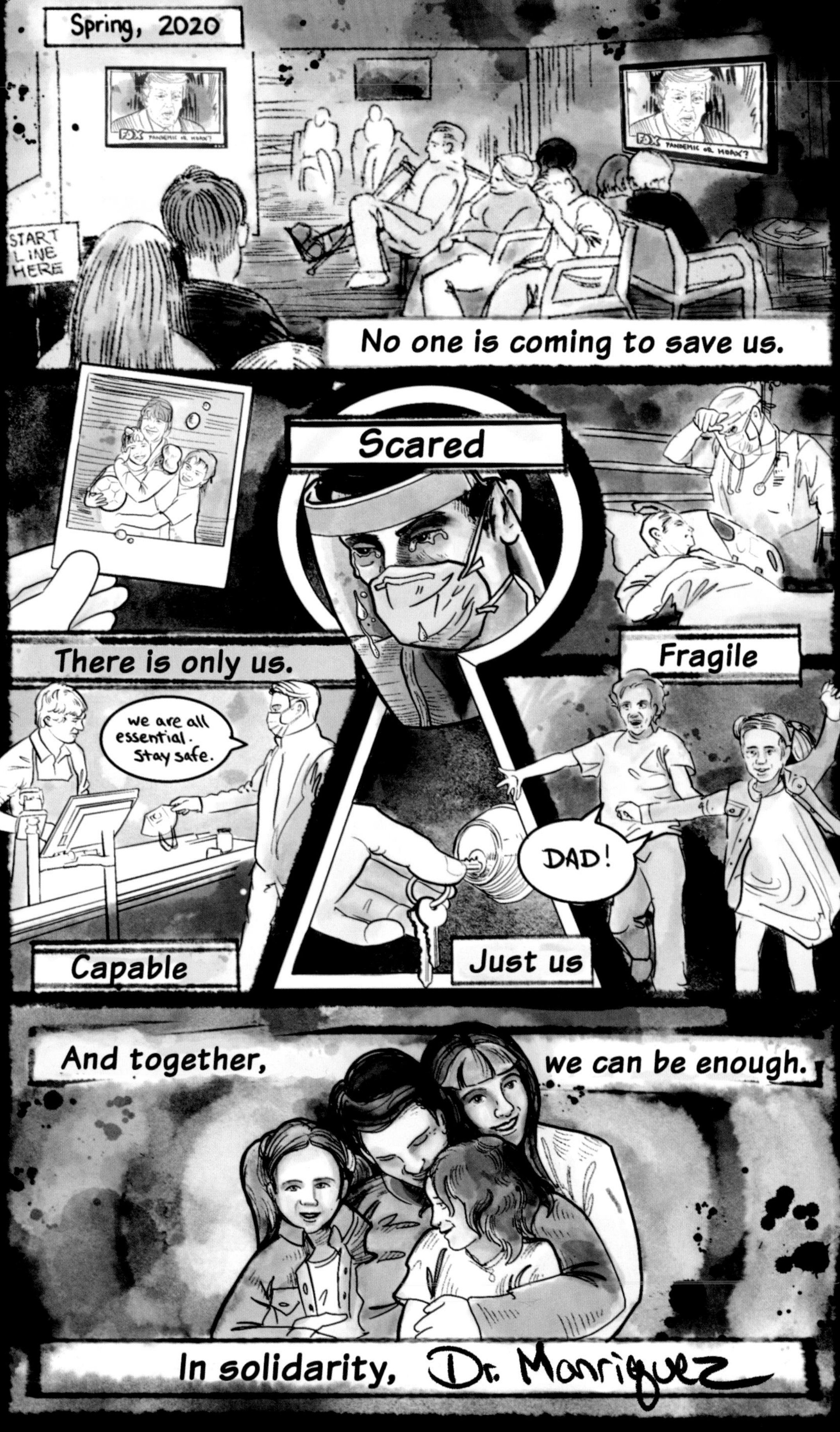

Spring, 2020
FOX PANDEMIC OR HOAX?
START LINE HERE
FOX PANDEMIC OR HOAX?
No one is coming to save us.
Scared
There is only us.
Fragile
we are all essential. Stay safe.
DAD!
Capable
Just us
And together,
we can be enough.
In solidarity, Dr. Manriquez

THE HERO IN MY HEART

STORY: KANG JING
ART: KANG JING
COLOURS: PAVITH C.

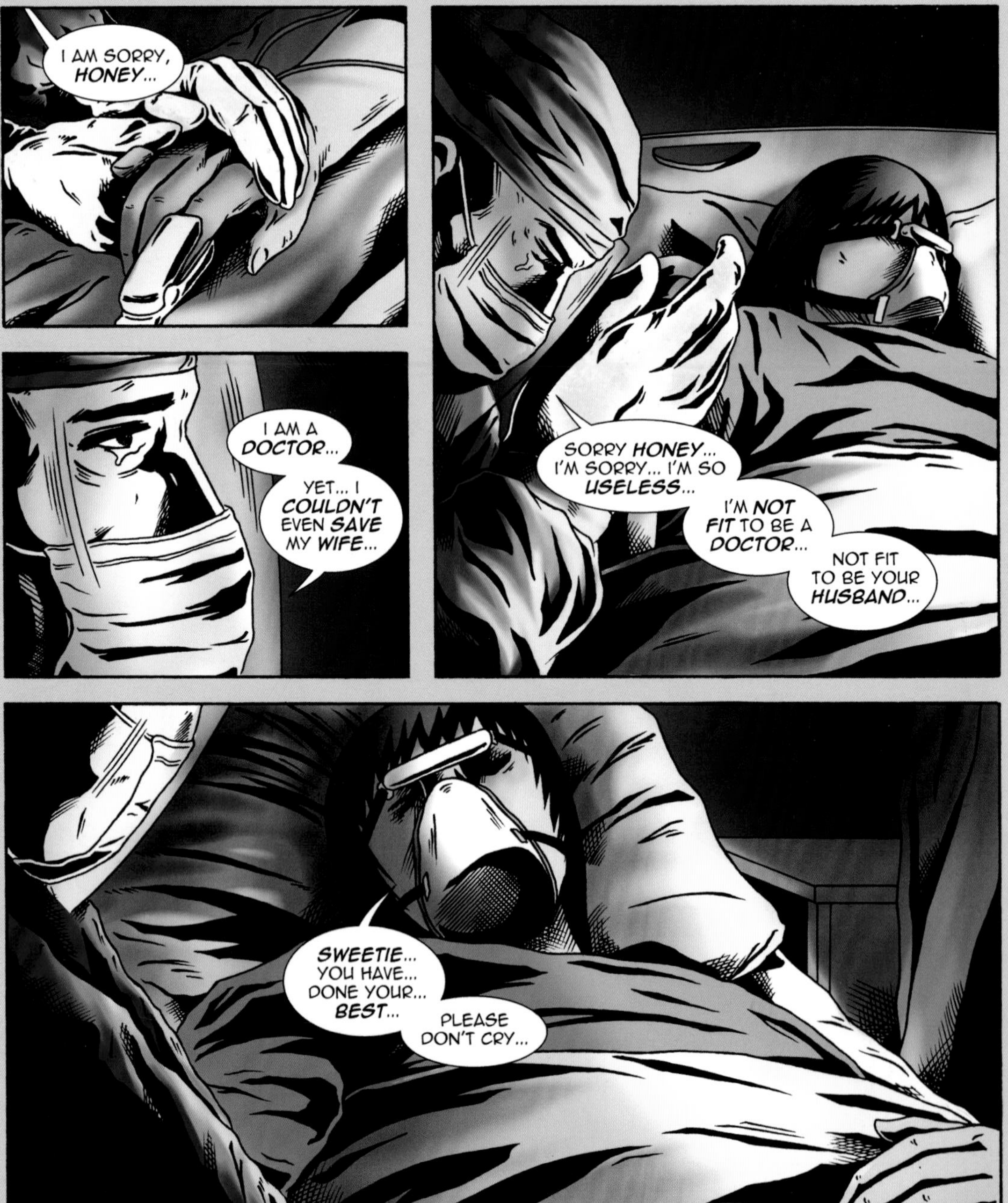
I AM SORRY, HONEY...
I AM A DOCTOR...
YET... I COULDN'T EVEN SAVE MY WIFE...
SORRY HONEY... I'M SORRY... I'M SO USELESS...
I'M NOT FIT TO BE A DOCTOR...
NOT FIT TO BE YOUR HUSBAND...
SWEETIE... YOU HAVE... DONE YOUR... BEST...
PLEASE DON'T CRY...

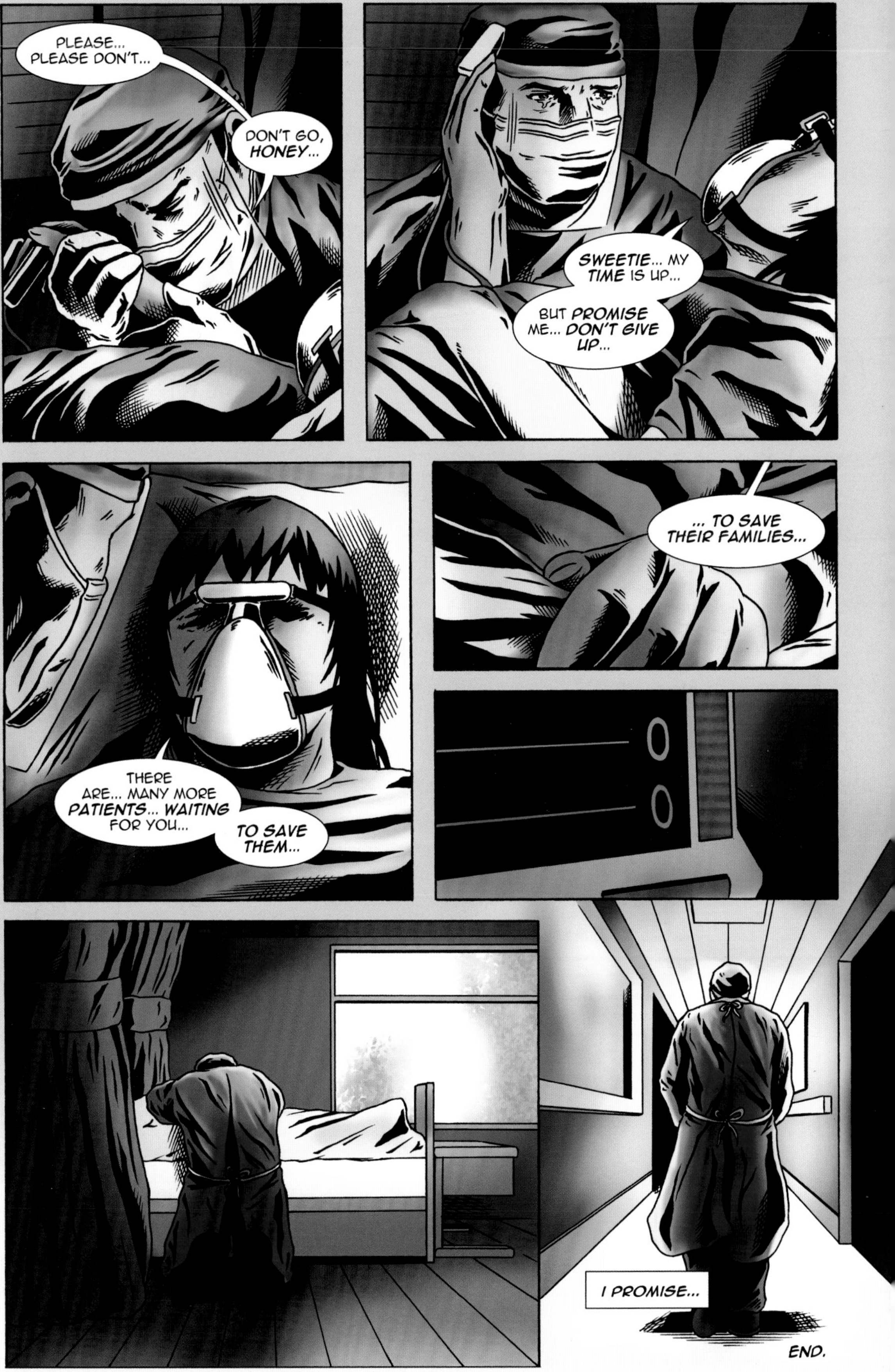
PLEASE... PLEASE DON'T...
DON'T GO, HONEY...
SWEETIE... MY TIME IS UP...
BUT PROMISE ME... DON'T GIVE UP...
THERE ARE... MANY MORE PATIENTS... WAITING FOR YOU...
TO SAVE THEM...
... TO SAVE THEIR FAMILIES...
I PROMISE...
END.

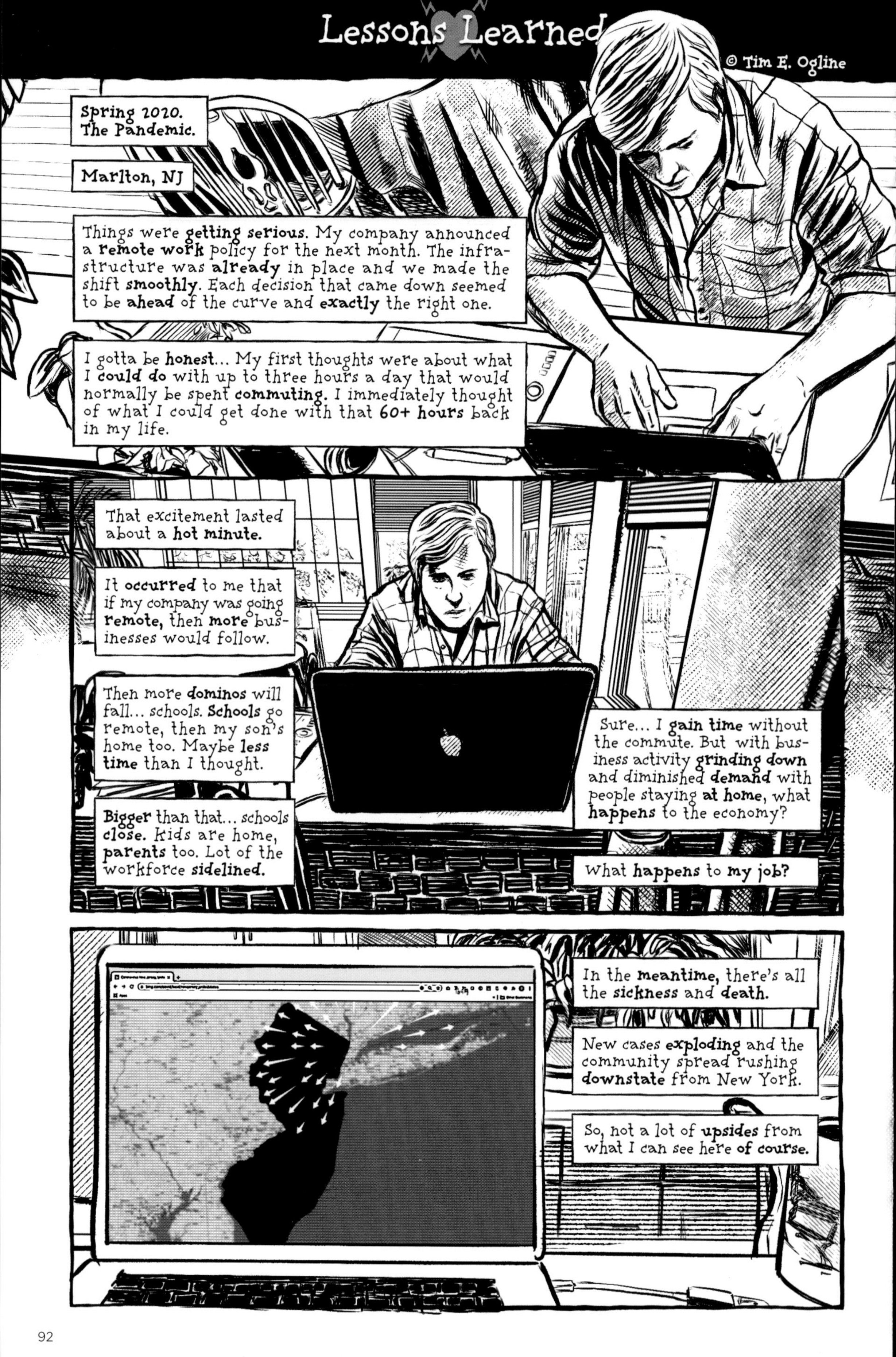
Lessons Learned
© Tim E. Ogline
Spring 2020. The Pandemic.
Marlton, NJ
Things were getting serious. My company announced a remote work policy for the next month. The infrastructure was already in place and we made the shift smoothly. Each decision that came down seemed to be ahead of the curve and exactly the right one.
I gotta be honest... My first thoughts were about what I could do with up to three hours a day that would normally be spent commuting. I immediately thought of what I could get done with that 60+ hours back in my life.
That excitement lasted about a hot minute.
It occurred to me that if my company was going remote, then more businesses would follow.
Then more dominos will fall... schools. Schools go remote, then my son's home too. Maybe less time than I thought.
Bigger than that... schools close. Kids are home, parents too. Lot of the workforce sidelined.
Sure... I gain time without the commute. But with business activity grinding down and diminished demand with people staying at home, what happens to the economy?
What happens to my job?
In the meantime, there's all the sickness and death.
New cases exploding and the community spread rushing downstate from New York.
So, not a lot of upsides from what I can see here of course.

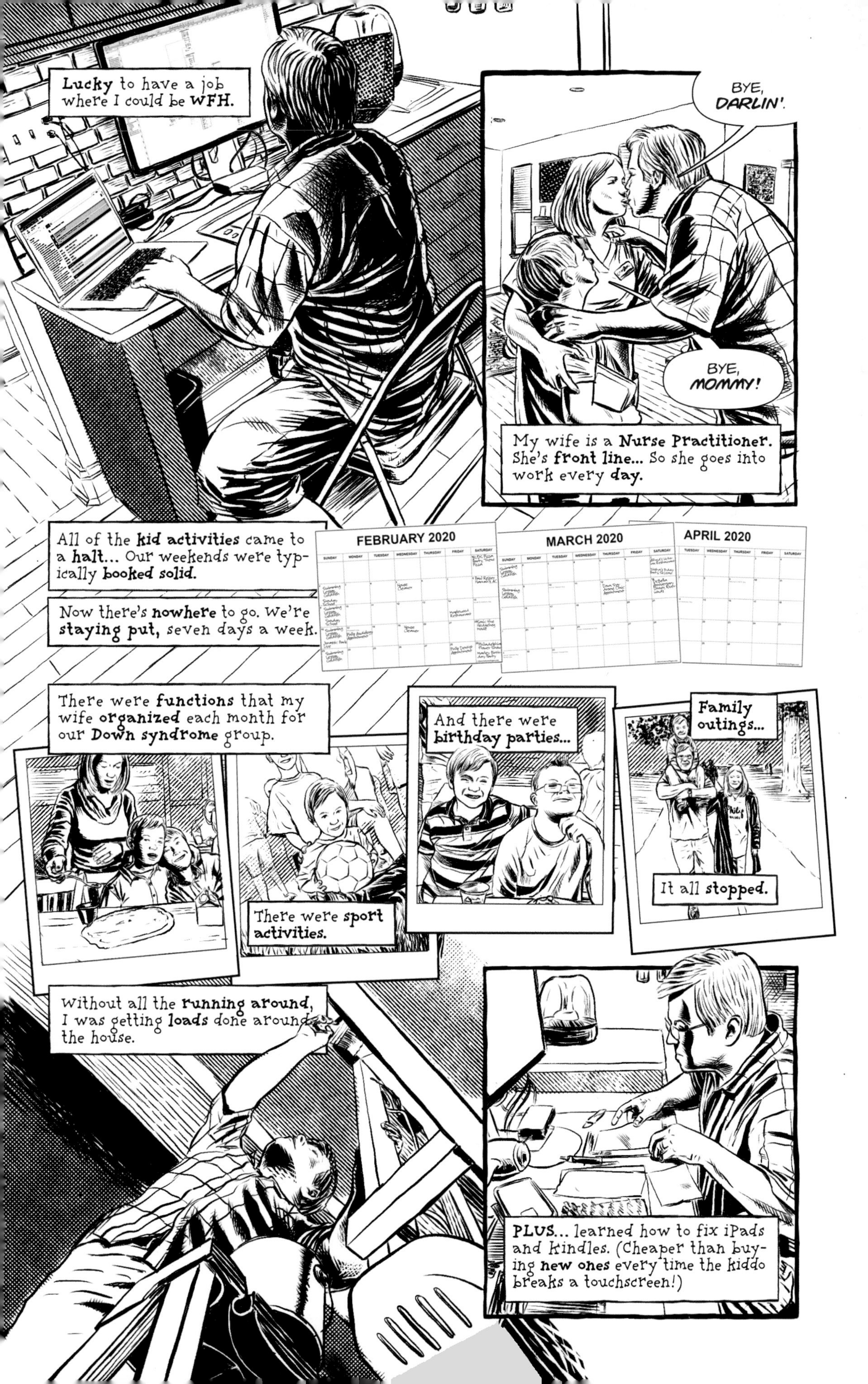

Lucky to have a job where I could be WFH.
BYE, DARLIN'.
BYE, MOMMY!
My wife is a Nurse Practitioner. She's front line... So she goes into work every day.
All of the kid activities came to a halt... Our weekends were typically booked solid.
Now there's nowhere to go. We're staying put, seven days a week.
FEBRUARY 2020
MARCH 2020
APRIL 2020
There were functions that my wife organized each month for our Down syndrome group.
There were sport activities.
And there were birthday parties...
Family outings...
It all stopped.
Without all the running around, I was getting loads done around the house.
PLUS... learned how to fix iPads and Kindles. (Cheaper than buying new ones every time the kiddo breaks a touchscreen!)

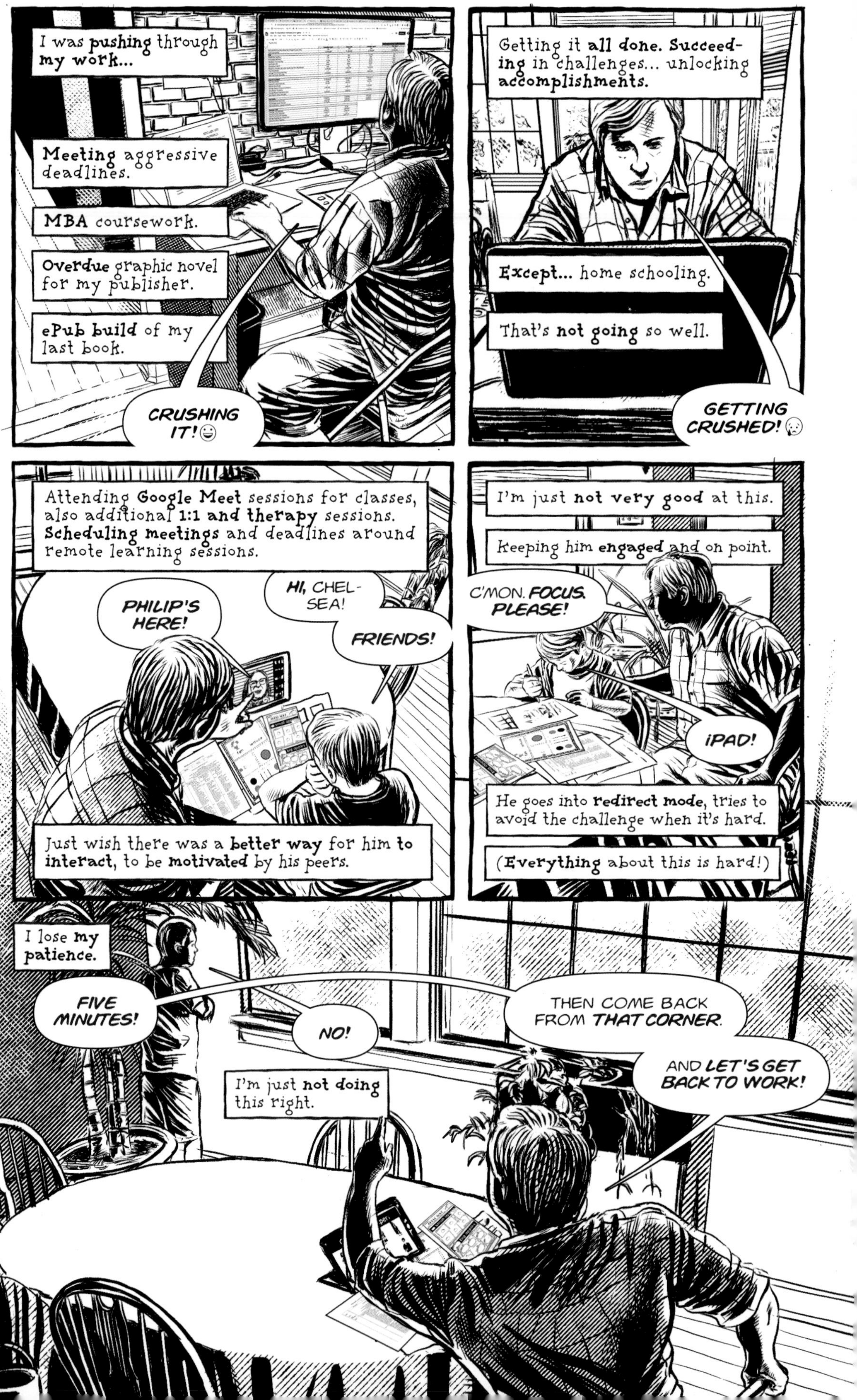
I was **pushing** through **my work...**
Meeting aggressive deadlines.
MBA coursework.
Overdue graphic novel for my publisher.
ePub build of my last book.
CRUSHING IT!
Getting it **all done. Succeeding** in challenges... unlocking **accomplishments.**
Except... home schooling.
That's **not going** so well.
GETTING CRUSHED!
Attending **Google Meet** sessions for classes, also additional **1:1 and therapy** sessions. **Scheduling meetings** and deadlines around remote learning sessions.
PHILIP'S HERE!
HI, CHELSEA!
FRIENDS!
Just wish there was a **better way** for him **to interact**, to be **motivated** by his peers.
I'm just **not very good** at this.
Keeping him **engaged** and on point.
C'MON. FOCUS. PLEASE!
iPAD!
He goes into **redirect mode**, tries to avoid the challenge when it's hard.
(**Everything** about this is hard!)
I lose **my patience.**
FIVE MINUTES!
NO!
THEN COME BACK FROM THAT CORNER.
AND LET'S GET BACK TO WORK!
I'm just **not doing** this right.

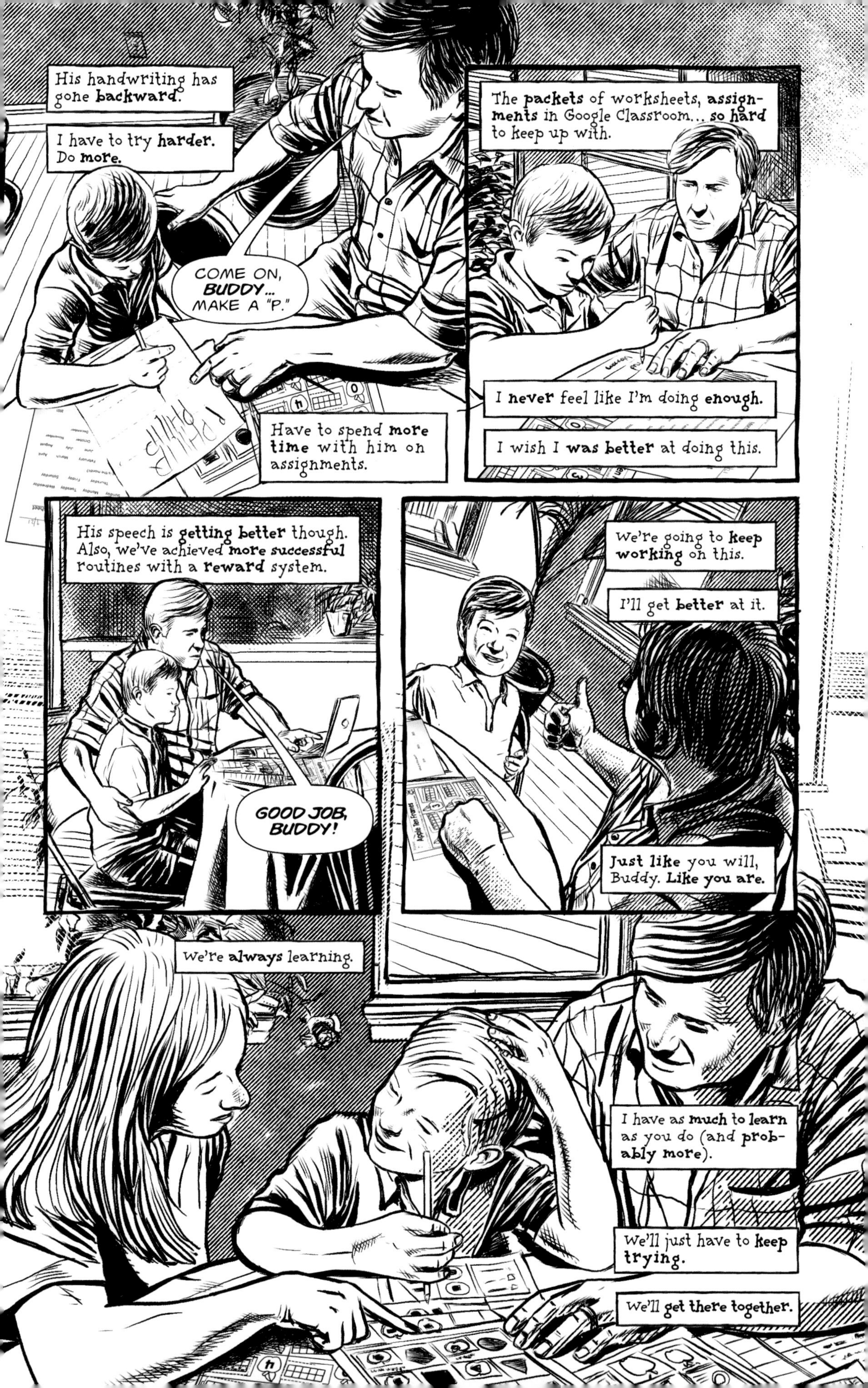
His handwriting has gone **backward**.
I have to try **harder**. Do **more**.
COME ON, BUDDY... MAKE A "P."
Have to spend **more time** with him on assignments.
The **packets** of worksheets, **assignments** in Google Classroom... **so hard** to keep up with.
I **never** feel like I'm doing **enough**.
I wish I **was better** at doing this.
His speech is **getting better** though. Also, we've achieved **more successful** routines with a **reward** system.
GOOD JOB, BUDDY!
We're going to **keep working** on this.
I'll get **better** at it.
Just like you will, Buddy. **Like you are**.
We're **always** learning.
I have as **much to learn** as you do (and **probably more**).
We'll just have to **keep trying**.
We'll **get there together**.

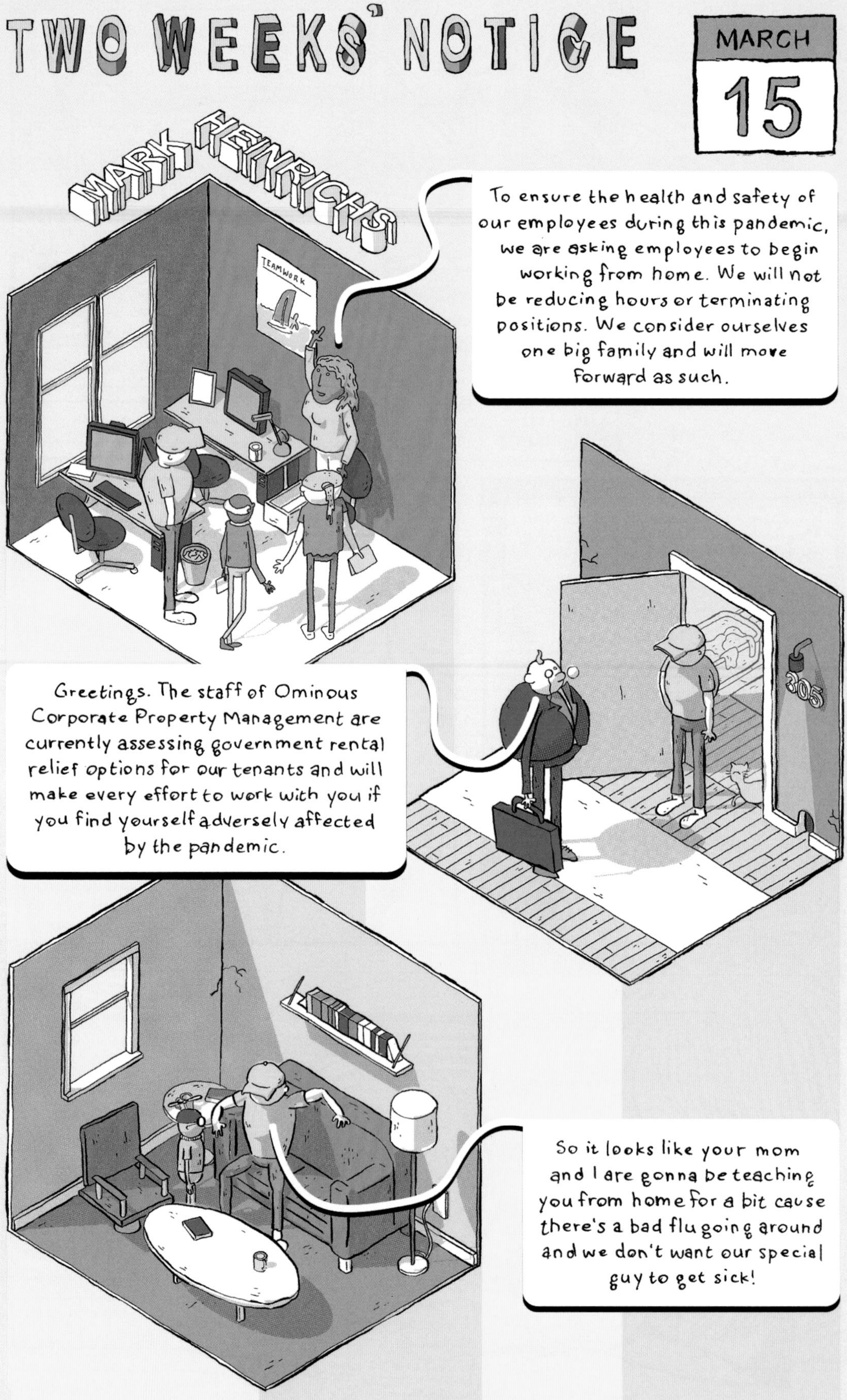
TWO WEEKS' NOTICE
MARCH 15
MARK HEINRICHS
TEAMWORK
To ensure the health and safety of our employees during this pandemic, we are asking employees to begin working from home. We will not be reducing hours or terminating positions. We consider ourselves one big family and will move forward as such.
Greetings. The staff of Ominous Corporate Property Management are currently assessing government rental relief options for our tenants and will make every effort to work with you if you find yourself adversely affected by the pandemic.
305
So it looks like your mom and I are gonna be teaching you from home for a bit cause there's a bad flu going around and we don't want our special guy to get sick!

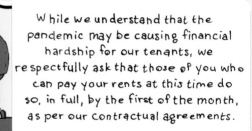

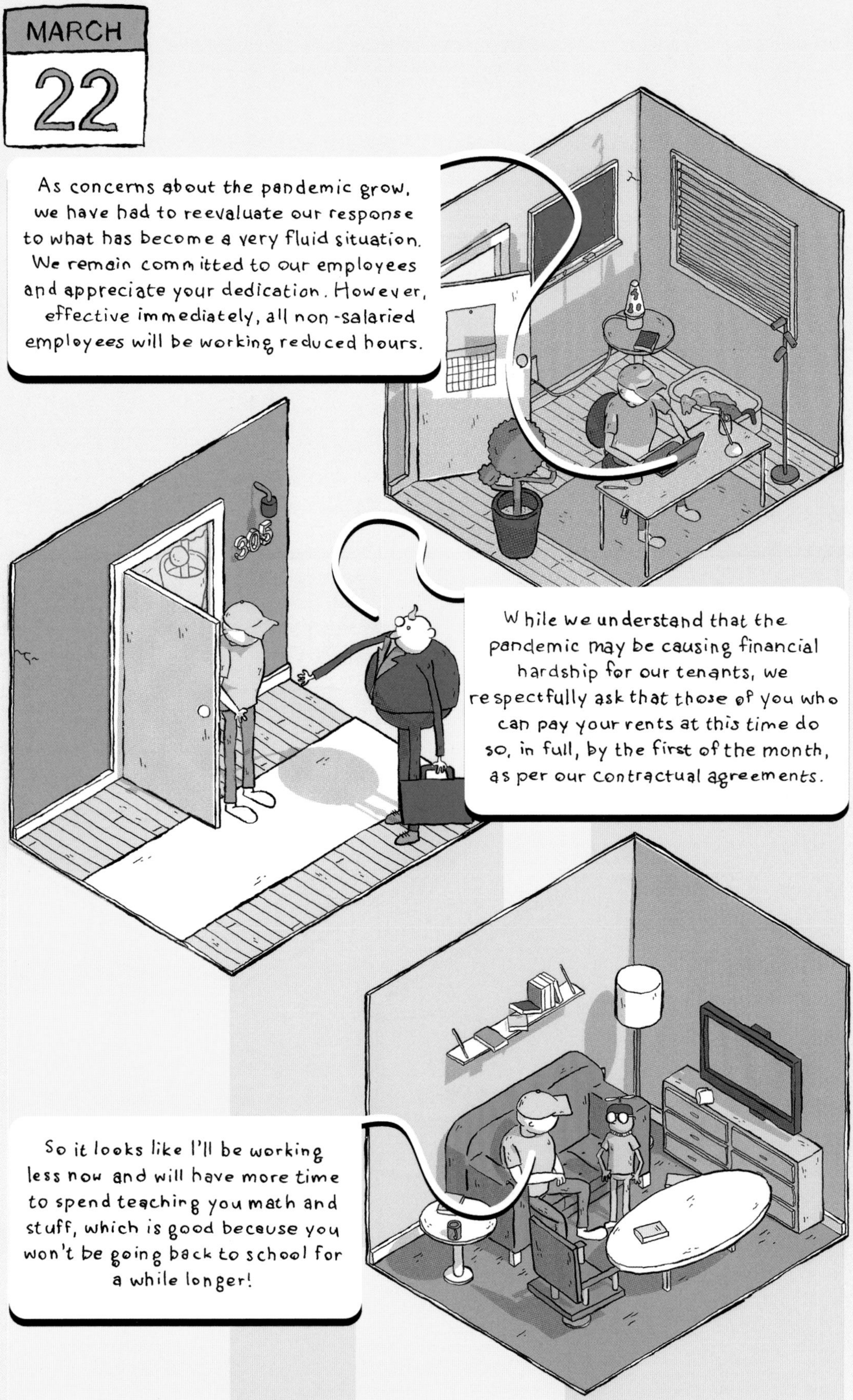

MARCH
22

As concerns about the pandemic grow, we have had to reevaluate our response to what has become a very fluid situation. We remain committed to our employees and appreciate your dedication. However, effective immediately, all non-salaried employees will be working reduced hours.

While we understand that the pandemic may be causing financial hardship for our tenants, we respectfully ask that those of you who can pay your rents at this time do so, in full, by the first of the month, as per our contractual agreements.

So it looks like I'll be working less now and will have more time to spend teaching you math and stuff, which is good because you won't be going back to school for a while longer!

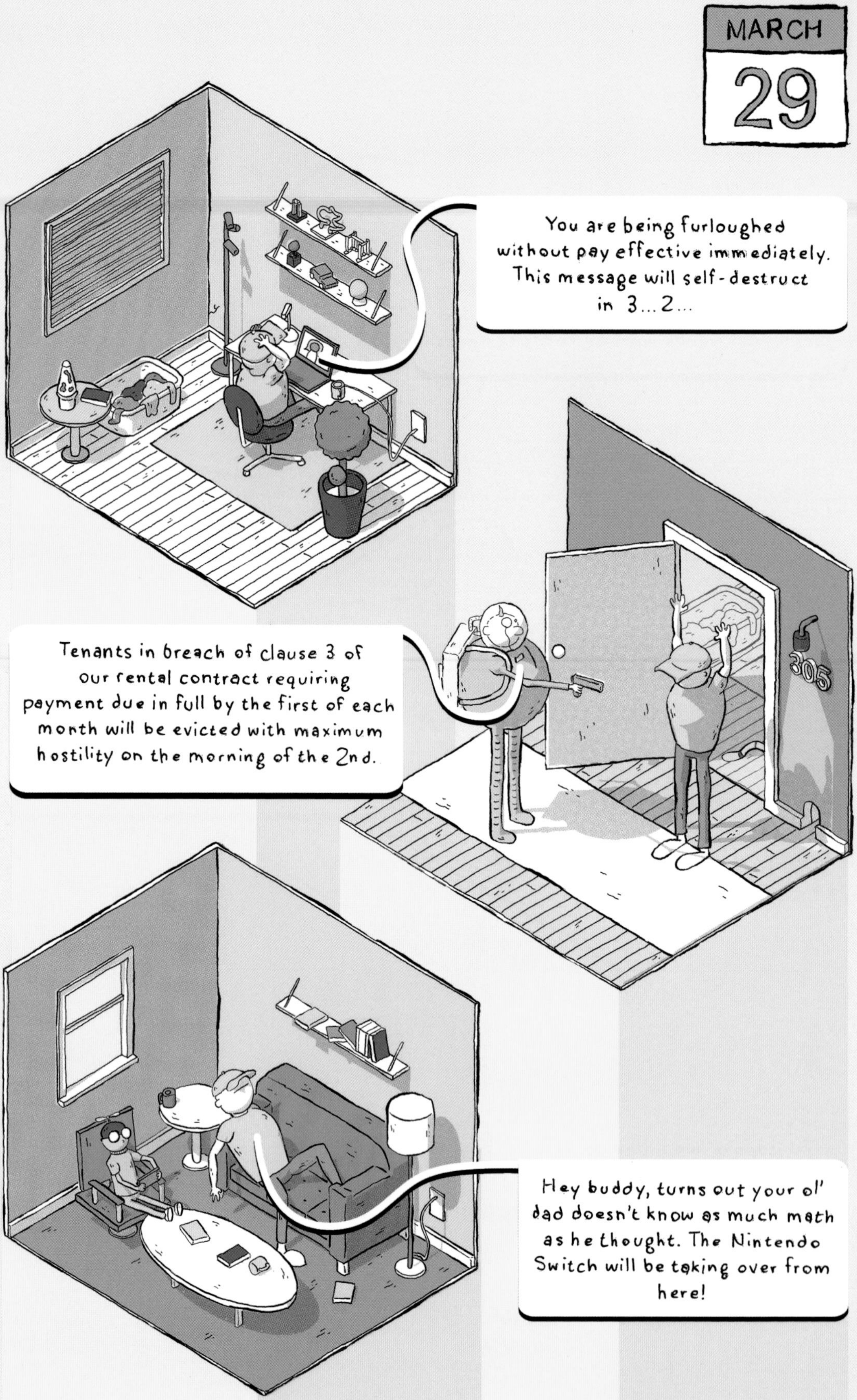
MARCH
29
You are being furloughed without pay effective immediately. This message will self-destruct in 3... 2...
Tenants in breach of clause 3 of our rental contract requiring payment due in full by the first of each month will be evicted with maximum hostility on the morning of the 2nd.
305
Hey buddy, turns out your ol' dad doesn't know as much math as he thought. The Nintendo Switch will be taking over from here!

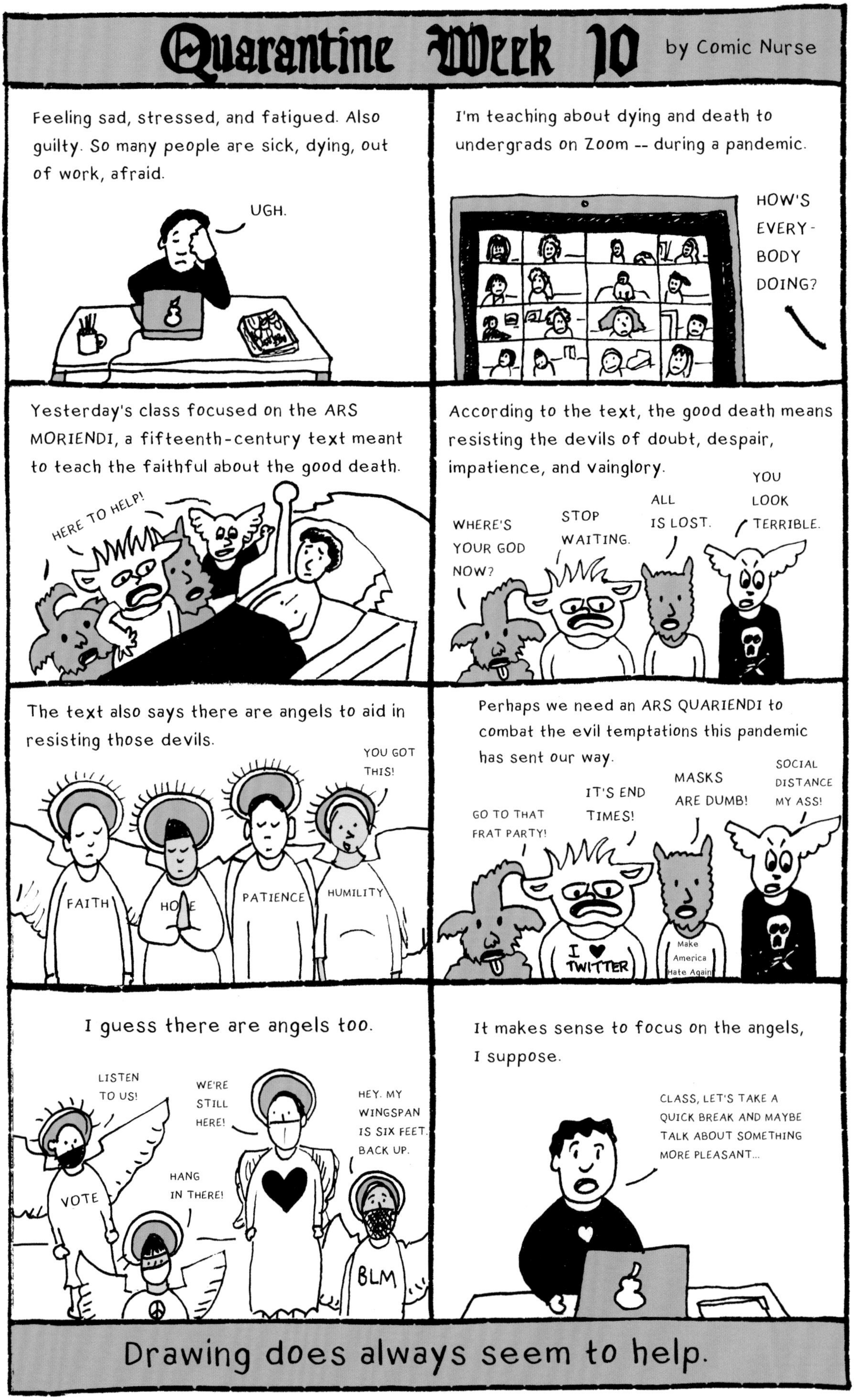
Quarantine Week 10
by Comic Nurse
Feeling sad, stressed, and fatigued. Also guilty. So many people are sick, dying, out of work, afraid.
UGH.
I'm teaching about dying and death to undergrads on Zoom -- during a pandemic.
HOW'S EVERY-BODY DOING?
Yesterday's class focused on the ARS MORIENDI, a fifteenth-century text meant to teach the faithful about the good death.
HERE TO HELP!
According to the text, the good death means resisting the devils of doubt, despair, impatience, and vainglory.
WHERE'S YOUR GOD NOW?
STOP WAITING.
ALL IS LOST.
YOU LOOK TERRIBLE.
The text also says there are angels to aid in resisting those devils.
FAITH
HOPE
PATIENCE
HUMILITY
YOU GOT THIS!
Perhaps we need an ARS QUARIENDI to combat the evil temptations this pandemic has sent our way.
GO TO THAT FRAT PARTY!
IT'S END TIMES!
MASKS ARE DUMB!
SOCIAL DISTANCE MY ASS!
I ♥ TWITTER
Make America Hate Again
I guess there are angels too.
LISTEN TO US!
VOTE
HANG IN THERE!
WE'RE STILL HERE!
HEY. MY WINGSPAN IS SIX FEET. BACK UP.
BLM
It makes sense to focus on the angels, I suppose.
CLASS, LET'S TAKE A QUICK BREAK AND MAYBE TALK ABOUT SOMETHING MORE PLEASANT...
Drawing does always seem to help.

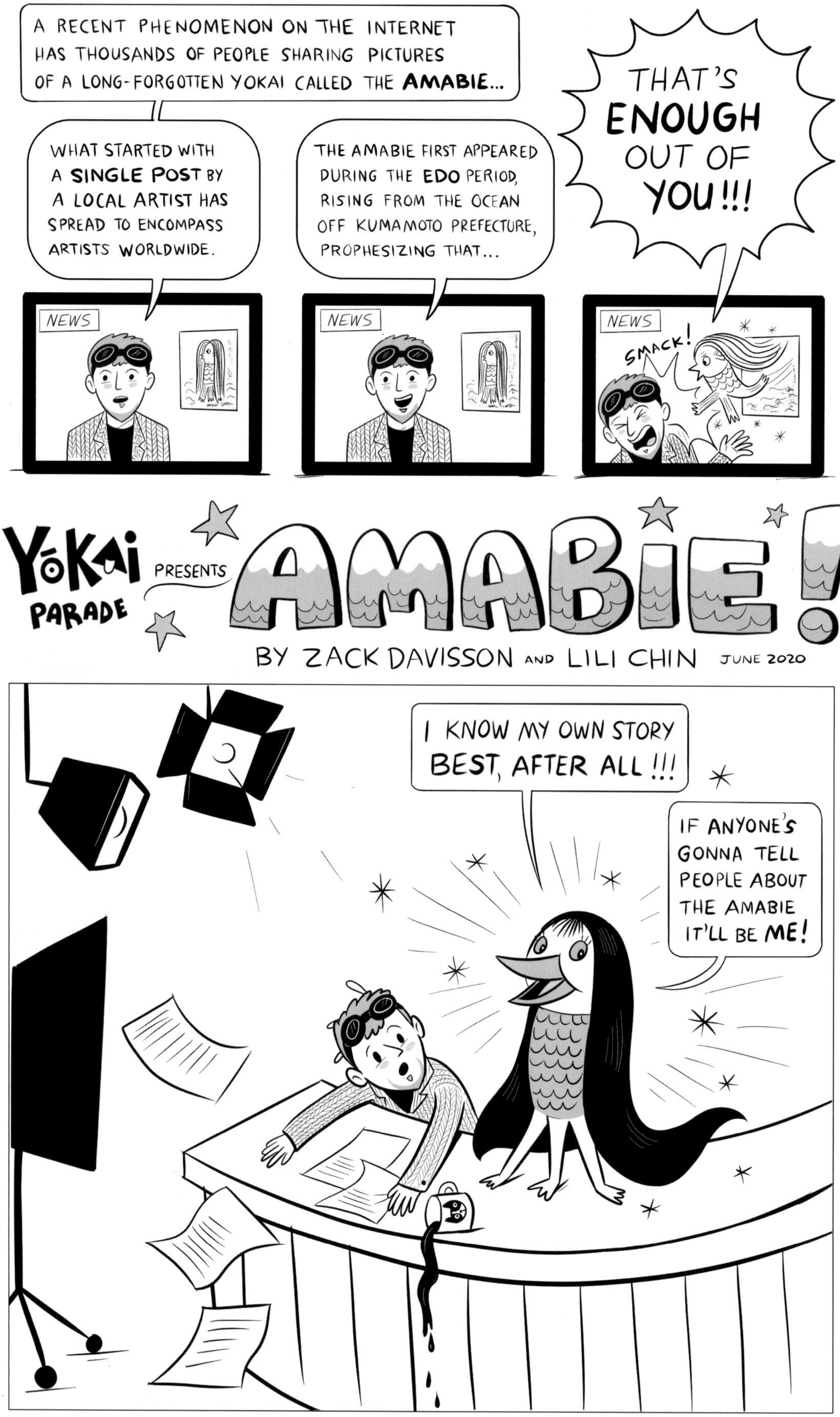
A RECENT PHENOMENON ON THE INTERNET HAS THOUSANDS OF PEOPLE SHARING PICTURES OF A LONG-FORGOTTEN YOKAI CALLED THE AMABIE...
WHAT STARTED WITH A SINGLE POST BY A LOCAL ARTIST HAS SPREAD TO ENCOMPASS ARTISTS WORLDWIDE.
NEWS
THE AMABIE FIRST APPEARED DURING THE EDO PERIOD, RISING FROM THE OCEAN OFF KUMAMOTO PREFECTURE, PROPHESIZING THAT...
NEWS
THAT'S ENOUGH OUT OF YOU!!!
NEWS
SMACK!
YŌKAI PARADE PRESENTS AMABIE!
BY ZACK DAVISSON AND LILI CHIN JUNE 2020
I KNOW MY OWN STORY BEST, AFTER ALL!!!
IF ANYONE'S GONNA TELL PEOPLE ABOUT THE AMABIE IT'LL BE ME!

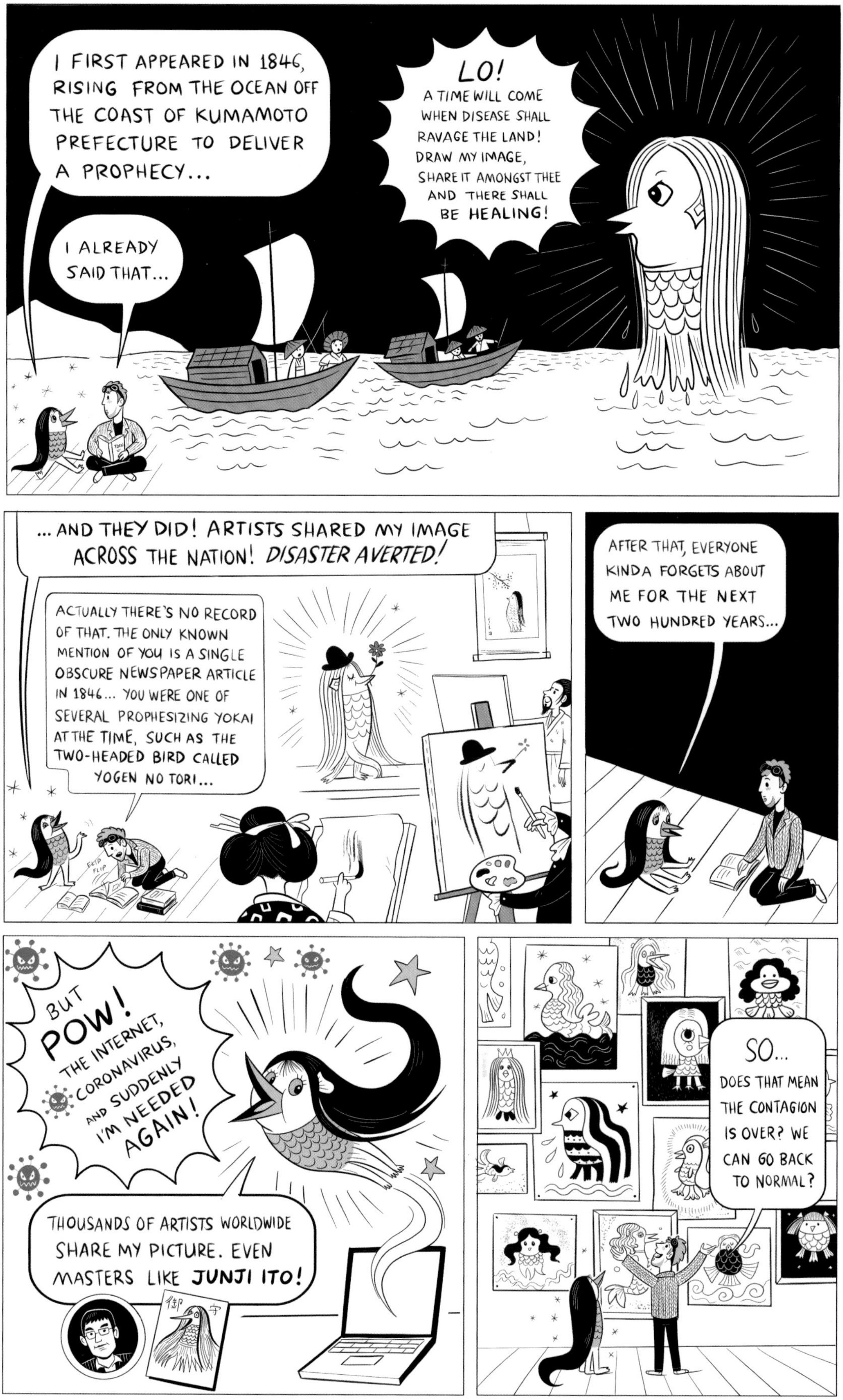
I FIRST APPEARED IN 1846, RISING FROM THE OCEAN OFF THE COAST OF KUMAMOTO PREFECTURE TO DELIVER A PROPHECY...
LO! A TIME WILL COME WHEN DISEASE SHALL RAVAGE THE LAND! DRAW MY IMAGE, SHARE IT AMONGST THEE AND THERE SHALL BE HEALING!
I ALREADY SAID THAT...
...AND THEY DID! ARTISTS SHARED MY IMAGE ACROSS THE NATION! DISASTER AVERTED!
ACTUALLY THERE'S NO RECORD OF THAT. THE ONLY KNOWN MENTION OF YOU IS A SINGLE OBSCURE NEWSPAPER ARTICLE IN 1846... YOU WERE ONE OF SEVERAL PROPHESIZING YOKAI AT THE TIME, SUCH AS THE TWO-HEADED BIRD CALLED YOGEN NO TORI...
FLIP FLIP
AFTER THAT, EVERYONE KINDA FORGETS ABOUT ME FOR THE NEXT TWO HUNDRED YEARS...
BUT POW! THE INTERNET, CORONAVIRUS, AND SUDDENLY I'M NEEDED AGAIN!
THOUSANDS OF ARTISTS WORLDWIDE SHARE MY PICTURE. EVEN MASTERS LIKE JUNJI ITO!
御 字
SO... DOES THAT MEAN THE CONTAGION IS OVER? WE CAN GO BACK TO NORMAL?

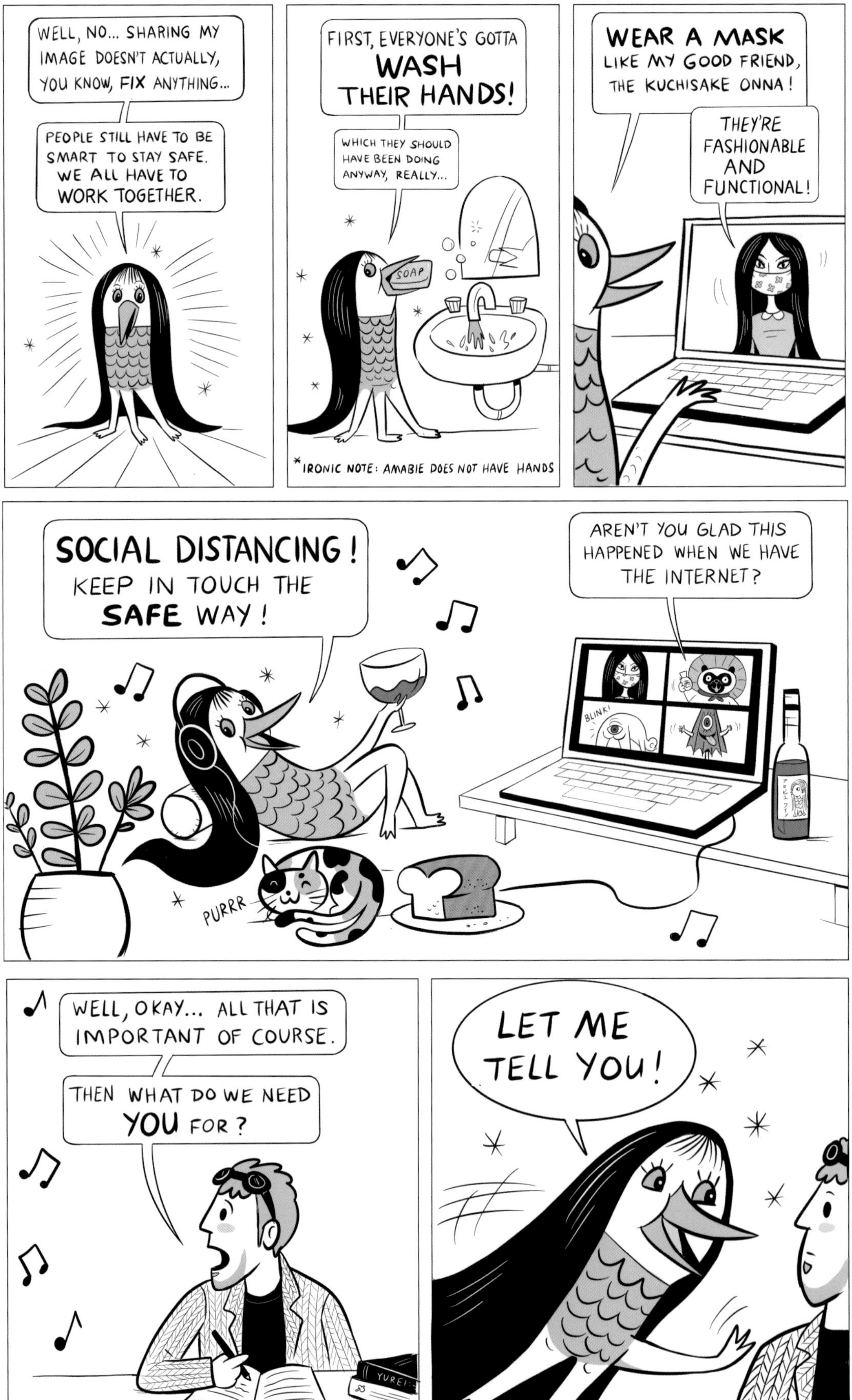
WELL, NO... SHARING MY IMAGE DOESN'T ACTUALLY, YOU KNOW, FIX ANYTHING...
PEOPLE STILL HAVE TO BE SMART TO STAY SAFE. WE ALL HAVE TO WORK TOGETHER.
FIRST, EVERYONE'S GOTTA WASH THEIR HANDS!
WHICH THEY SHOULD HAVE BEEN DOING ANYWAY, REALLY...
SOAP
*IRONIC NOTE: AMABIE DOES NOT HAVE HANDS
WEAR A MASK LIKE MY GOOD FRIEND, THE KUCHISAKE ONNA!
THEY'RE FASHIONABLE AND FUNCTIONAL!
SOCIAL DISTANCING! KEEP IN TOUCH THE SAFE WAY!
AREN'T YOU GLAD THIS HAPPENED WHEN WE HAVE THE INTERNET?
BLINK!
PURRR
WELL, OKAY... ALL THAT IS IMPORTANT OF COURSE.
THEN WHAT DO WE NEED YOU FOR?
YUREI
LET ME TELL YOU!

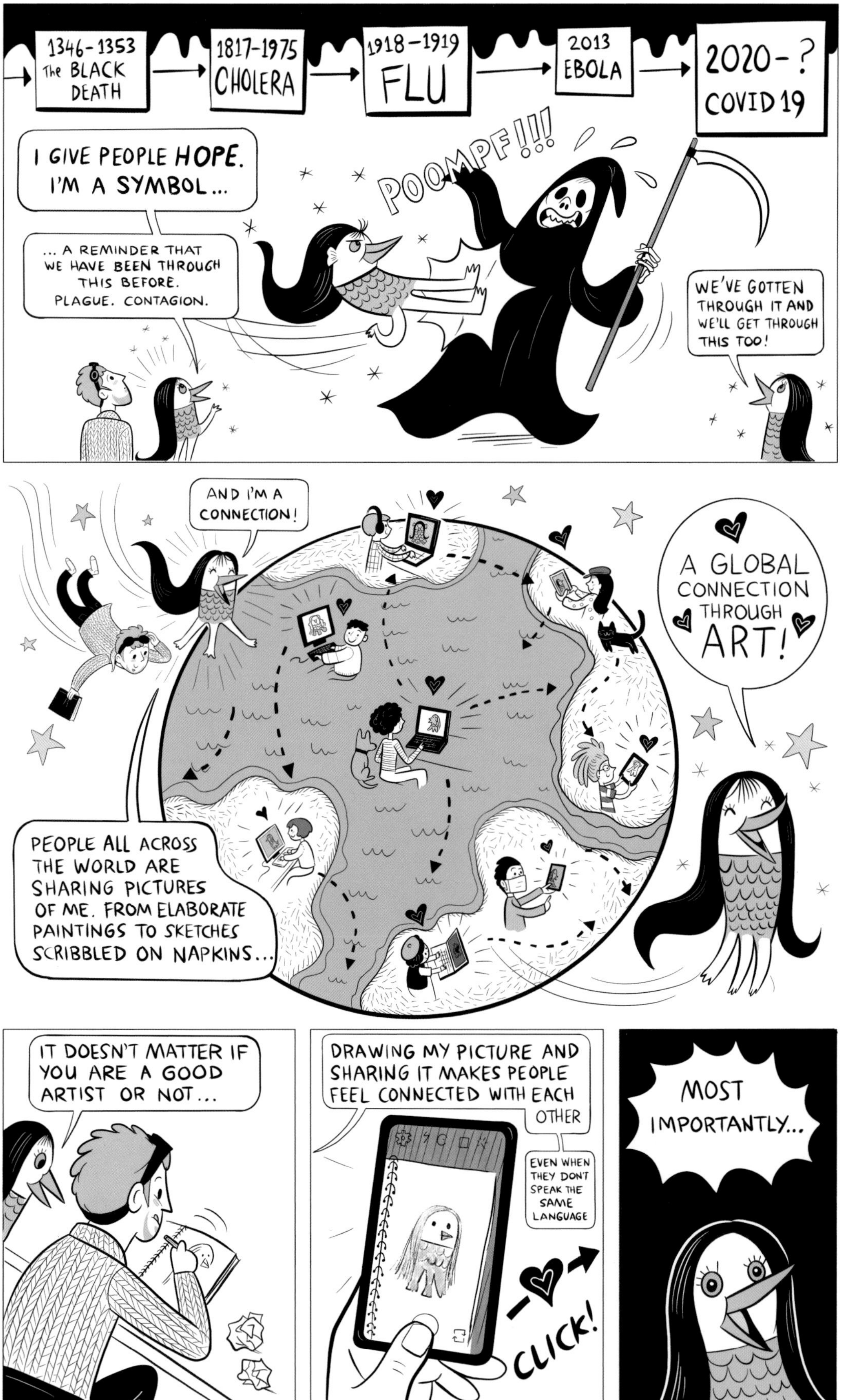
1346-1353 The BLACK DEATH
1817-1975 CHOLERA
1918-1919 FLU
2013 EBOLA
2020-? COVID 19
I GIVE PEOPLE HOPE. I'M A SYMBOL...
... A REMINDER THAT WE HAVE BEEN THROUGH THIS BEFORE. PLAGUE. CONTAGION.
POOMPF!!!
WE'VE GOTTEN THROUGH IT AND WE'LL GET THROUGH THIS TOO!
AND I'M A CONNECTION!
A GLOBAL CONNECTION THROUGH ART!
PEOPLE ALL ACROSS THE WORLD ARE SHARING PICTURES OF ME. FROM ELABORATE PAINTINGS TO SKETCHES SCRIBBLED ON NAPKINS...
IT DOESN'T MATTER IF YOU ARE A GOOD ARTIST OR NOT...
DRAWING MY PICTURE AND SHARING IT MAKES PEOPLE FEEL CONNECTED WITH EACH OTHER
EVEN WHEN THEY DON'T SPEAK THE SAME LANGUAGE
CLICK!
MOST IMPORTANTLY...

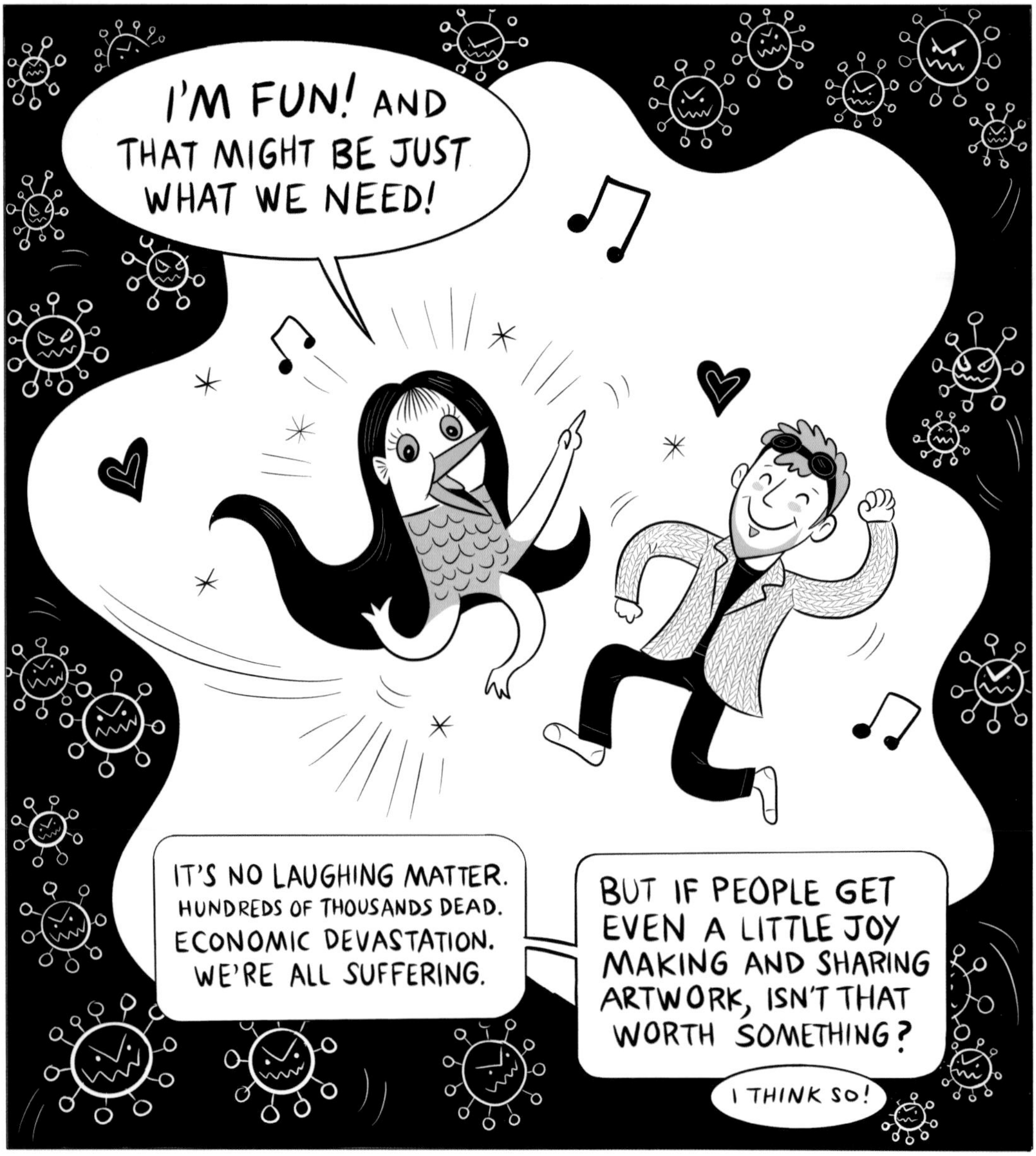
I'M FUN! AND THAT MIGHT BE JUST WHAT WE NEED!
IT'S NO LAUGHING MATTER. HUNDREDS OF THOUSANDS DEAD. ECONOMIC DEVASTATION. WE'RE ALL SUFFERING.
BUT IF PEOPLE GET EVEN A LITTLE JOY MAKING AND SHARING ARTWORK, ISN'T THAT WORTH SOMETHING?
I THINK SO!

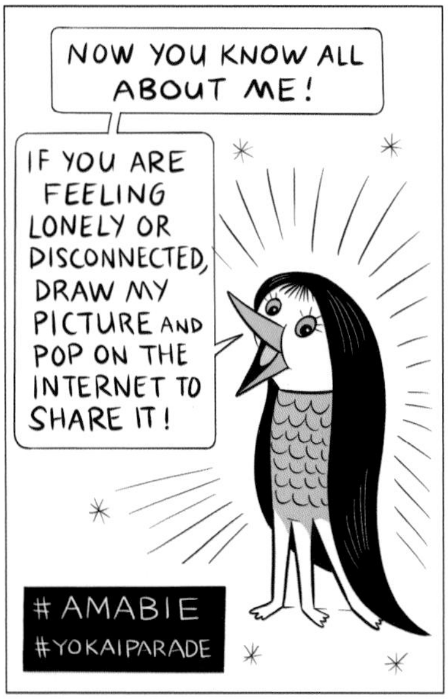
NOW YOU KNOW ALL ABOUT ME!
IF YOU ARE FEELING LONELY OR DISCONNECTED, DRAW MY PICTURE AND POP ON THE INTERNET TO SHARE IT!
#AMABIE
#YOKAIPARADE

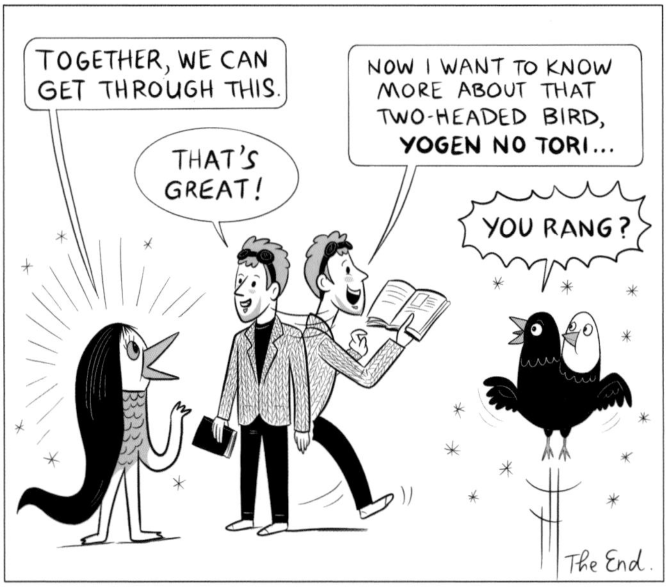
TOGETHER, WE CAN GET THROUGH THIS.
THAT'S GREAT!
NOW I WANT TO KNOW MORE ABOUT THAT TWO-HEADED BIRD, YOGEN NO TORI...
YOU RANG?
The End.

How to Have a Powwow in a Pandemic

Native communities in North America have been particularly hard-hit by COVID-19.

This isn't the first time.

Words by
S.I. ROSENBAUM

Art by
ARIGON STARR

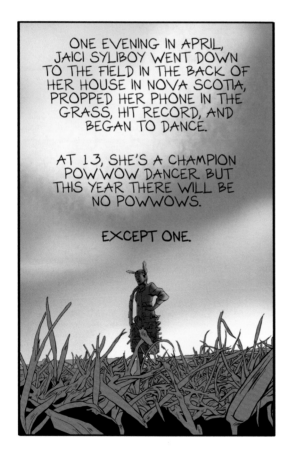

ONE EVENING IN APRIL, JAICI SYLIBOY WENT DOWN TO THE FIELD IN THE BACK OF HER HOUSE IN NOVA SCOTIA, PROPPED HER PHONE IN THE GRASS, HIT RECORD, AND BEGAN TO DANCE.

AT 13, SHE'S A CHAMPION POWWOW DANCER BUT THIS YEAR THERE WILL BE NO POWWOWS.

EXCEPT ONE.

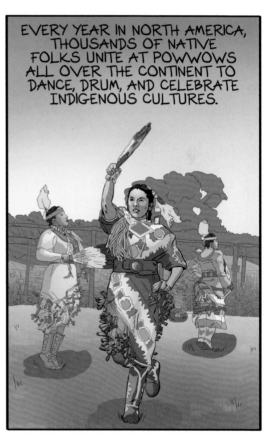

EVERY YEAR IN NORTH AMERICA, THOUSANDS OF NATIVE FOLKS UNITE AT POWWOWS ALL OVER THE CONTINENT TO DANCE, DRUM, AND CELEBRATE INDIGENOUS CULTURES.

In 2020, COVID-19 swept in just as Powwow season was beginning.

Native American communities would be among the hardest hit.

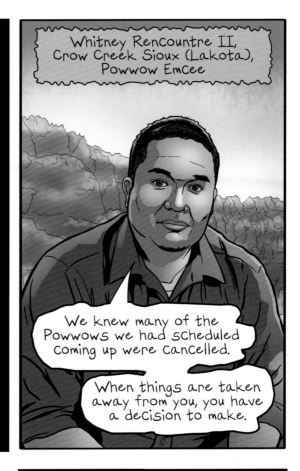

Whitney Rencountre II, Crow Creek Sioux (Lakota), Powwow Emcee

We knew many of the Powwows we had scheduled coming up were cancelled.

When things are taken away from you, you have a decision to make.

I was sitting on the couch, just depressed.

What can be done? How can dancers lift their spirits?

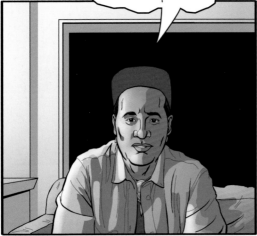

Dan Simonds, Mashantucket Pequot, artisan and Powwow vendor

NATIVE PEOPLE HAVE ENDURED PANDEMICS BEFORE. NATIVE RECORDS FROM THAT TIME TELL THE STORY:

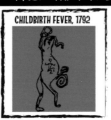
CHILDBIRTH FEVER, 1792

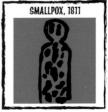
SMALLPOX, 1811

BY THE LATE 1800S, TRIBES HAD ENDURED WAVE UPON WAVE OF PANDEMICS...

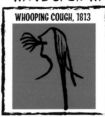
WHOOPING COUGH, 1813

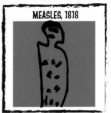
MEASLES, 1818

...THAT WOULD WORSEN WITH THE DEPRIVATION AND FORCED MARCHES OF THE GOVERNMENT'S INDIAN REMOVAL PROGRAM

THE NATIVE PEOPLE WHO SURVIVED — THE 1900 CENSUS RECORDED ONLY 237,000, WHERE THERE HAD BEEN MILLIONS A FEW GENERATIONS BEFORE — WERE INTERNED IN RESERVATIONS, STARVING, THEIR SACRED DANCES OUTLAWED.

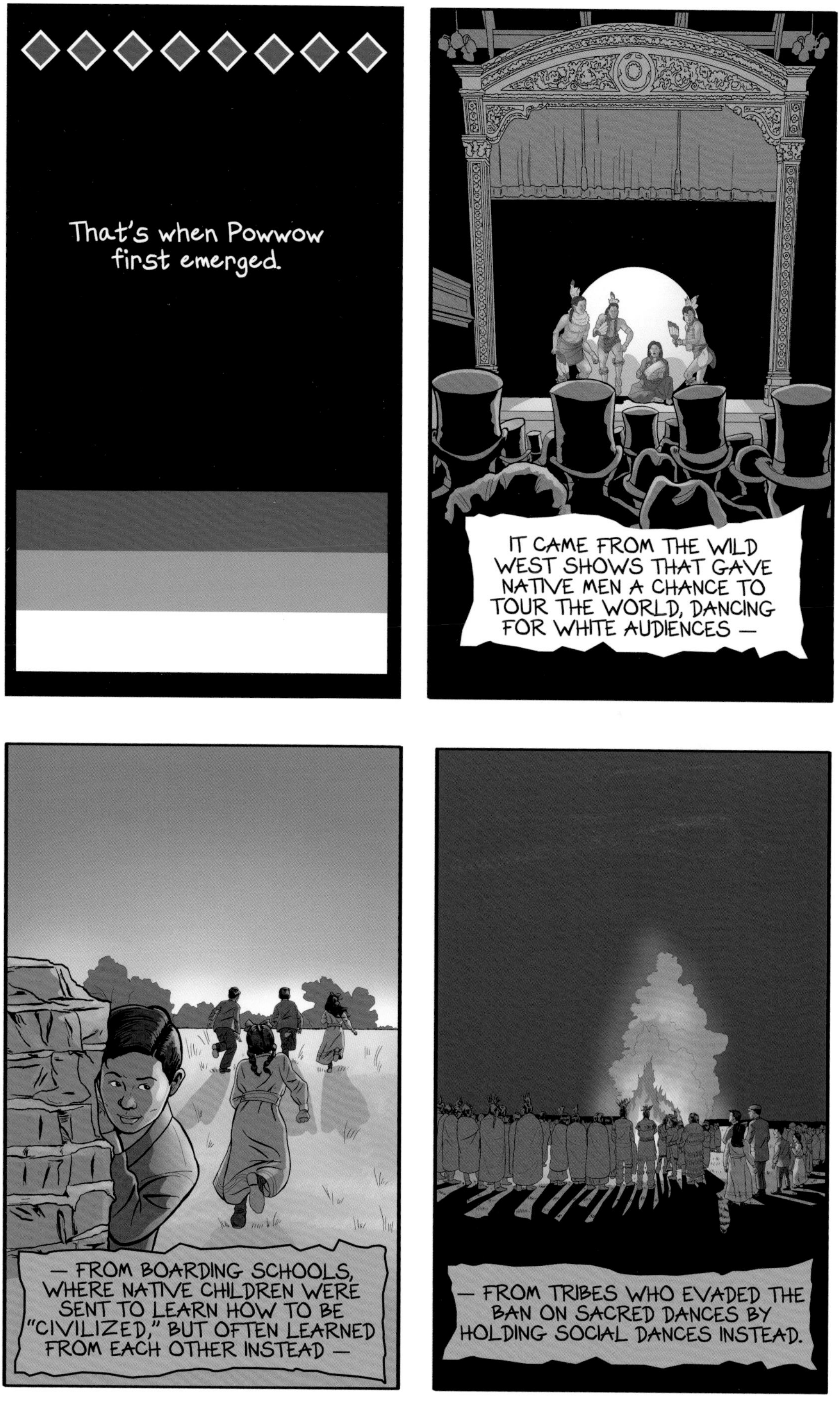
That's when Powwow first emerged.
IT CAME FROM THE WILD WEST SHOWS THAT GAVE NATIVE MEN A CHANCE TO TOUR THE WORLD, DANCING FOR WHITE AUDIENCES —
— FROM BOARDING SCHOOLS, WHERE NATIVE CHILDREN WERE SENT TO LEARN HOW TO BE "CIVILIZED," BUT OFTEN LEARNED FROM EACH OTHER INSTEAD —
— FROM TRIBES WHO EVADED THE BAN ON SACRED DANCES BY HOLDING SOCIAL DANCES INSTEAD.

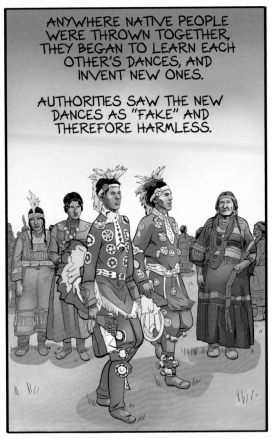

ANYWHERE NATIVE PEOPLE WERE THROWN TOGETHER, THEY BEGAN TO LEARN EACH OTHER'S DANCES, AND INVENT NEW ONES.

AUTHORITIES SAW THE NEW DANCES AS "FAKE" AND THEREFORE HARMLESS.

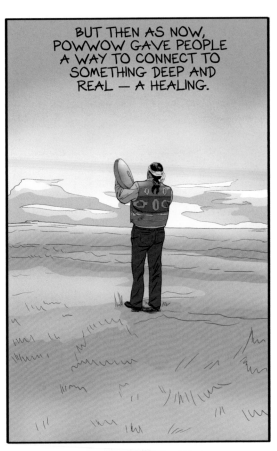

BUT THEN AS NOW, POWWOW GAVE PEOPLE A WAY TO CONNECT TO SOMETHING DEEP AND REAL — A HEALING.

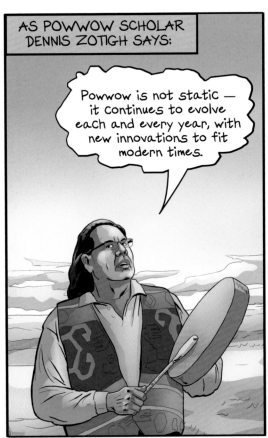

AS POWWOW SCHOLAR DENNIS ZOTIGH SAYS:

Powwow is not static — it continues to evolve each and every year, with new innovations to fit modern times.

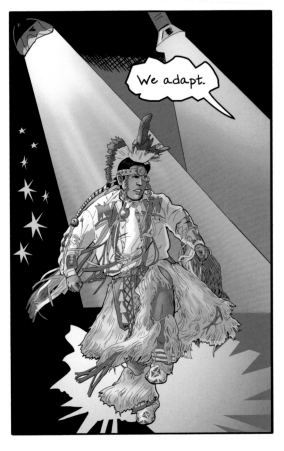

We adapt.

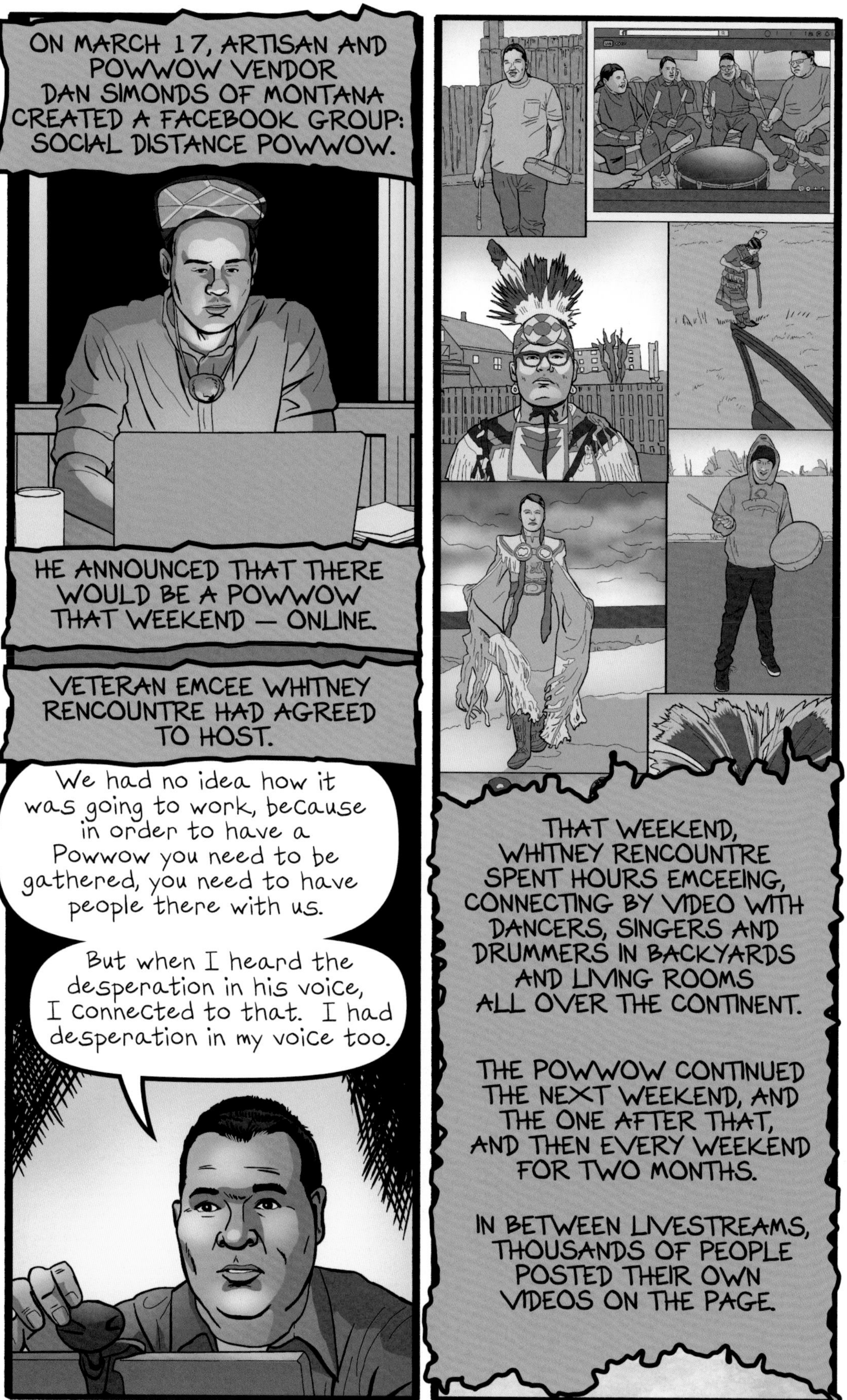
ON MARCH 17, ARTISAN AND POWWOW VENDOR DAN SIMONDS OF MONTANA CREATED A FACEBOOK GROUP: SOCIAL DISTANCE POWWOW.
HE ANNOUNCED THAT THERE WOULD BE A POWWOW THAT WEEKEND — ONLINE.
VETERAN EMCEE WHITNEY RENCOUNTRE HAD AGREED TO HOST.
We had no idea how it was going to work, because in order to have a Powwow you need to be gathered, you need to have people there with us.
But when I heard the desperation in his voice, I connected to that. I had desperation in my voice too.
THAT WEEKEND, WHITNEY RENCOUNTRE SPENT HOURS EMCEEING, CONNECTING BY VIDEO WITH DANCERS, SINGERS AND DRUMMERS IN BACKYARDS AND LIVING ROOMS ALL OVER THE CONTINENT.
THE POWWOW CONTINUED THE NEXT WEEKEND, AND THE ONE AFTER THAT, AND THEN EVERY WEEKEND FOR TWO MONTHS.
IN BETWEEN LIVESTREAMS, THOUSANDS OF PEOPLE POSTED THEIR OWN VIDEOS ON THE PAGE.

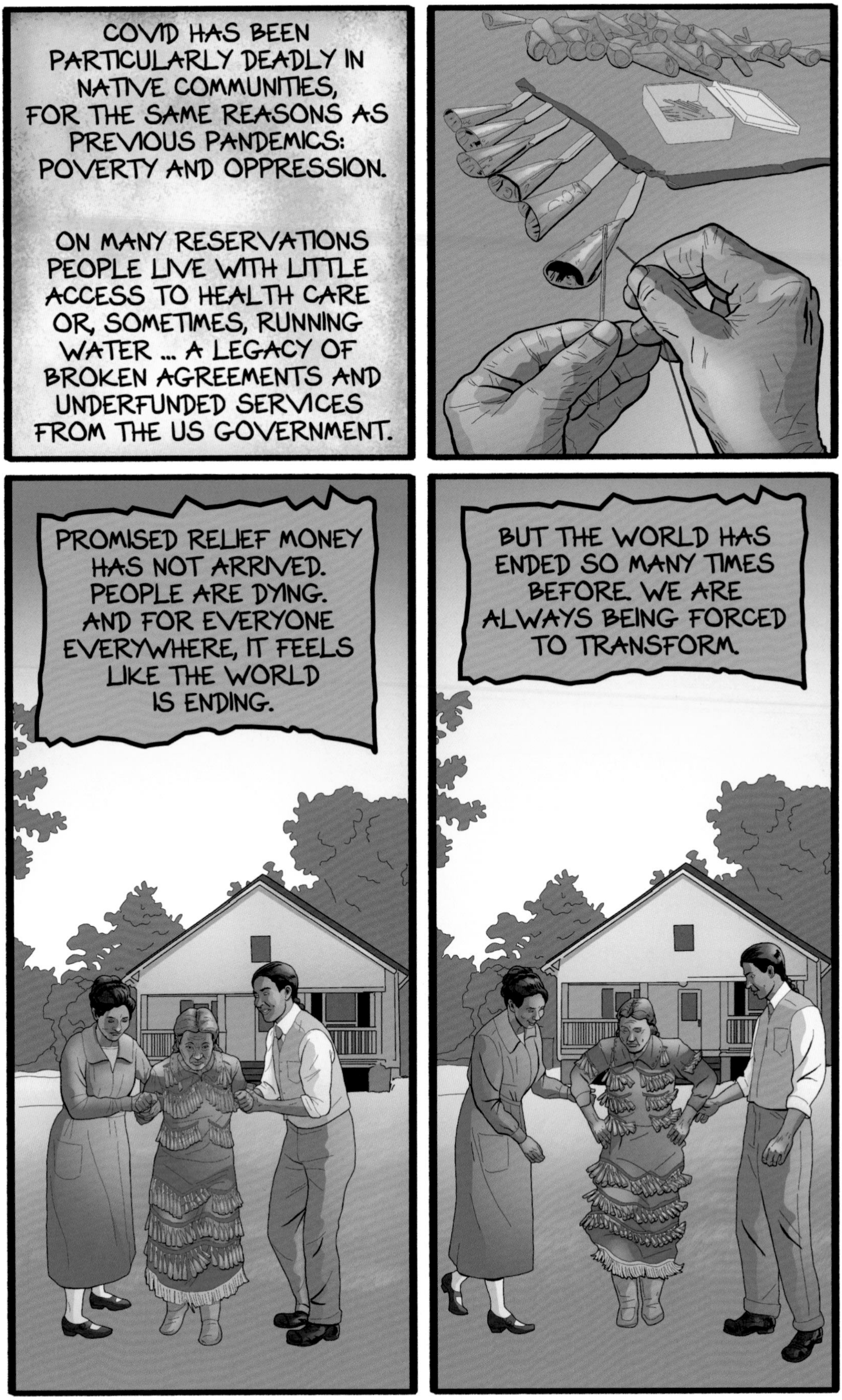
COVID HAS BEEN PARTICULARLY DEADLY IN NATIVE COMMUNITIES, FOR THE SAME REASONS AS PREVIOUS PANDEMICS: POVERTY AND OPPRESSION.
ON MANY RESERVATIONS PEOPLE LIVE WITH LITTLE ACCESS TO HEALTH CARE OR, SOMETIMES, RUNNING WATER ... A LEGACY OF BROKEN AGREEMENTS AND UNDERFUNDED SERVICES FROM THE US GOVERNMENT.
PROMISED RELIEF MONEY HAS NOT ARRIVED. PEOPLE ARE DYING. AND FOR EVERYONE EVERYWHERE, IT FEELS LIKE THE WORLD IS ENDING.
BUT THE WORLD HAS ENDED SO MANY TIMES BEFORE. WE ARE ALWAYS BEING FORCED TO TRANSFORM.

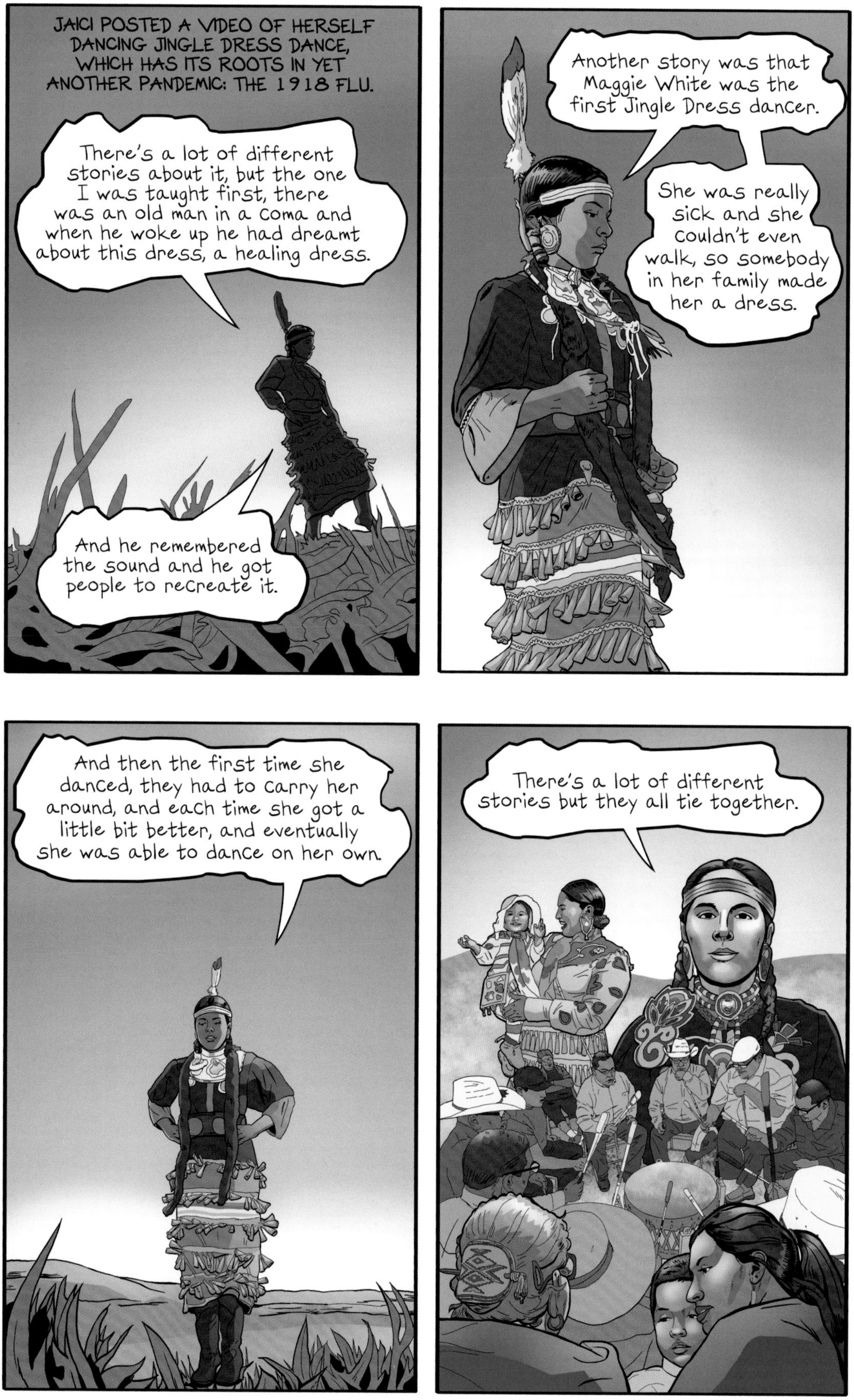
JAICI POSTED A VIDEO OF HERSELF DANCING JINGLE DRESS DANCE, WHICH HAS ITS ROOTS IN YET ANOTHER PANDEMIC: THE 1918 FLU.
There's a lot of different stories about it, but the one I was taught first, there was an old man in a coma and when he woke up he had dreamt about this dress, a healing dress.
And he remembered the sound and he got people to recreate it.
Another story was that Maggie White was the first Jingle Dress dancer.
She was really sick and she couldn't even walk, so somebody in her family made her a dress.
And then the first time she danced, they had to carry her around, and each time she got a little bit better, and eventually she was able to dance on her own.
There's a lot of different stories but they all tie together.

NO DOGS
?!
?!
?!
We didn't get far...

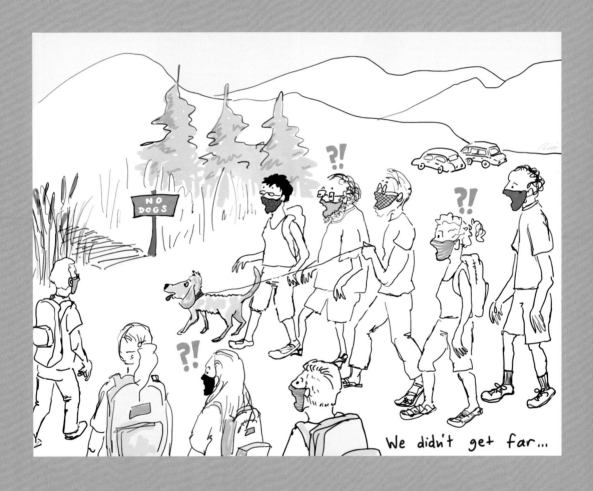

KATIE'S CORONAVIRUS DIARY!

Creator/Writer: Tom K. Mason · Artist: Eduardo Garcia · Letterer: Kurt Hathaway · Colorist: Chris Summers

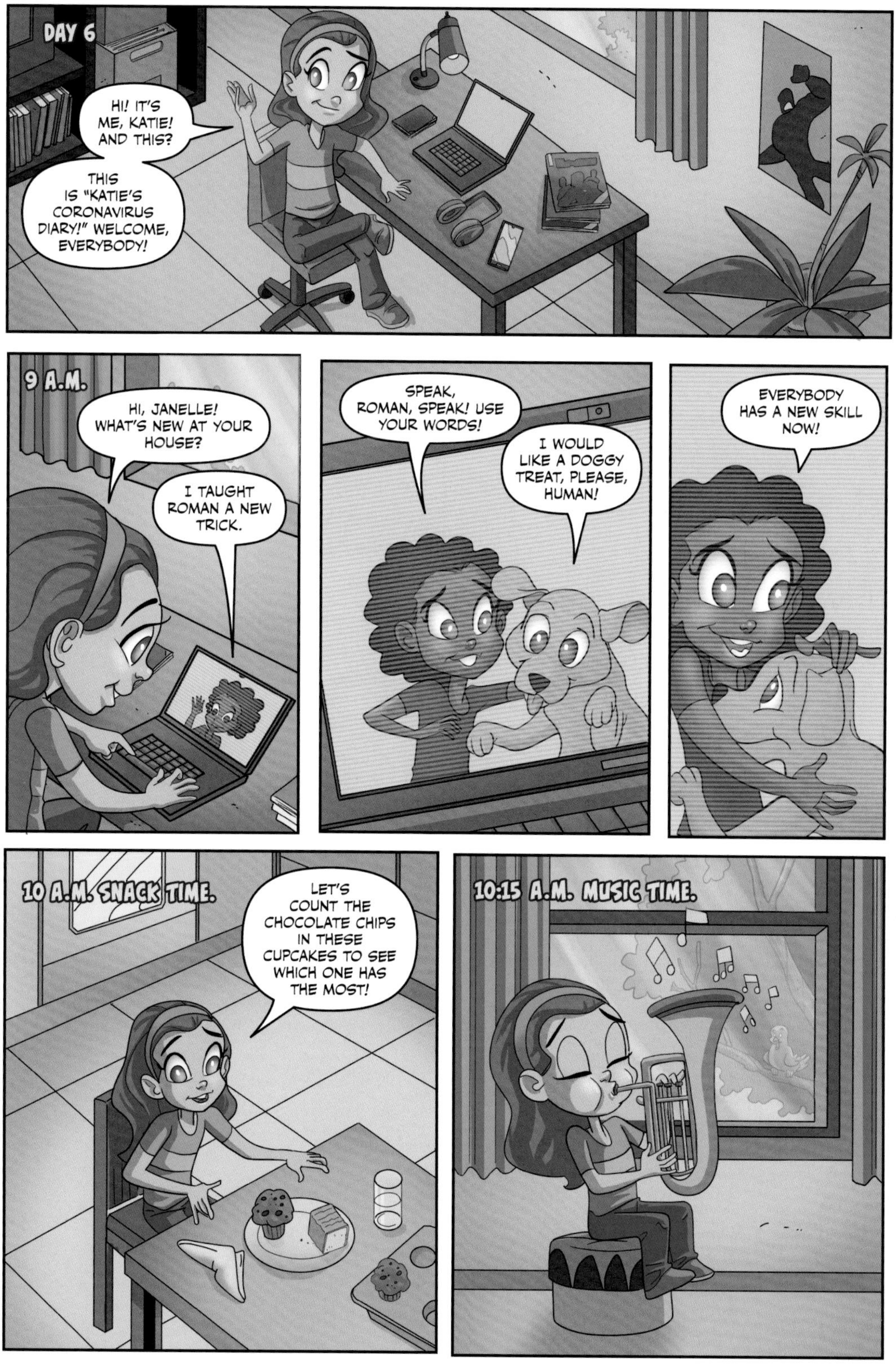
DAY 6
HI! IT'S ME, KATIE! AND THIS?
THIS IS "KATIE'S CORONAVIRUS DIARY!" WELCOME, EVERYBODY!
9 A.M.
HI, JANELLE! WHAT'S NEW AT YOUR HOUSE?
I TAUGHT ROMAN A NEW TRICK.
SPEAK, ROMAN, SPEAK! USE YOUR WORDS!
I WOULD LIKE A DOGGY TREAT, PLEASE, HUMAN!
EVERYBODY HAS A NEW SKILL NOW!
10 A.M. SNACK TIME.
LET'S COUNT THE CHOCOLATE CHIPS IN THESE CUPCAKES TO SEE WHICH ONE HAS THE MOST!
10:15 A.M. MUSIC TIME.

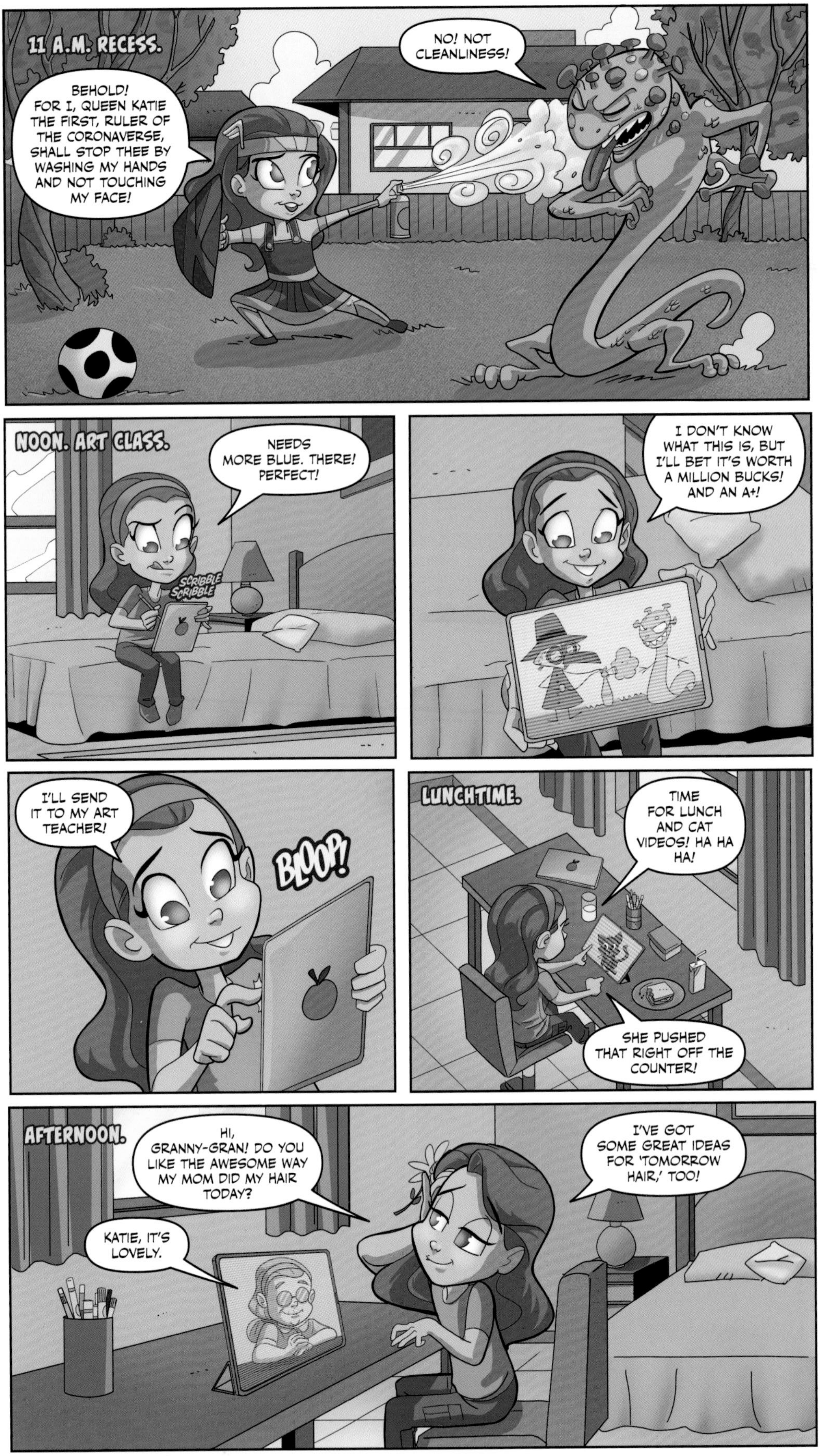
11 A.M. RECESS.
BEHOLD! FOR I, QUEEN KATIE THE FIRST, RULER OF THE CORONAVERSE, SHALL STOP THEE BY WASHING MY HANDS AND NOT TOUCHING MY FACE!
NO! NOT CLEANLINESS!
NOON. ART CLASS.
NEEDS MORE BLUE. THERE! PERFECT!
SCRIBBLE SCRIBBLE
I DON'T KNOW WHAT THIS IS, BUT I'LL BET IT'S WORTH A MILLION BUCKS! AND AN A+!
I'LL SEND IT TO MY ART TEACHER!
BLOOP!
LUNCHTIME.
TIME FOR LUNCH AND CAT VIDEOS! HA HA HA!
SHE PUSHED THAT RIGHT OFF THE COUNTER!
AFTERNOON.
HI, GRANNY-GRAN! DO YOU LIKE THE AWESOME WAY MY MOM DID MY HAIR TODAY?
I'VE GOT SOME GREAT IDEAS FOR 'TOMORROW HAIR,' TOO!
KATIE, IT'S LOVELY.

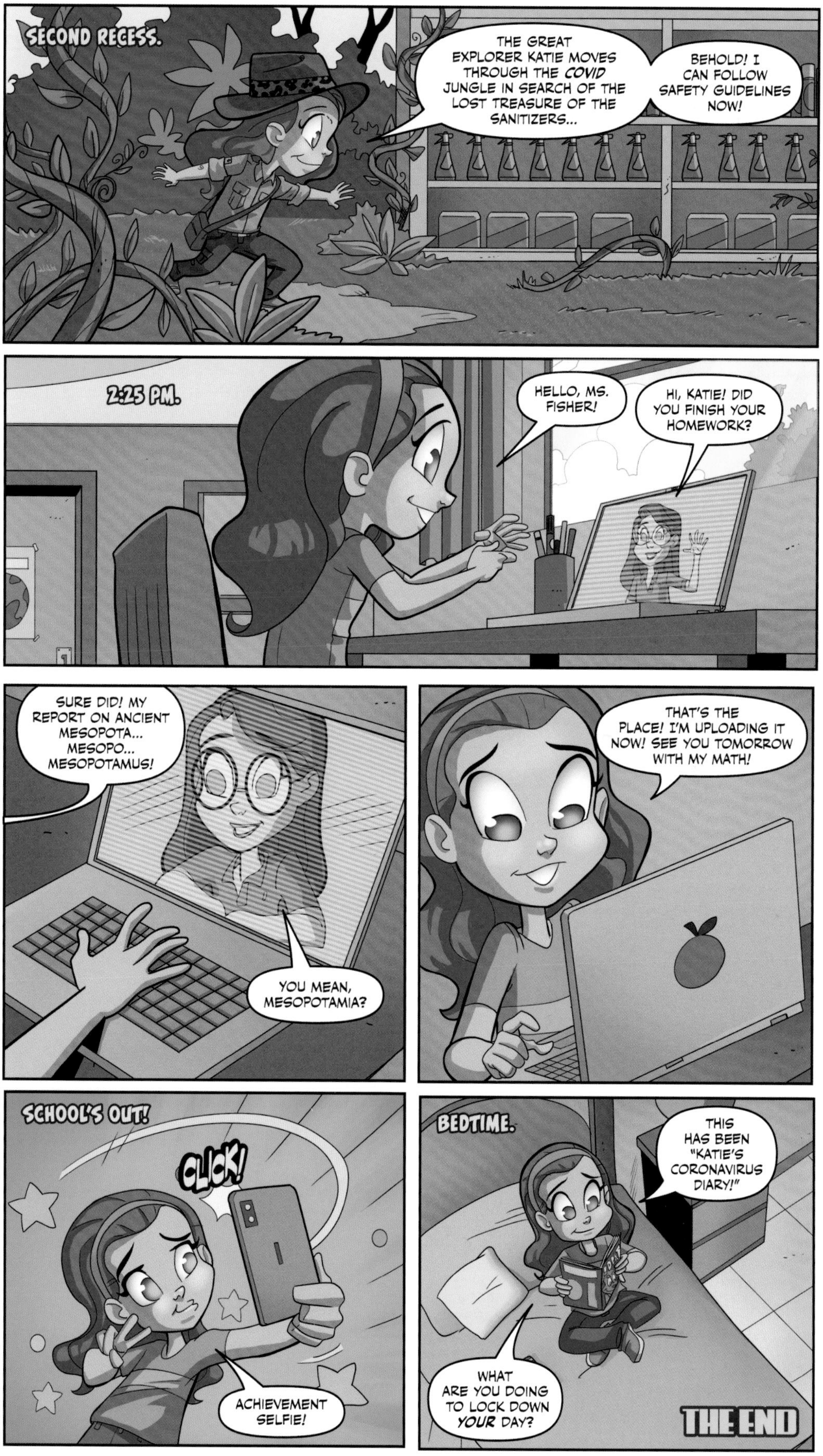
SECOND RECESS.
THE GREAT EXPLORER KATIE MOVES THROUGH THE *COVID* JUNGLE IN SEARCH OF THE LOST TREASURE OF THE SANITIZERS...
BEHOLD! I CAN FOLLOW SAFETY GUIDELINES NOW!
2:25 PM.
HELLO, MS. FISHER!
HI, KATIE! DID YOU FINISH YOUR HOMEWORK?
SURE DID! MY REPORT ON ANCIENT MESOPOTA... MESOPO... MESOPOTAMUS!
YOU MEAN, MESOPOTAMIA?
THAT'S THE PLACE! I'M UPLOADING IT NOW! SEE YOU TOMORROW WITH MY MATH!
SCHOOL'S OUT!
CLICK!
ACHIEVEMENT SELFIE!
BEDTIME.
THIS HAS BEEN "KATIE'S CORONAVIRUS DIARY!"
WHAT ARE YOU DOING TO LOCK DOWN *YOUR* DAY?
THE END

PAW Patrol to the coronavirus rescue…

by Sage Stossel

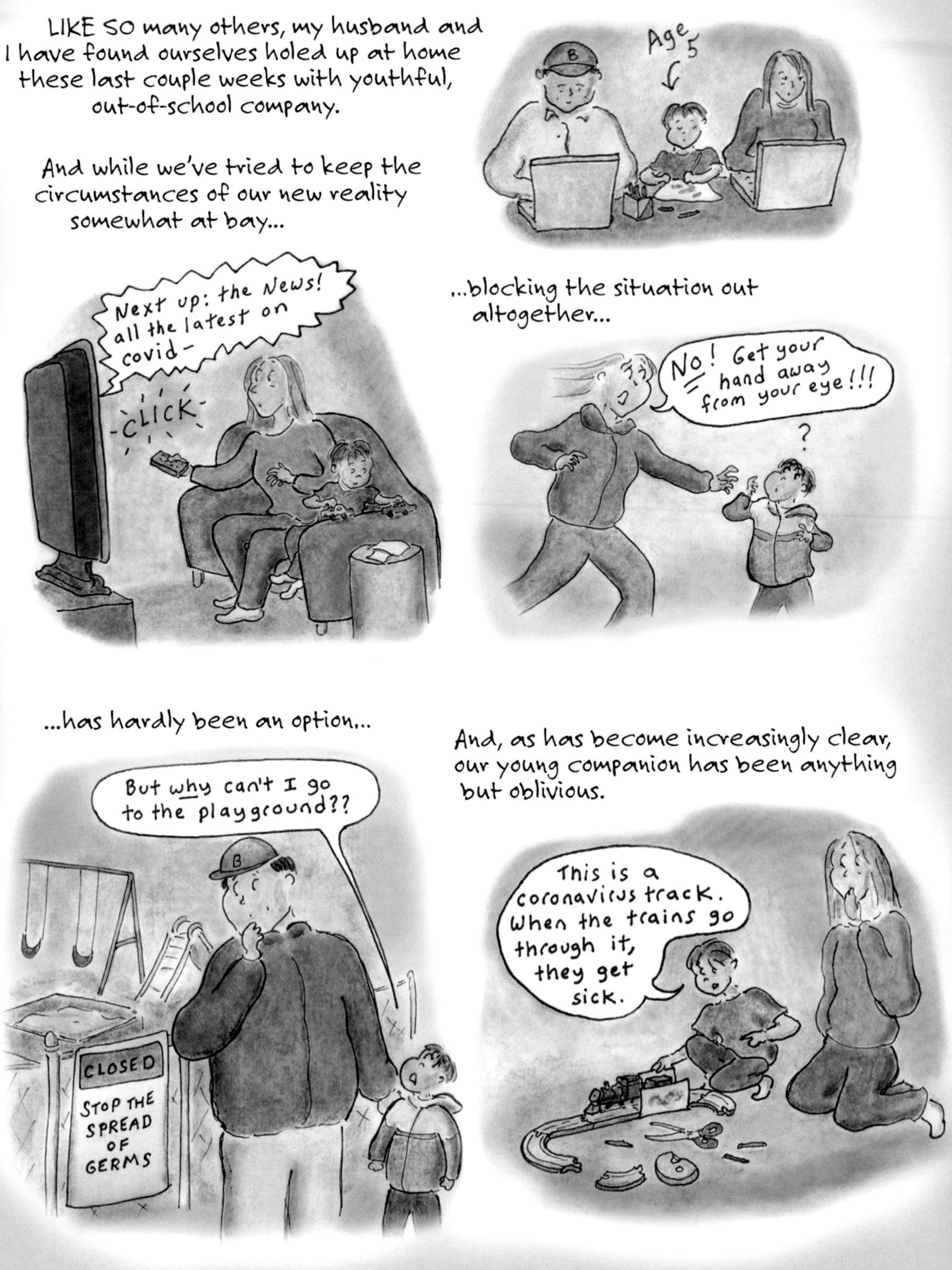
LIKE SO many others, my husband and I have found ourselves holed up at home these last couple weeks with youthful, out-of-school company.
Age 5
And while we've tried to keep the circumstances of our new reality somewhat at bay…
Next up: the News! all the latest on covid–
CLICK
…blocking the situation out altogether…
No! Get your hand away from your eye!!!
?
…has hardly been an option…
But why can't I go to the playground??
CLOSED
STOP THE SPREAD OF GERMS
And, as has become increasingly clear, our young companion has been anything but oblivious.
This is a coronavirus track. When the trains go through it, they get sick.

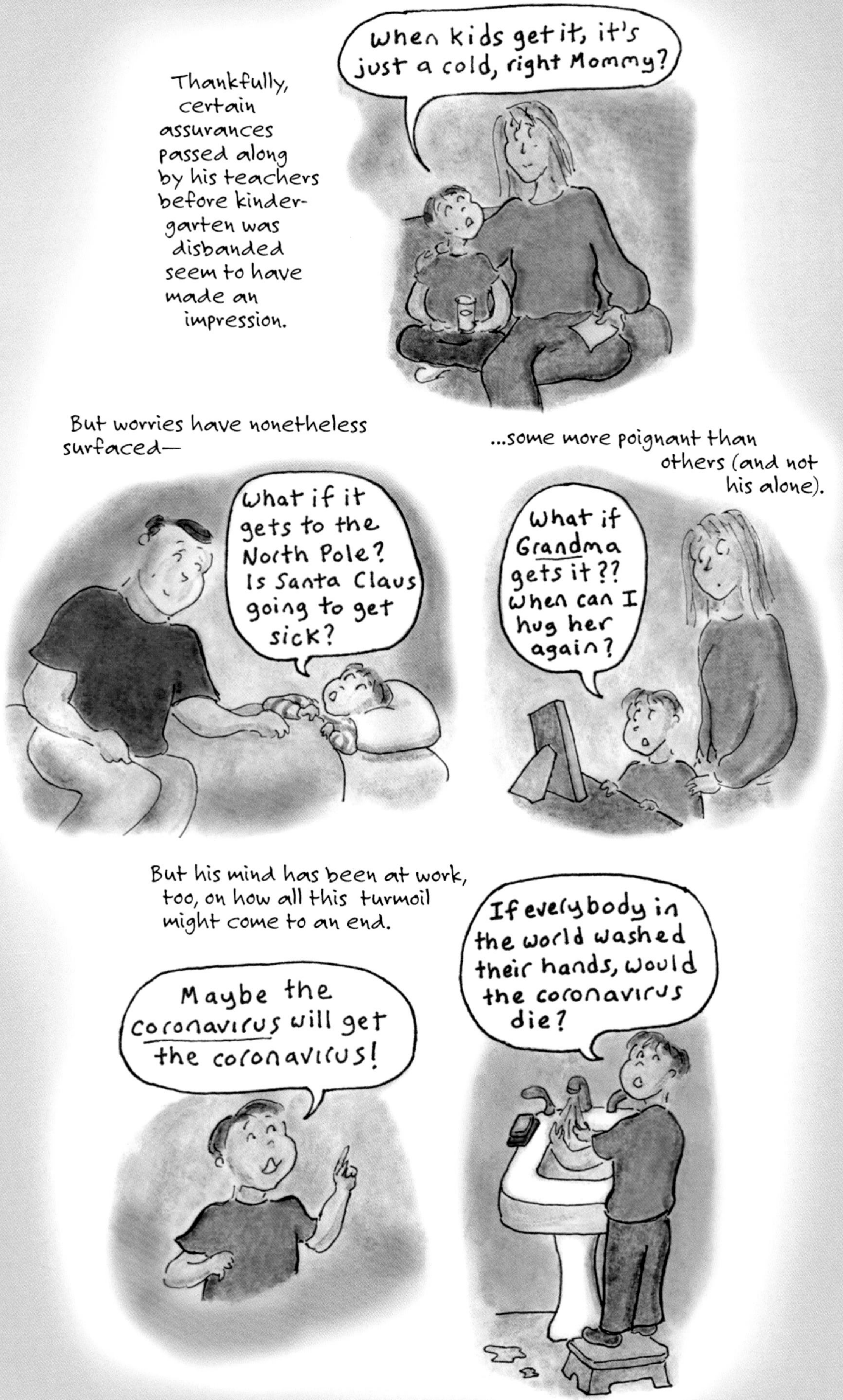
Thankfully, certain assurances passed along by his teachers before kinder-garten was disbanded seem to have made an impression.
When kids get it, it's just a cold, right Mommy?
But worries have nonetheless surfaced—
What if it gets to the North Pole? Is Santa Claus going to get sick?
...some more poignant than others (and not his alone).
What if Grandma gets it?? When can I hug her again?
But his mind has been at work, too, on how all this turmoil might come to an end.
Maybe the coronavirus will get the coronavirus!
If everybody in the world washed their hands, would the coronavirus die?

We've even had occasion to wonder if he might be hoping to do something about it himself...

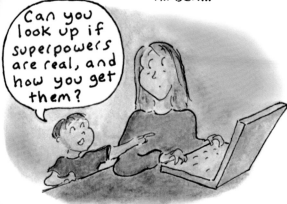

Can you look up if superpowers are real, and how you get them?

(...or, at the very least, to feel less at the mercy of forces beyond his control).

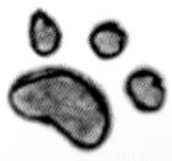

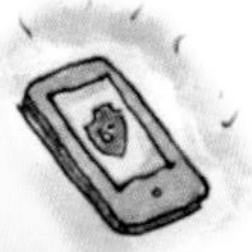

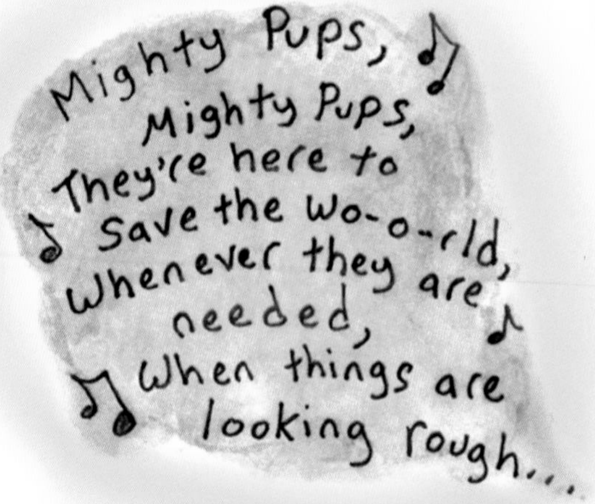

...one can't help but wonder if what he's really hoping for is rescue from above by powerful figures in charge.

A childish fantasy, perhaps.

But who among us can't relate?

And given what we've seen so far from our **real-world** powers-that-be...

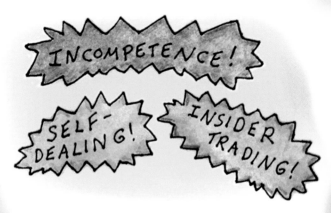

INCOMPETENCE!

SELF-DEALING!

INSIDER TRADING!

Judging, though, by the number of times we've heard the PAW Patrol "Mighty Pups" theme song blasting from various devices during Screen Time...

Mighty Pups, ♪ Mighty Pups, ♪ They're here to Save the Wo-o-rld, Whenever they are needed, ♪ When things are looking rough...

...we should **all** be so lucky as to hold out hope that Ryder and his team of pups might be coming to save the day.

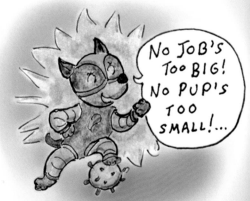

No Job's Too Big! No Pup's Too Small!...

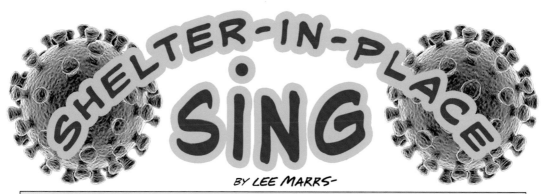

SHELTER-IN-PLACE SING

BY LEE MARRS-

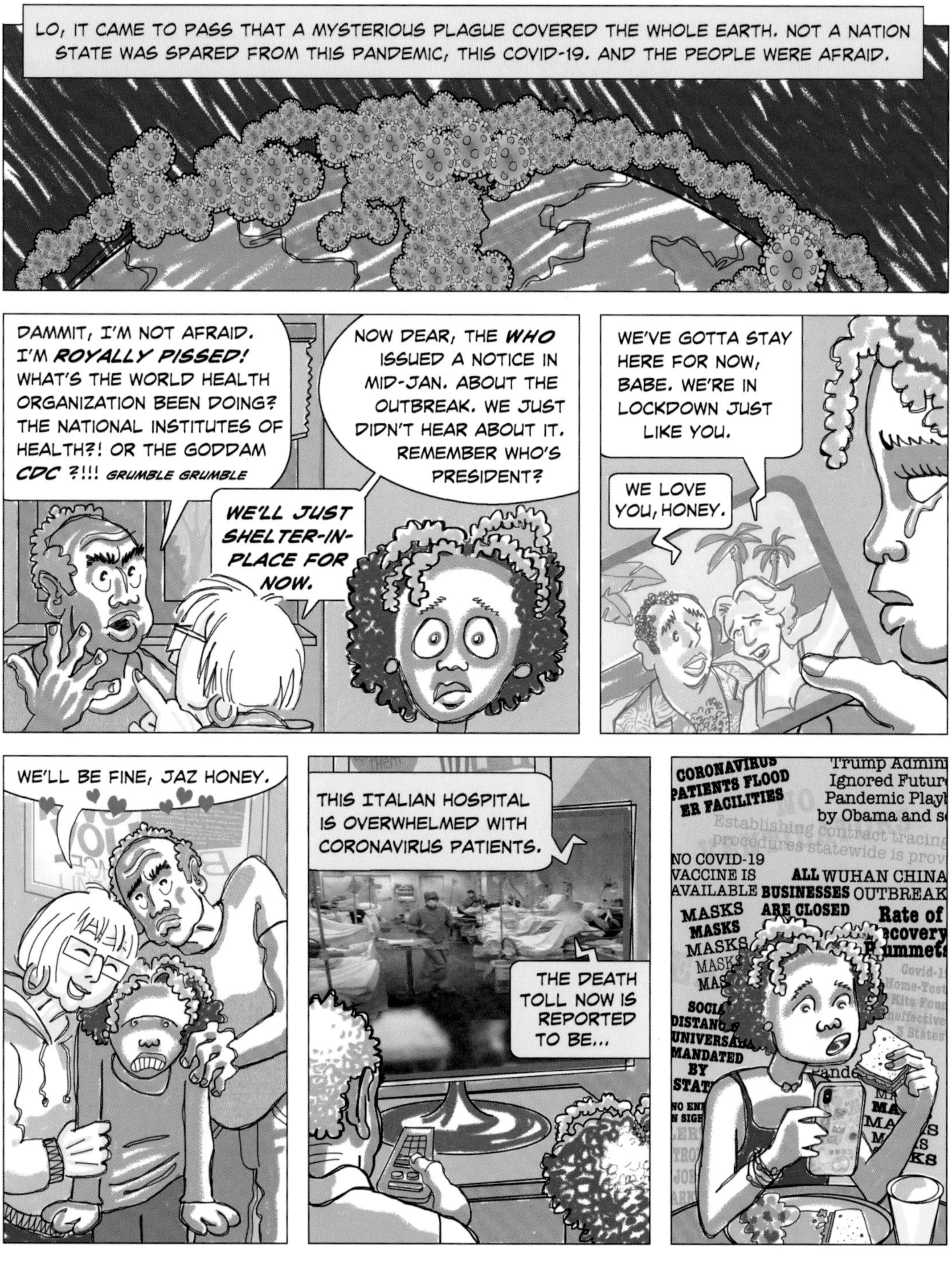
LO, IT CAME TO PASS THAT A MYSTERIOUS PLAGUE COVERED THE WHOLE EARTH. NOT A NATION STATE WAS SPARED FROM THIS PANDEMIC, THIS COVID-19. AND THE PEOPLE WERE AFRAID.
DAMMIT, I'M NOT AFRAID. I'M ROYALLY PISSED! WHAT'S THE WORLD HEALTH ORGANIZATION BEEN DOING? THE NATIONAL INSTITUTES OF HEALTH?! OR THE GODDAM CDC ?!!! GRUMBLE GRUMBLE
WE'LL JUST SHELTER-IN-PLACE FOR NOW.
NOW DEAR, THE WHO ISSUED A NOTICE IN MID-JAN. ABOUT THE OUTBREAK. WE JUST DIDN'T HEAR ABOUT IT. REMEMBER WHO'S PRESIDENT?
WE'VE GOTTA STAY HERE FOR NOW, BABE. WE'RE IN LOCKDOWN JUST LIKE YOU.
WE LOVE YOU, HONEY.
WE'LL BE FINE, JAZ HONEY.
THIS ITALIAN HOSPITAL IS OVERWHELMED WITH CORONAVIRUS PATIENTS.
THE DEATH TOLL NOW IS REPORTED TO BE...
CORONAVIRUS PATIENTS FLOOD ER FACILITIES
NO COVID-19 VACCINE IS AVAILABLE
ALL BUSINESSES ARE CLOSED
MASKS
MASKS
MASKS

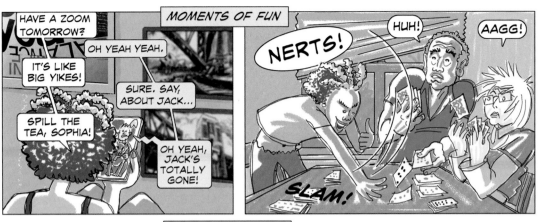

MOMENTS OF FUN

HAVE A ZOOM TOMORROW?

OH YEAH YEAH.

IT'S LIKE BIG YIKES!

SURE. SAY, ABOUT JACK...

SPILL THE TEA, SOPHIA!

OH YEAH, JACK'S TOTALLY GONE!

NERTS!

HUH!

AAGG!

SLAM!

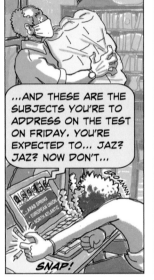

SOME NOT SO FUN

...AND THESE ARE THE SUBJECTS YOU'RE TO ADDRESS ON THE TEST ON FRIDAY. YOU'RE EXPECTED TO... JAZ? JAZ? NOW DON'T...

SNAP!

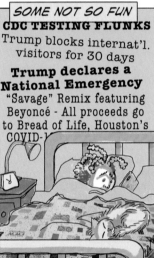

CDC TESTING FLUNKS

Trump blocks internat'l. visitors for 30 days

Trump declares a National Emergency

"Savage" Remix featuring Beyoncé - All proceeds go to Bread of Life, Houston's COVID-1

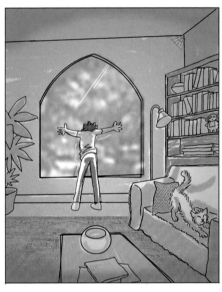

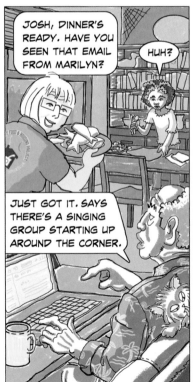

JOSH, DINNER'S READY. HAVE YOU SEEN THAT EMAIL FROM MARILYN?

HUH?

JUST GOT IT. SAYS THERE'S A SINGING GROUP STARTING UP AROUND THE CORNER.

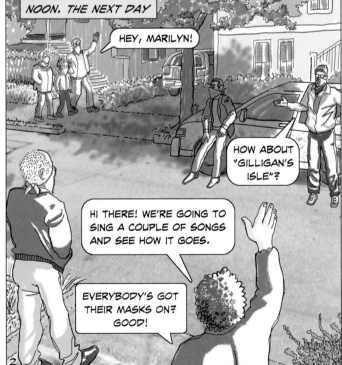

NOON. THE NEXT DAY

HEY, MARILYN!

HOW ABOUT "GILLIGAN'S ISLE"?

HI THERE! WE'RE GOING TO SING A COUPLE OF SONGS AND SEE HOW IT GOES.

EVERYBODY'S GOT THEIR MASKS ON? GOOD!

2

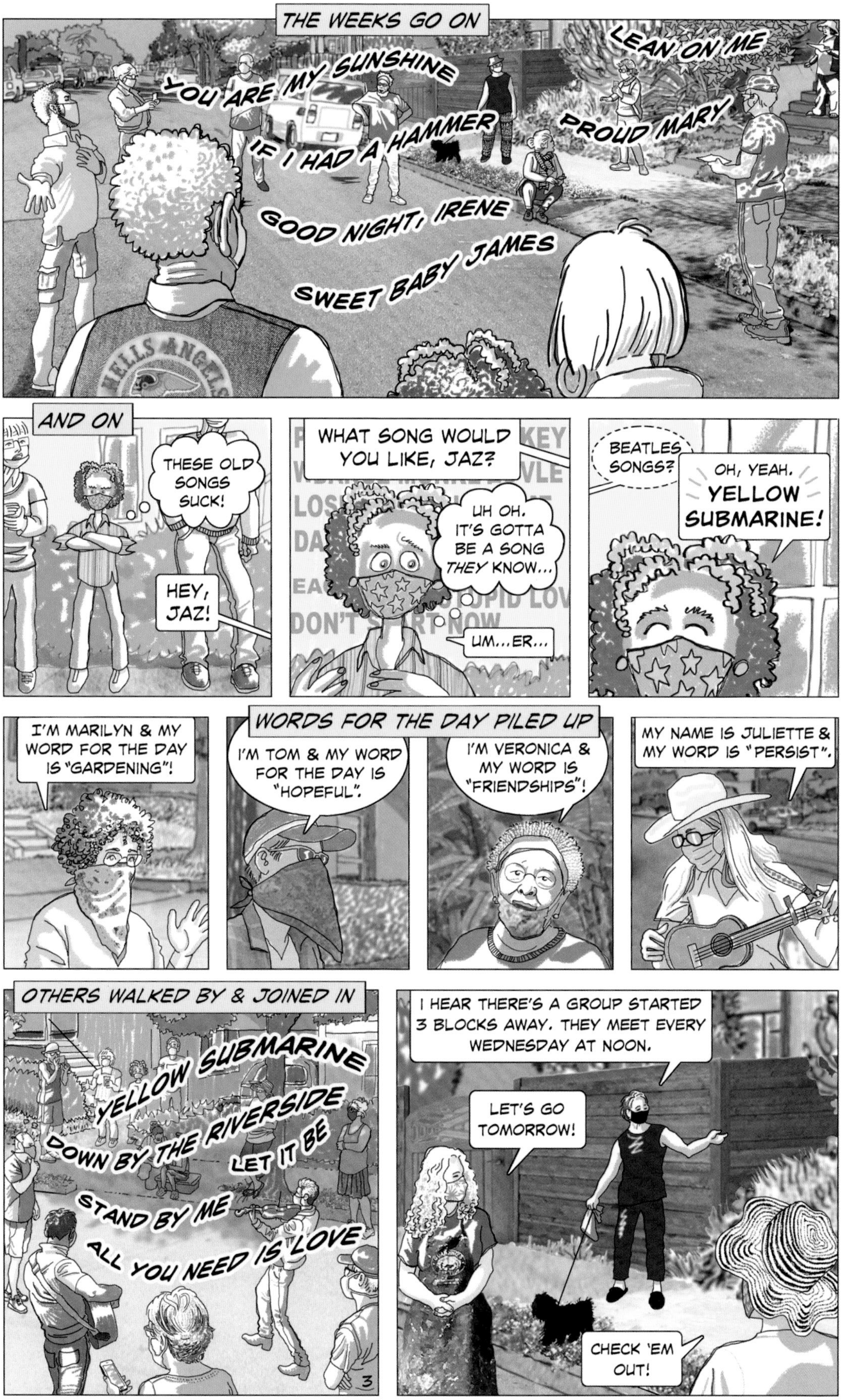
THE WEEKS GO ON
YOU ARE MY SUNSHINE
IF I HAD A HAMMER
GOOD NIGHT, IRENE
SWEET BABY JAMES
LEAN ON ME
PROUD MARY
AND ON
THESE OLD SONGS SUCK!
HEY, JAZ!
WHAT SONG WOULD YOU LIKE, JAZ?
UH OH. IT'S GOTTA BE A SONG THEY KNOW...
UM...ER...
BEATLES SONGS?
OH, YEAH. YELLOW SUBMARINE!
WORDS FOR THE DAY PILED UP
I'M MARILYN & MY WORD FOR THE DAY IS "GARDENING"!
I'M TOM & MY WORD FOR THE DAY IS "HOPEFUL".
I'M VERONICA & MY WORD IS "FRIENDSHIPS"!
MY NAME IS JULIETTE & MY WORD IS "PERSIST".
OTHERS WALKED BY & JOINED IN
YELLOW SUBMARINE
DOWN BY THE RIVERSIDE
LET IT BE
STAND BY ME
ALL YOU NEED IS LOVE
I HEAR THERE'S A GROUP STARTED 3 BLOCKS AWAY. THEY MEET EVERY WEDNESDAY AT NOON.
LET'S GO TOMORROW!
CHECK 'EM OUT!

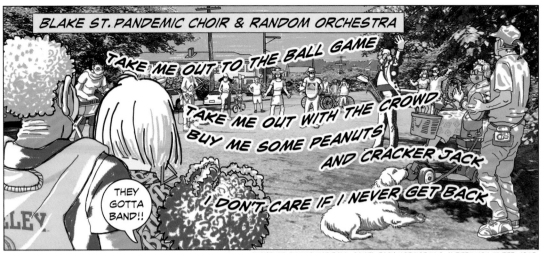

BLAKE ST. PANDEMIC CHOIR & RANDOM ORCHESTRA

TAKE ME OUT TO THE BALL GAME
TAKE ME OUT WITH THE CROWD
BUY ME SOME PEANUTS
AND CRACKER JACK
I DON'T CARE IF I NEVER GET BACK

THEY GOTTA BAND!!

"TAKE ME OUT TO THE BALL GAME" JACK NORWORTH & ALBERT VON TILZER 1908

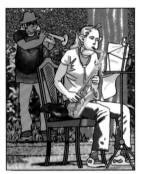
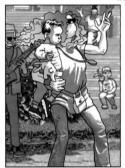
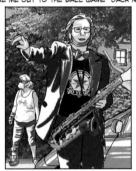
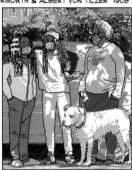

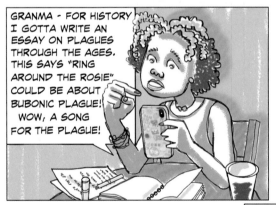

GRANMA - FOR HISTORY I GOTTA WRITE AN ESSAY ON PLAGUES THROUGH THE AGES. THIS SAYS "RING AROUND THE ROSIE" COULD BE ABOUT BUBONIC PLAGUE! WOW, A SONG FOR THE PLAGUE!

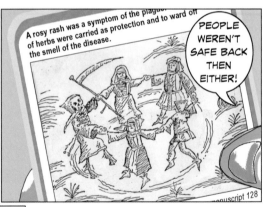

A rosy rash was a symptom of the plague. of herbs were carried as protection and to ward off the smell of the disease.

PEOPLE WEREN'T SAFE BACK THEN EITHER!

manuscript 128

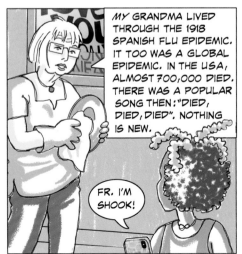

MY GRANDMA LIVED THROUGH THE 1918 SPANISH FLU EPIDEMIC. IT TOO WAS A GLOBAL EPIDEMIC. IN THE USA, ALMOST 700,000 DIED. THERE WAS A POPULAR SONG THEN: "DIED, DIED, DIED". NOTHING IS NEW.

FR. I'M SHOOK!

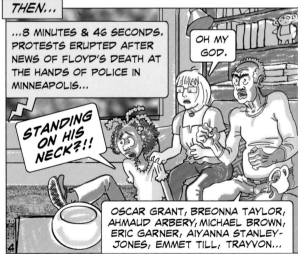

THEN...

...8 MINUTES & 46 SECONDS. PROTESTS ERUPTED AFTER NEWS OF FLOYD'S DEATH AT THE HANDS OF POLICE IN MINNEAPOLIS...

OH MY GOD.

STANDING ON HIS NECK?!!

OSCAR GRANT, BREONNA TAYLOR, AHMAUD ARBERY, MICHAEL BROWN, ERIC GARNER, AIYANNA STANLEY-JONES, EMMET TILL, TRAYVON...

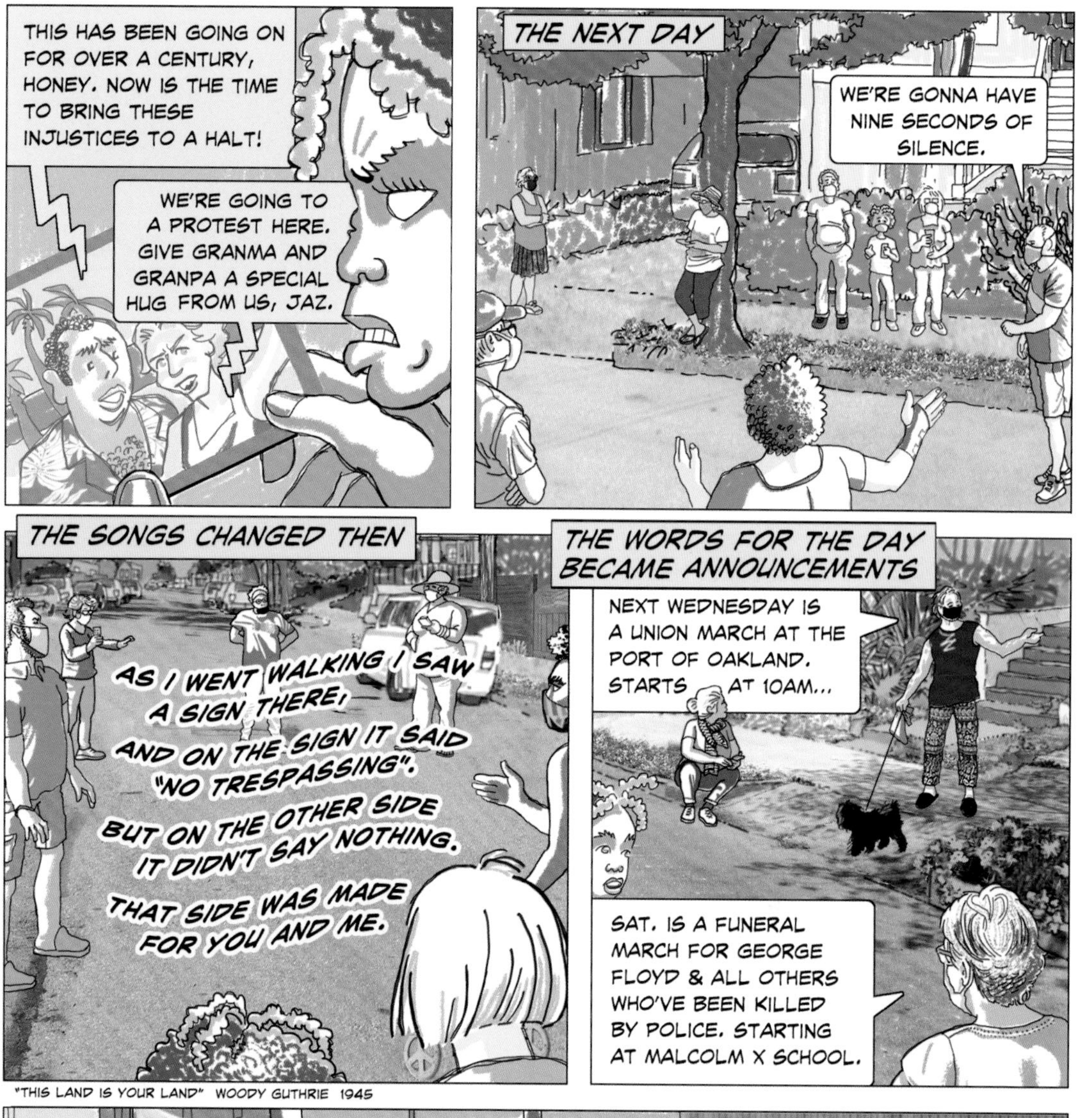
THIS HAS BEEN GOING ON FOR OVER A CENTURY, HONEY. NOW IS THE TIME TO BRING THESE INJUSTICES TO A HALT!
WE'RE GOING TO A PROTEST HERE. GIVE GRANMA AND GRANPA A SPECIAL HUG FROM US, JAZ.
THE NEXT DAY
WE'RE GONNA HAVE NINE SECONDS OF SILENCE.
THE SONGS CHANGED THEN
AS I WENT WALKING I SAW A SIGN THERE,
AND ON THE SIGN IT SAID "NO TRESPASSING".
BUT ON THE OTHER SIDE IT DIDN'T SAY NOTHING.
THAT SIDE WAS MADE FOR YOU AND ME.
THE WORDS FOR THE DAY BECAME ANNOUNCEMENTS
NEXT WEDNESDAY IS A UNION MARCH AT THE PORT OF OAKLAND. STARTS AT 10AM...
SAT. IS A FUNERAL MARCH FOR GEORGE FLOYD & ALL OTHERS WHO'VE BEEN KILLED BY POLICE. STARTING AT MALCOLM X SCHOOL.

"THIS LAND IS YOUR LAND" WOODY GUTHRIE 1945

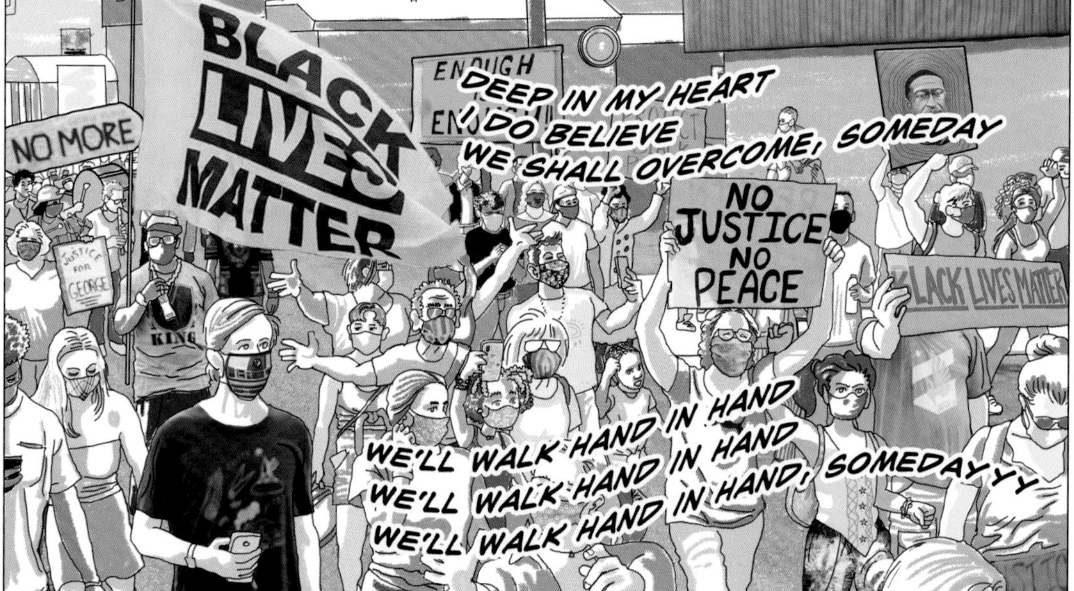
BLACK LIVES MATTER
NO MORE
ENOUGH
JUSTICE FOR GEORGE
DEEP IN MY HEART I DO BELIEVE WE SHALL OVERCOME, SOMEDAY
NO JUSTICE NO PEACE
BLACK LIVES MATTER
KING
WE'LL WALK HAND IN HAND
WE'LL WALK HAND IN HAND
WE'LL WALK HAND IN HAND, SOMEDAYYY
END

"WE SHALL OVERCOME" PETE SEEGER 1947

THANKS TO MONTSE & BEORN HARTWIG FOR TEEN SLANG.

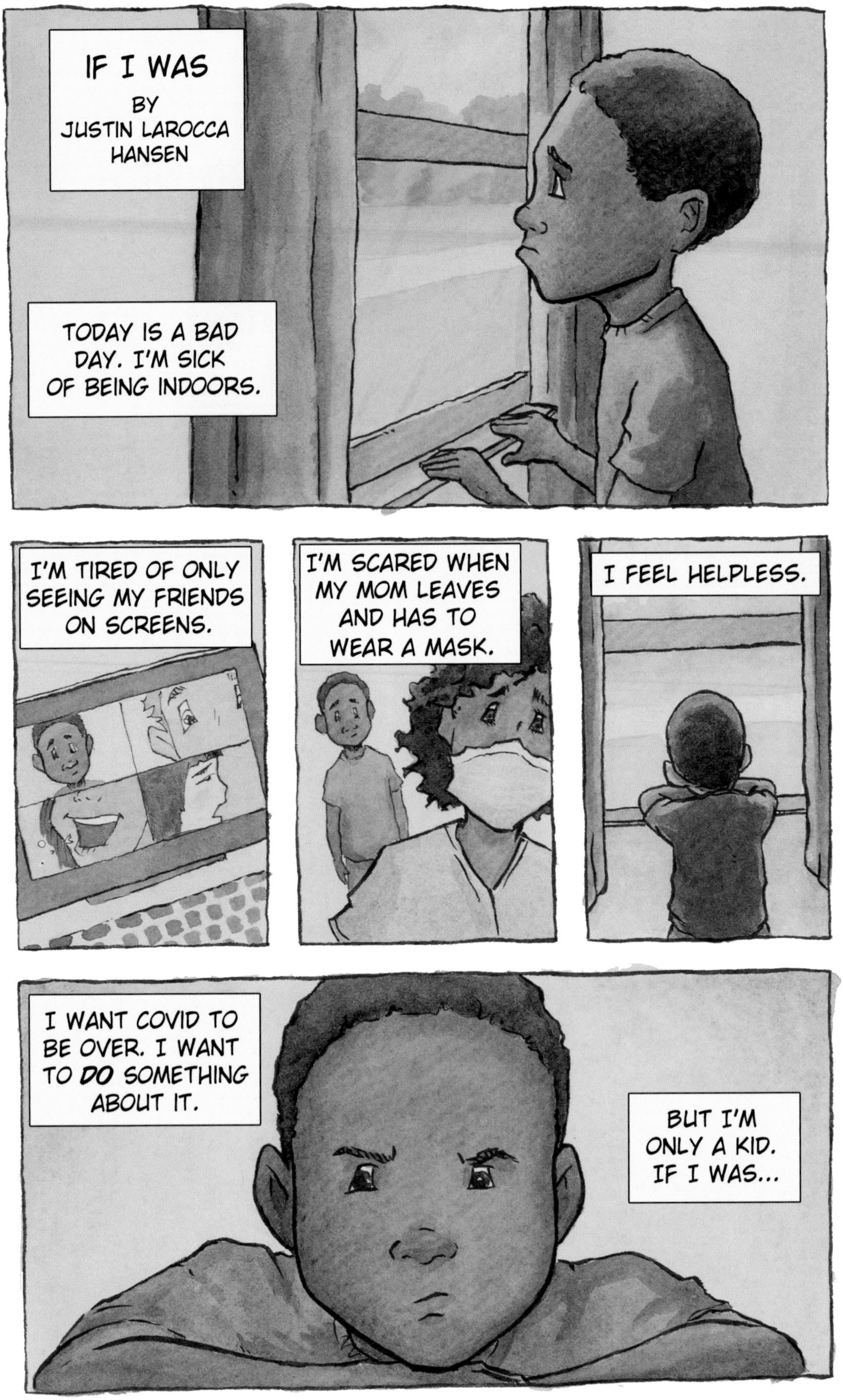
IF I WAS
BY
JUSTIN LAROCCA
HANSEN
TODAY IS A BAD DAY. I'M SICK OF BEING INDOORS.
I'M TIRED OF ONLY SEEING MY FRIENDS ON SCREENS.
I'M SCARED WHEN MY MOM LEAVES AND HAS TO WEAR A MASK.
I FEEL HELPLESS.
I WANT COVID TO BE OVER. I WANT TO DO SOMETHING ABOUT IT.
BUT I'M ONLY A KID. IF I WAS...

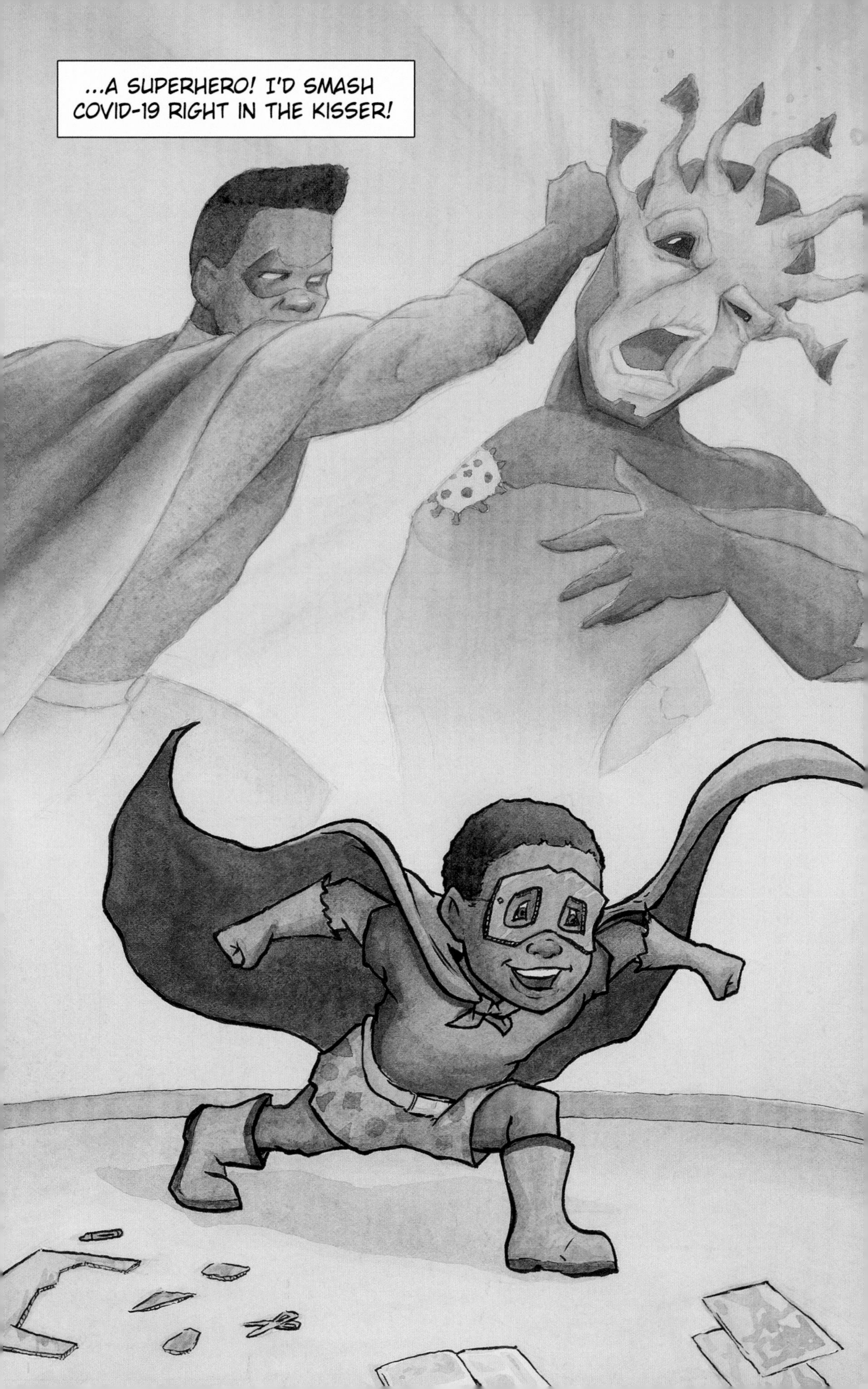
...A SUPERHERO! I'D SMASH COVID-19 RIGHT IN THE KISSER!

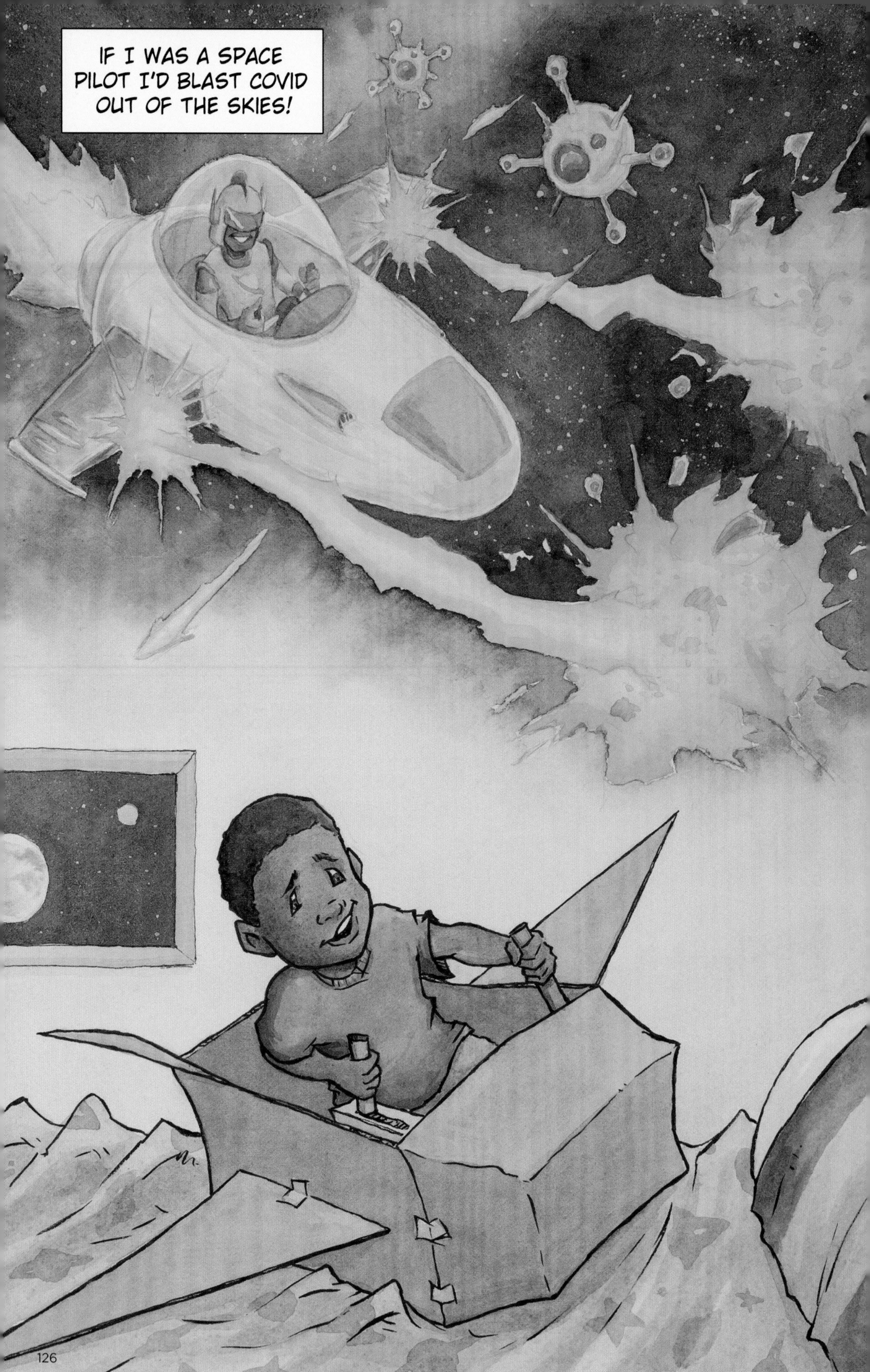
IF I WAS A SPACE PILOT I'D BLAST COVID OUT OF THE SKIES!

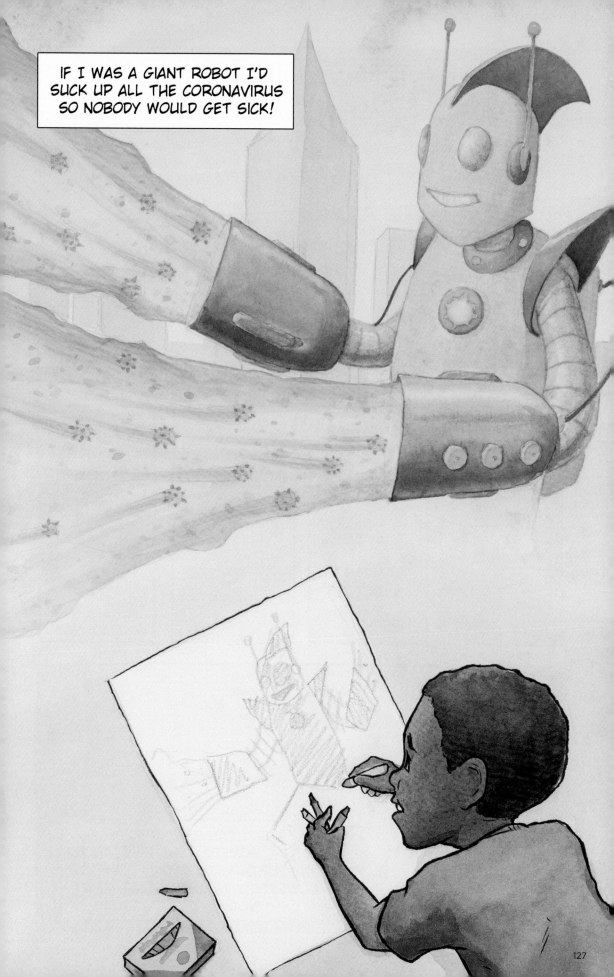

IF I WAS A GIANT ROBOT I'D SUCK UP ALL THE CORONAVIRUS SO NOBODY WOULD GET SICK!

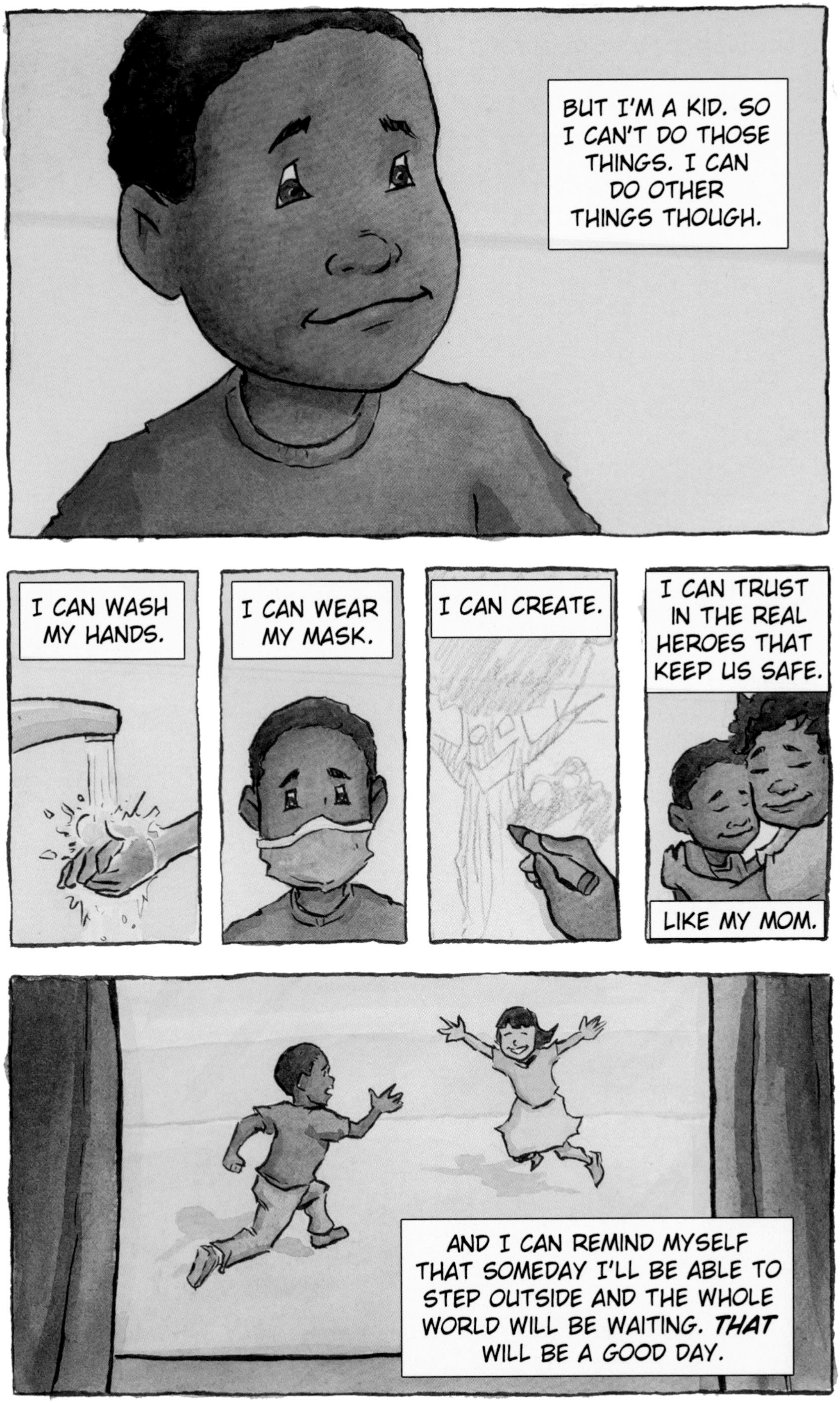
BUT I'M A KID. SO I CAN'T DO THOSE THINGS. I CAN DO OTHER THINGS THOUGH.
I CAN WASH MY HANDS.
I CAN WEAR MY MASK.
I CAN CREATE.
I CAN TRUST IN THE REAL HEROES THAT KEEP US SAFE.
LIKE MY MOM.
AND I CAN REMIND MYSELF THAT SOMEDAY I'LL BE ABLE TO STEP OUTSIDE AND THE WHOLE WORLD WILL BE WAITING. *THAT* WILL BE A GOOD DAY.

Librarying During a Pandemic

LIBRARY COMIC STRIPS BY GENE AMBAUM AND WILLOW PAYNE

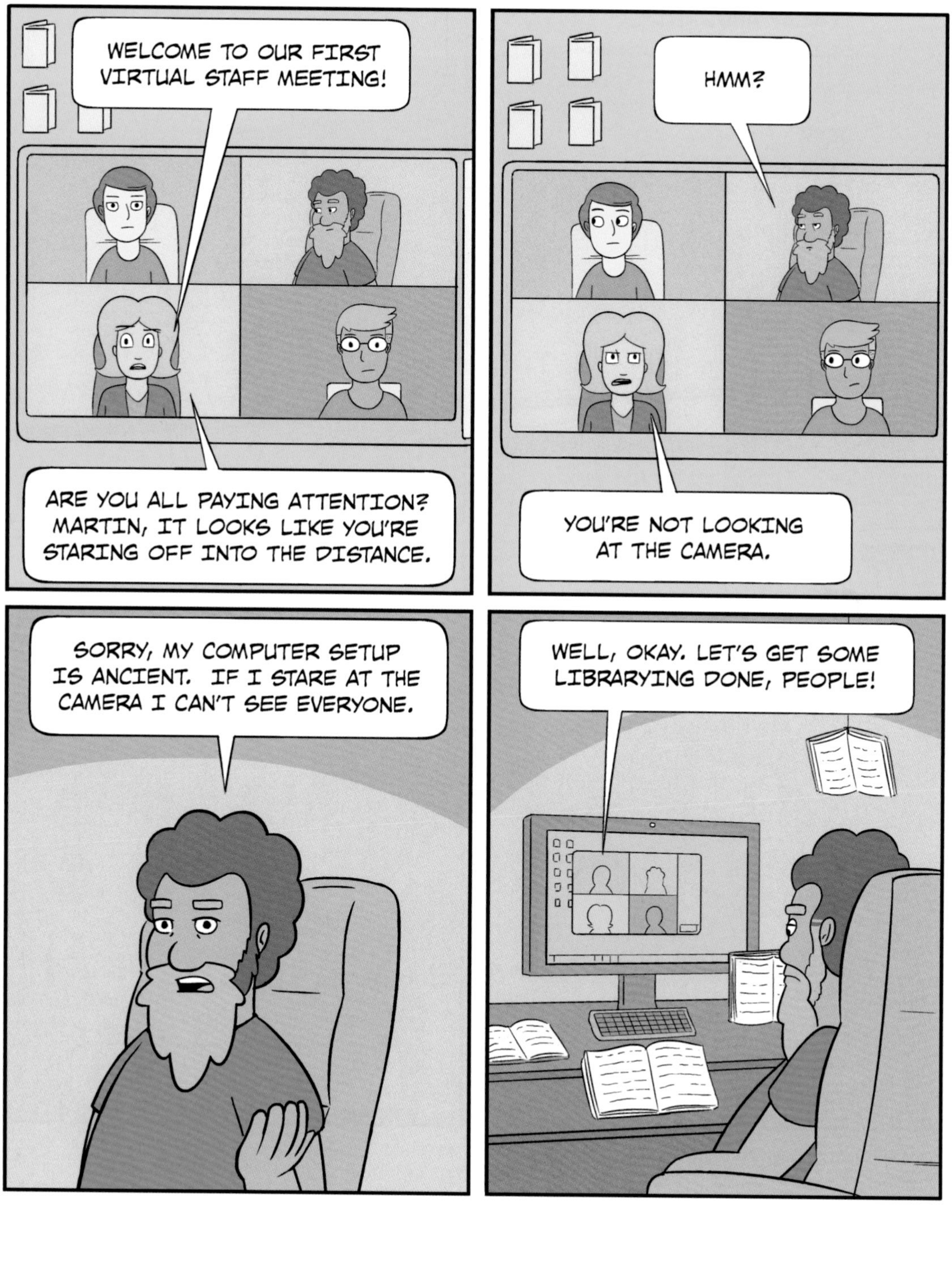
WELCOME TO OUR FIRST VIRTUAL STAFF MEETING!
ARE YOU ALL PAYING ATTENTION? MARTIN, IT LOOKS LIKE YOU'RE STARING OFF INTO THE DISTANCE.
HMM?
YOU'RE NOT LOOKING AT THE CAMERA.
SORRY, MY COMPUTER SETUP IS ANCIENT. IF I STARE AT THE CAMERA I CAN'T SEE EVERYONE.
WELL, OKAY. LET'S GET SOME LIBRARYING DONE, PEOPLE!

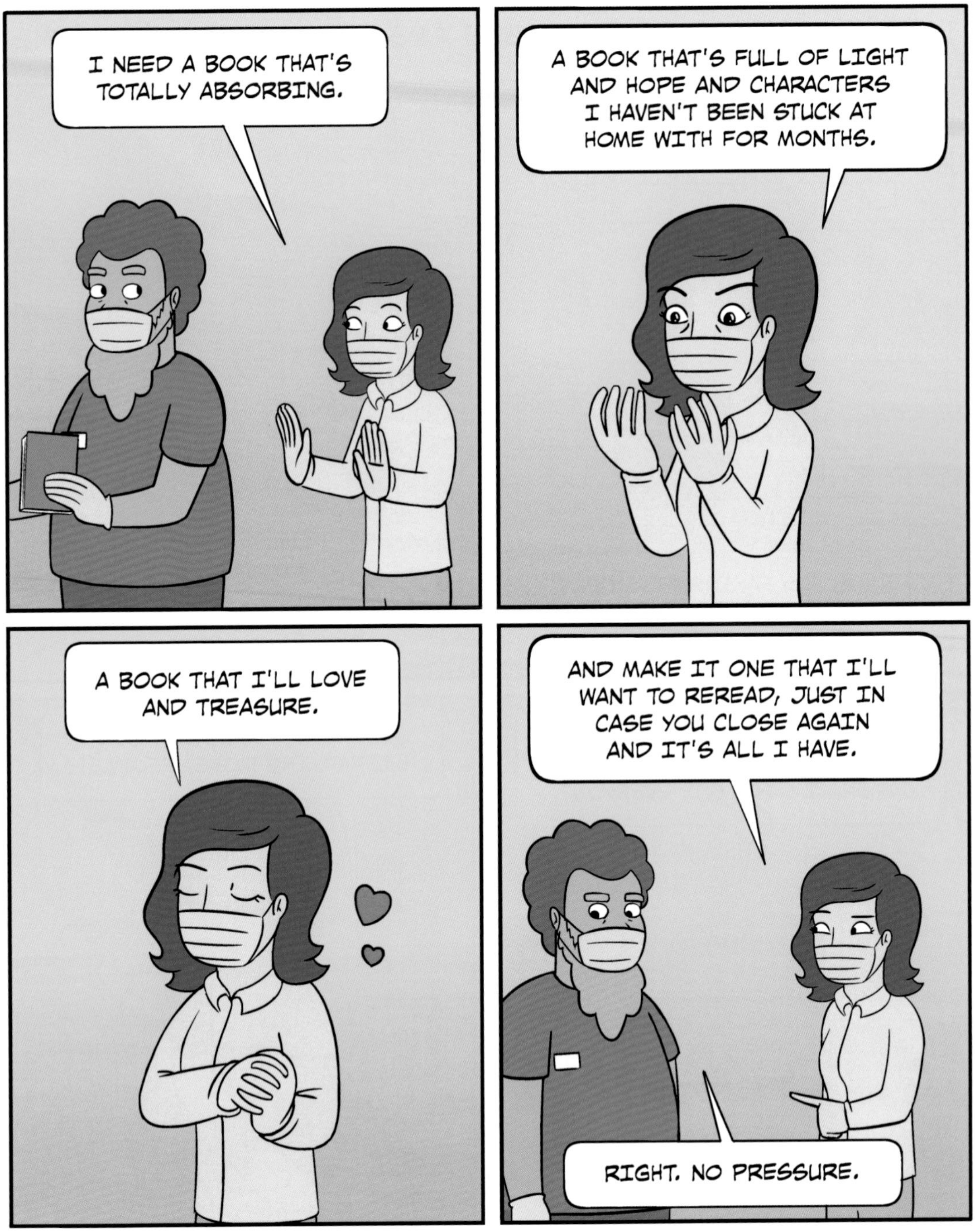
I NEED A BOOK THAT'S TOTALLY ABSORBING.
A BOOK THAT'S FULL OF LIGHT AND HOPE AND CHARACTERS I HAVEN'T BEEN STUCK AT HOME WITH FOR MONTHS.
A BOOK THAT I'LL LOVE AND TREASURE.
AND MAKE IT ONE THAT I'LL WANT TO REREAD, JUST IN CASE YOU CLOSE AGAIN AND IT'S ALL I HAVE.
RIGHT. NO PRESSURE.

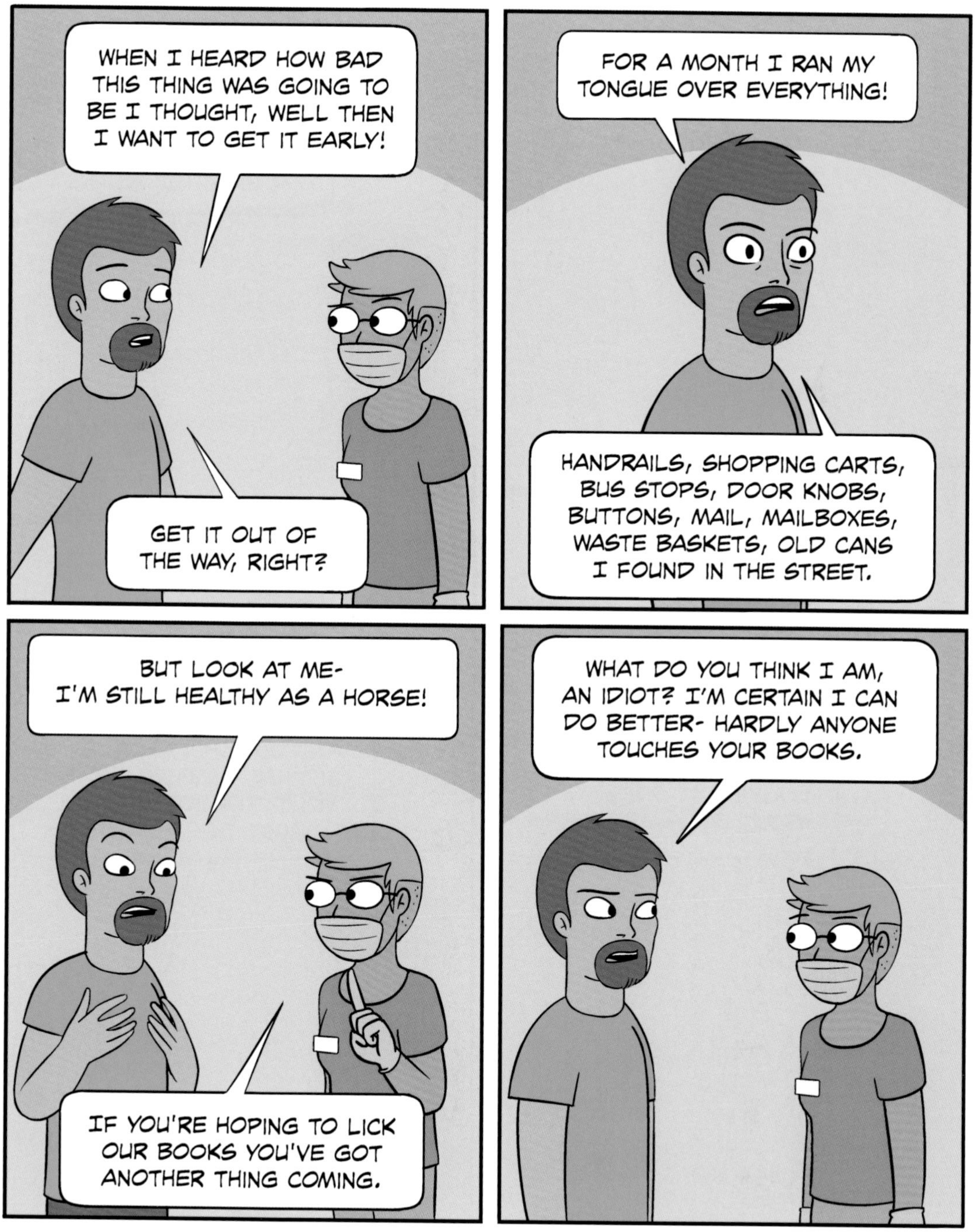
WHEN I HEARD HOW BAD THIS THING WAS GOING TO BE I THOUGHT, WELL THEN I WANT TO GET IT EARLY!
GET IT OUT OF THE WAY, RIGHT?
FOR A MONTH I RAN MY TONGUE OVER EVERYTHING!
HANDRAILS, SHOPPING CARTS, BUS STOPS, DOOR KNOBS, BUTTONS, MAIL, MAILBOXES, WASTE BASKETS, OLD CANS I FOUND IN THE STREET.
BUT LOOK AT ME- I'M STILL HEALTHY AS A HORSE!
IF YOU'RE HOPING TO LICK OUR BOOKS YOU'VE GOT ANOTHER THING COMING.
WHAT DO YOU THINK I AM, AN IDIOT? I'M CERTAIN I CAN DO BETTER- HARDLY ANYONE TOUCHES YOUR BOOKS.

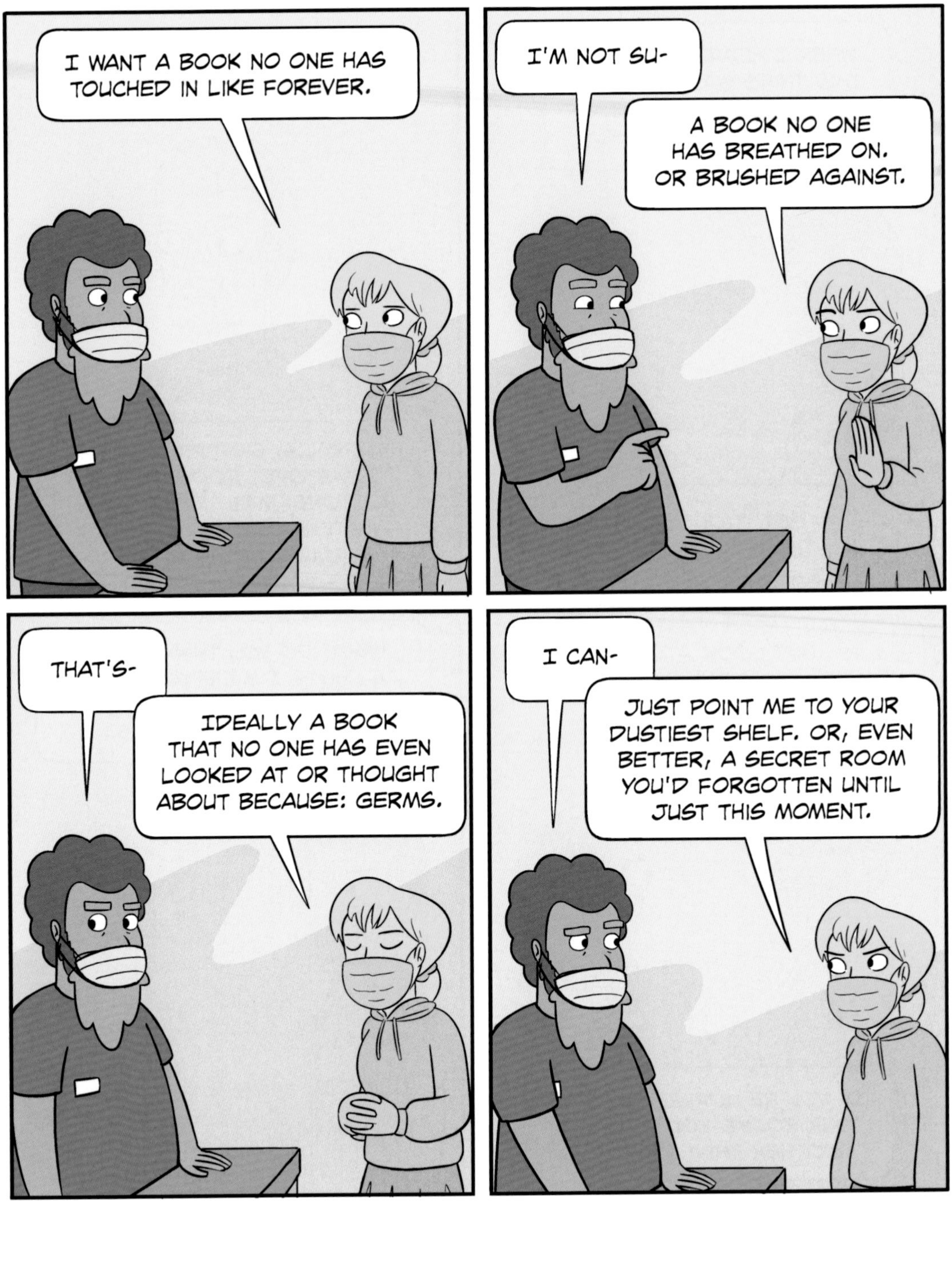
I WANT A BOOK NO ONE HAS TOUCHED IN LIKE FOREVER.
I'M NOT SU-
A BOOK NO ONE HAS BREATHED ON. OR BRUSHED AGAINST.
THAT'S-
IDEALLY A BOOK THAT NO ONE HAS EVEN LOOKED AT OR THOUGHT ABOUT BECAUSE: GERMS.
I CAN-
JUST POINT ME TO YOUR DUSTIEST SHELF. OR, EVEN BETTER, A SECRET ROOM YOU'D FORGOTTEN UNTIL JUST THIS MOMENT.

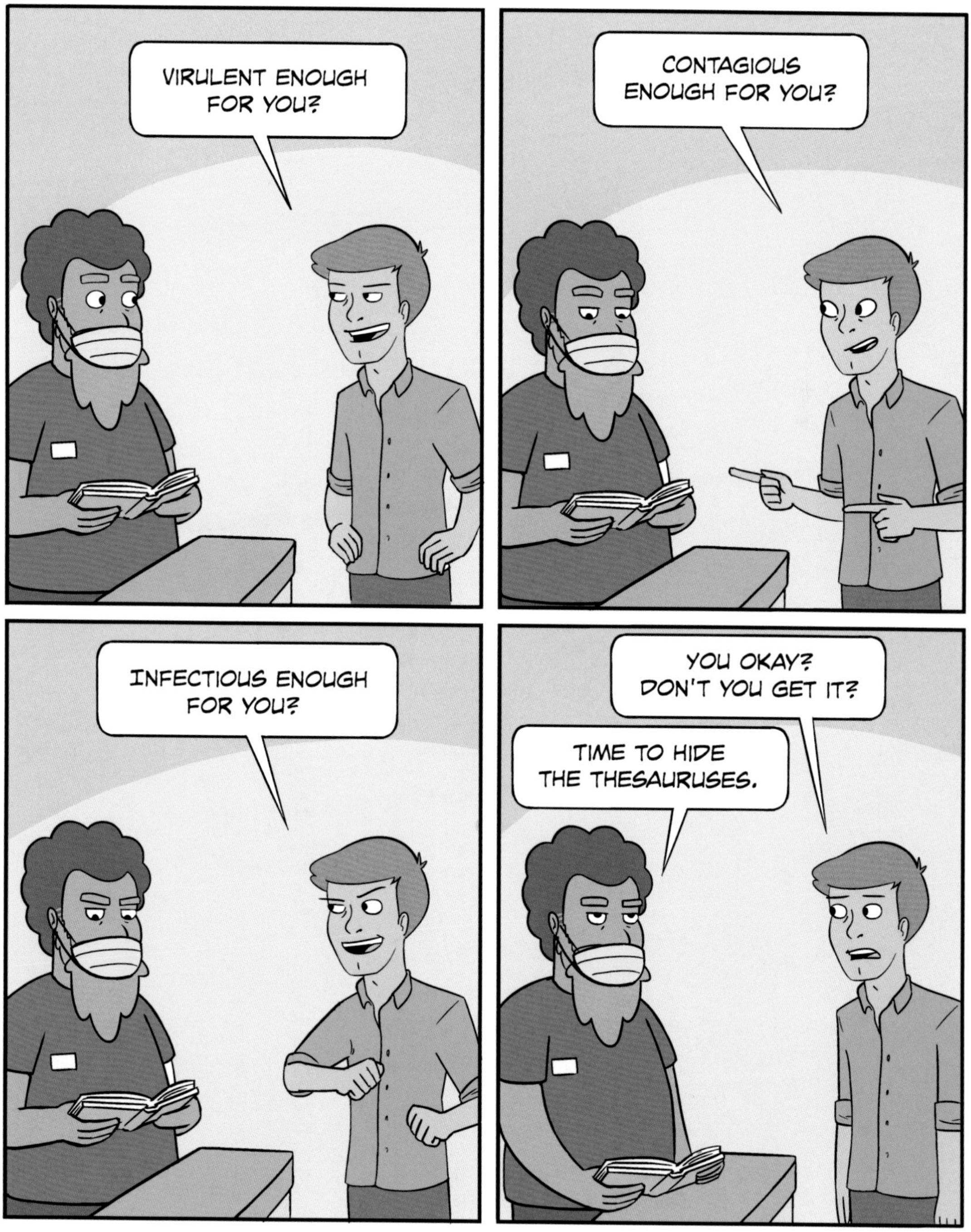
VIRULENT ENOUGH FOR YOU?
CONTAGIOUS ENOUGH FOR YOU?
INFECTIOUS ENOUGH FOR YOU?
YOU OKAY? DON'T YOU GET IT?
TIME TO HIDE THE THESAURUSES.

Hi Bill! Hi Jean. Watcha up to?
Just heading over to a friend's place for dinner. Of course, bringing our own cups, plates, utensils, food, chairs...

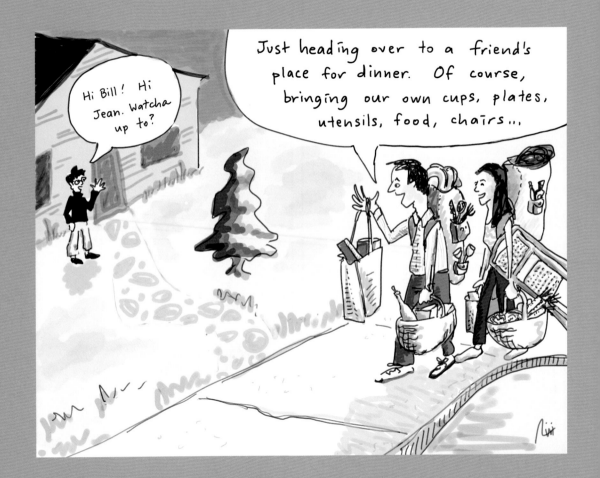

Small Acts

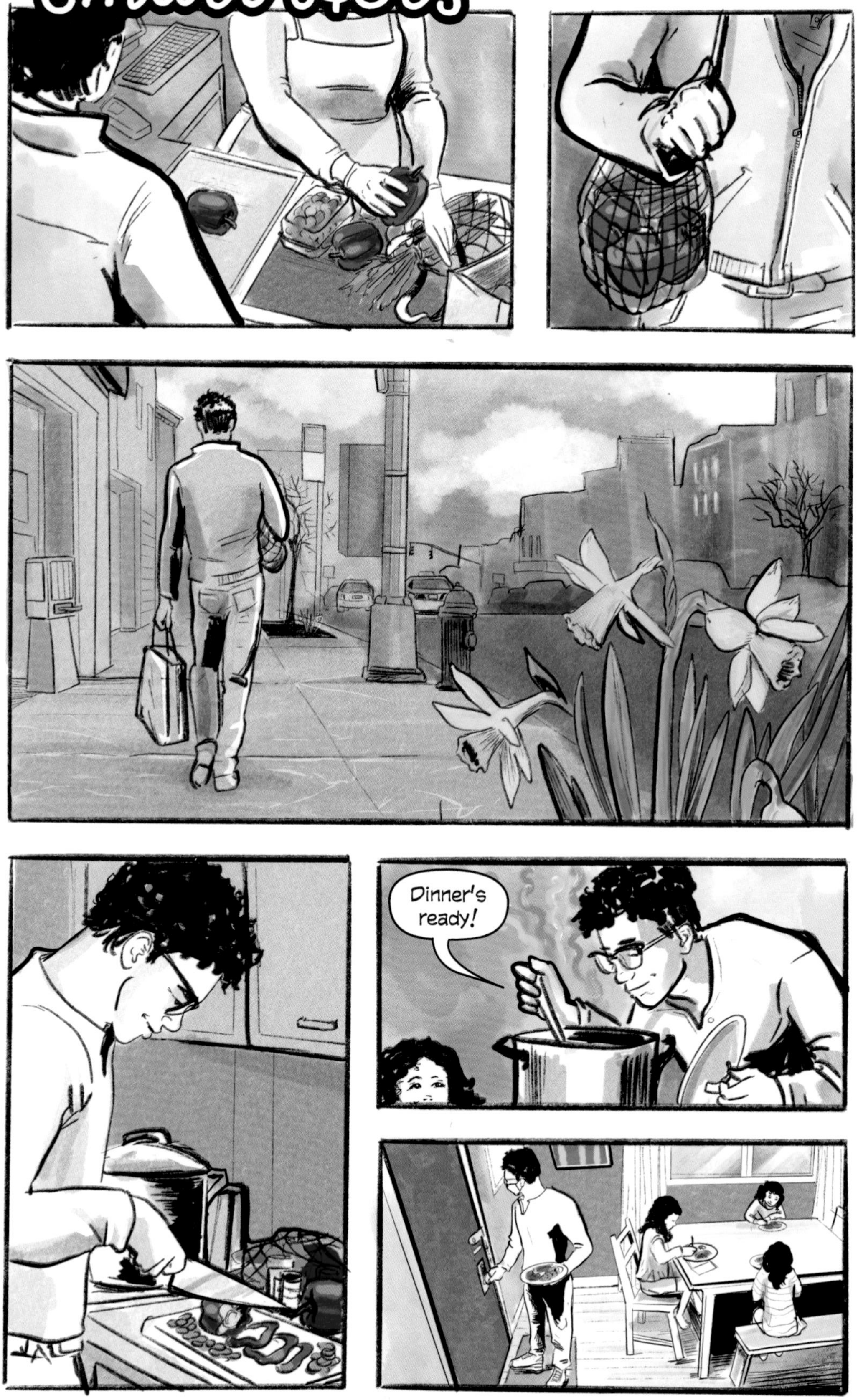

Dinner's ready!

WRITTEN BY STEPHANIE NINA PITSIRILOS ILLUSTRATED BY SETH MARTEL

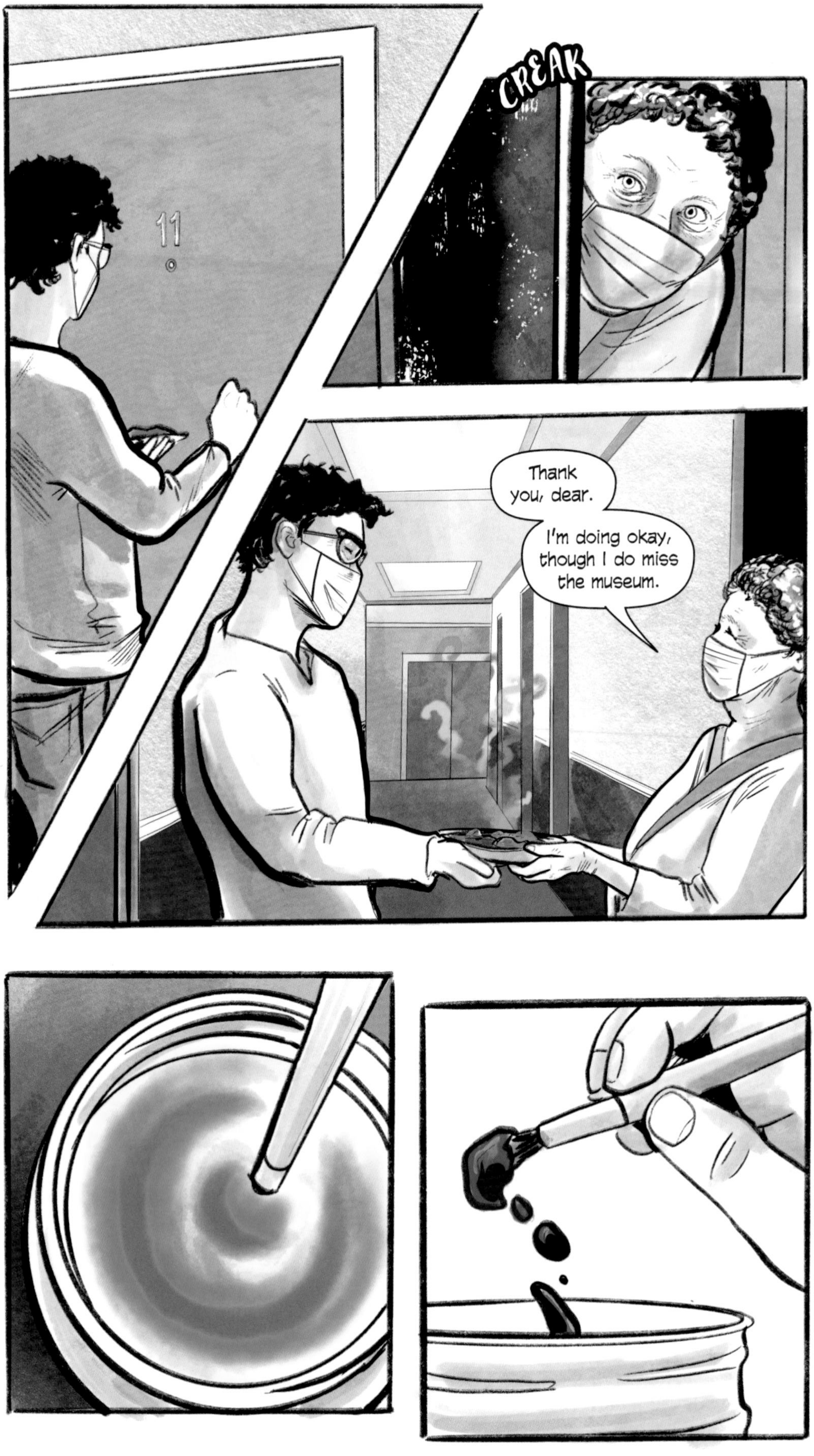

CREAK
Thank you, dear.
I'm doing okay, though I do miss the museum.

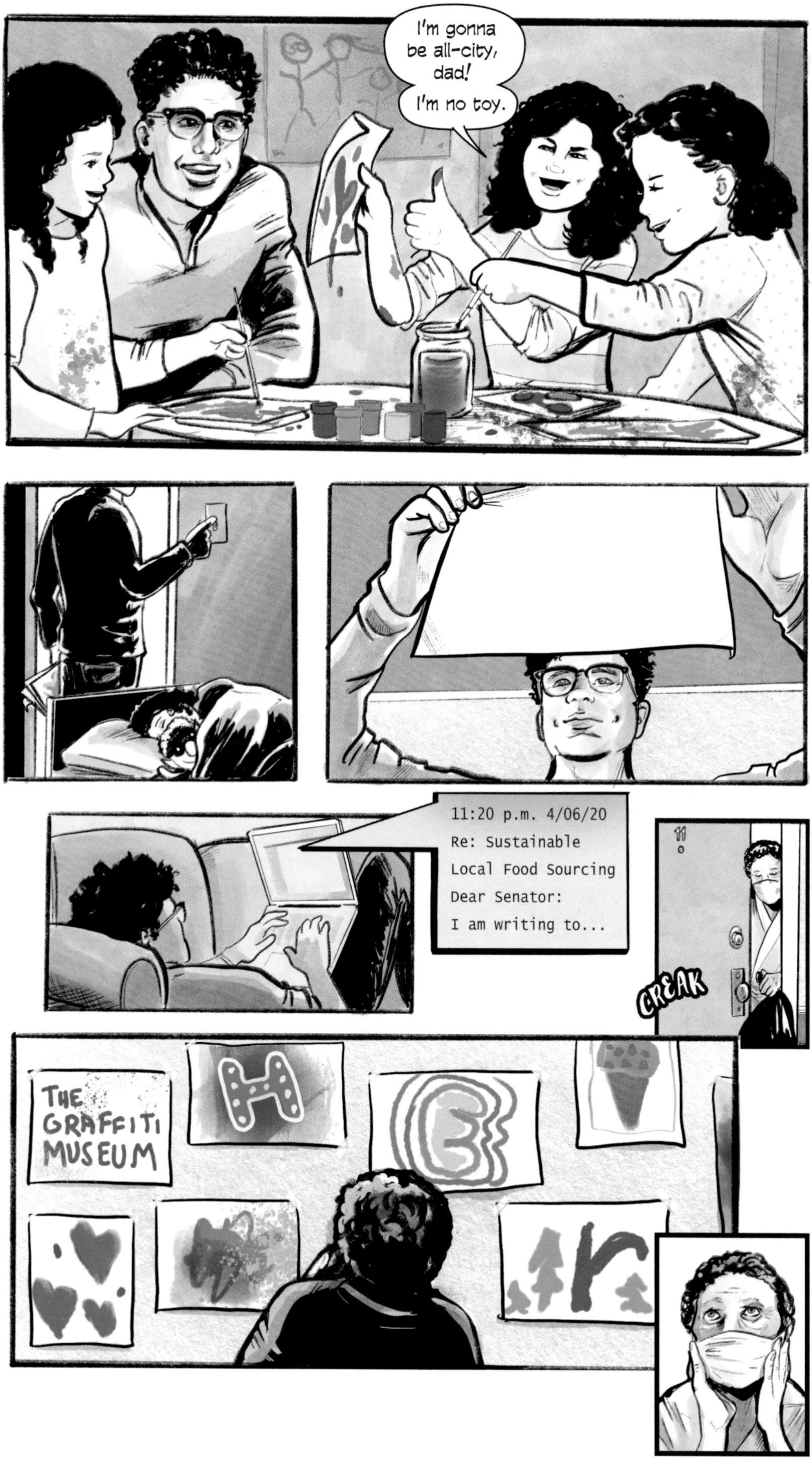
I'm gonna be all-city, dad!
I'm no toy.
11:20 p.m. 4/06/20
Re: Sustainable Local Food Sourcing
Dear Senator:
I am writing to...
CREAK
THE GRAFFITI MUSEUM

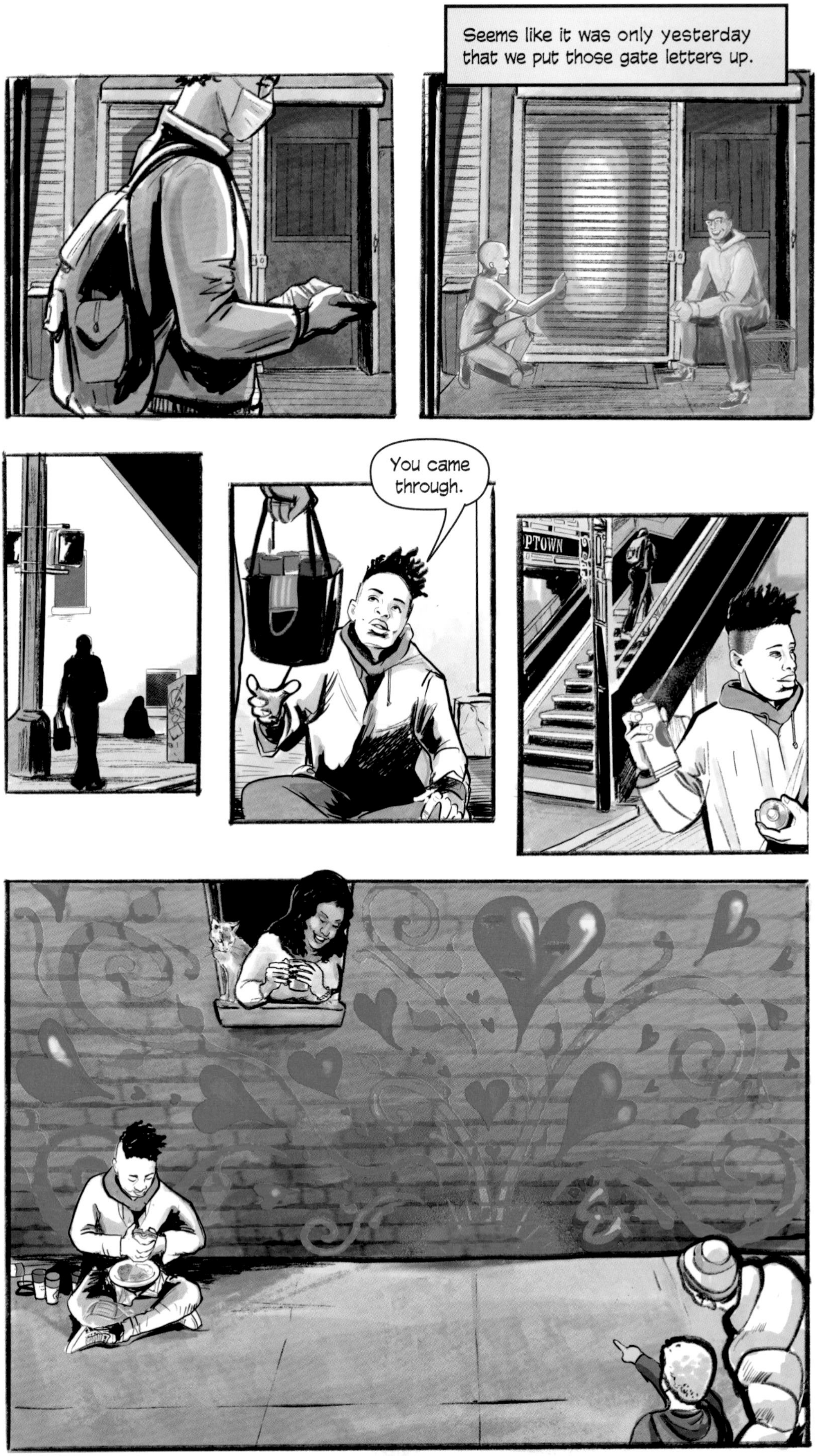
Seems like it was only yesterday that we put those gate letters up.
You came through.
UPTOWN

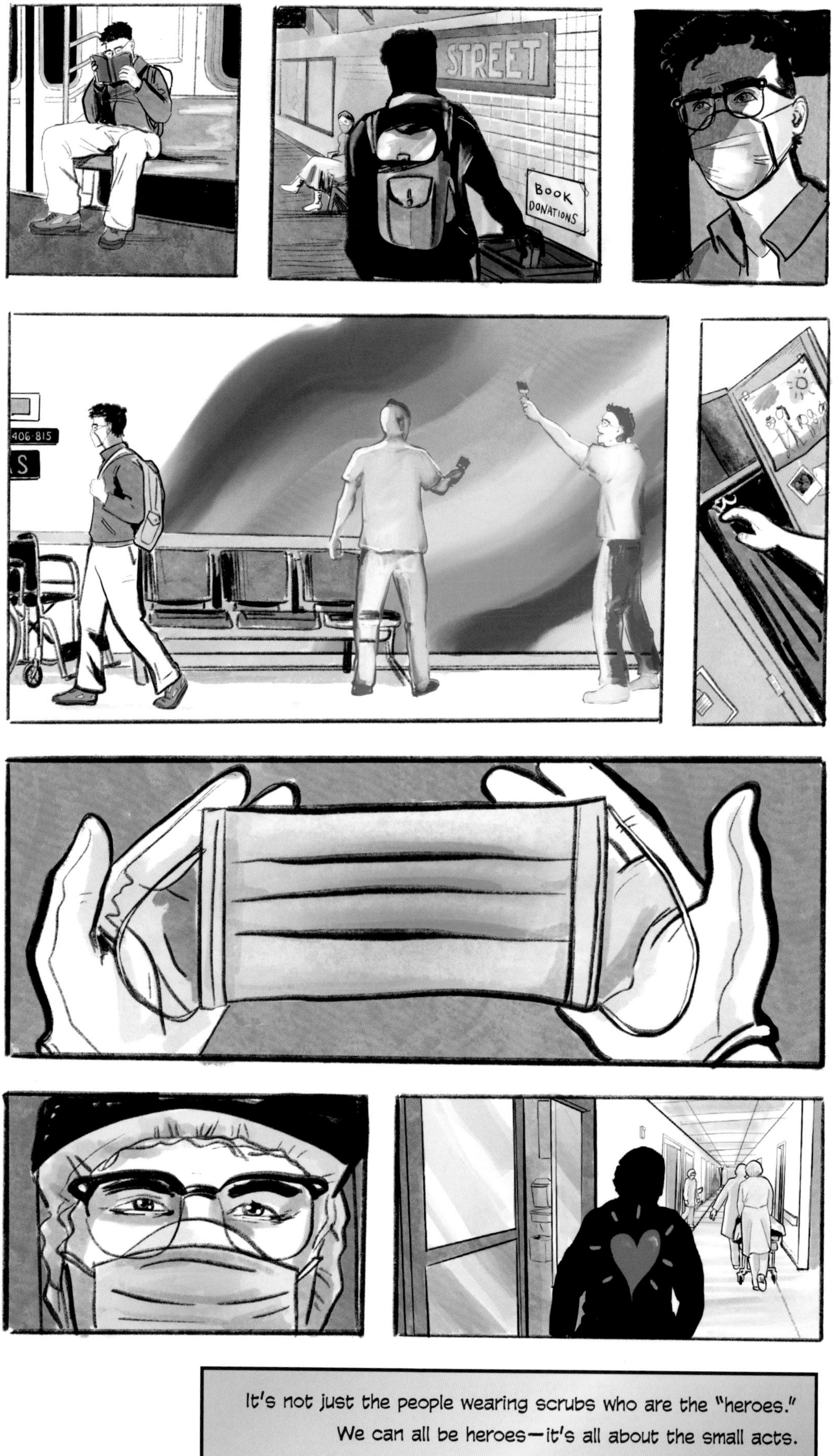
STREET
BOOK DONATIONS
406-815
S
It's not just the people wearing scrubs who are the "heroes."
We can all be heroes—it's all about the small acts.

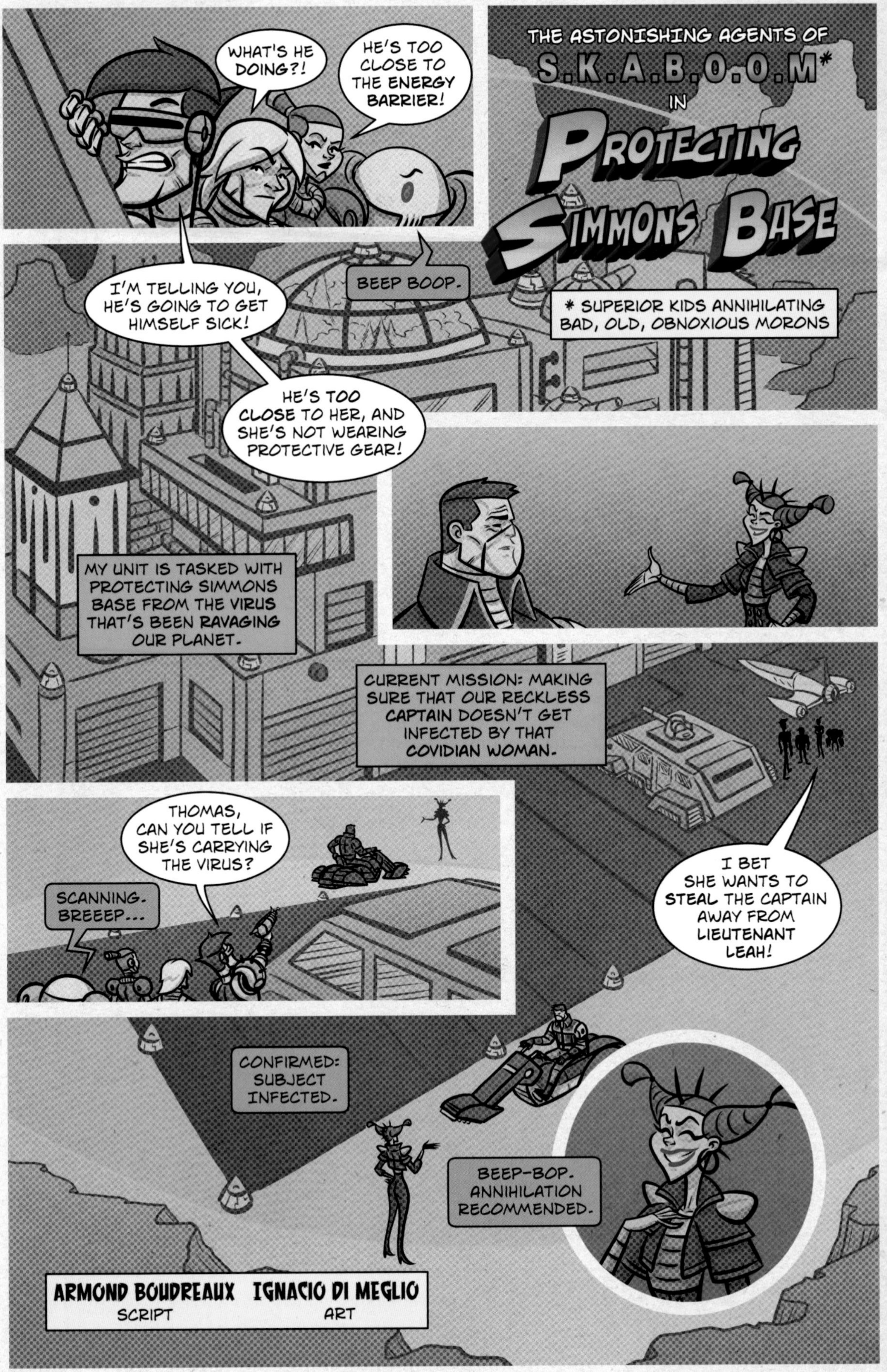
THE ASTONISHING AGENTS OF S.K.A.B.O.O.M* IN
PROTECTING SIMMONS BASE
* SUPERIOR KIDS ANNIHILATING BAD, OLD, OBNOXIOUS MORONS
WHAT'S HE DOING?!
HE'S TOO CLOSE TO THE ENERGY BARRIER!
I'M TELLING YOU, HE'S GOING TO GET HIMSELF SICK!
BEEP BOOP.
HE'S TOO CLOSE TO HER, AND SHE'S NOT WEARING PROTECTIVE GEAR!
MY UNIT IS TASKED WITH PROTECTING SIMMONS BASE FROM THE VIRUS THAT'S BEEN RAVAGING OUR PLANET.
CURRENT MISSION: MAKING SURE THAT OUR RECKLESS CAPTAIN DOESN'T GET INFECTED BY THAT COVIDIAN WOMAN.
THOMAS, CAN YOU TELL IF SHE'S CARRYING THE VIRUS?
SCANNING. BREEEP...
I BET SHE WANTS TO STEAL THE CAPTAIN AWAY FROM LIEUTENANT LEAH!
CONFIRMED: SUBJECT INFECTED.
BEEP-BOP. ANNIHILATION RECOMMENDED.
ARMOND BOUDREAUX SCRIPT
IGNACIO DI MEGLIO ART

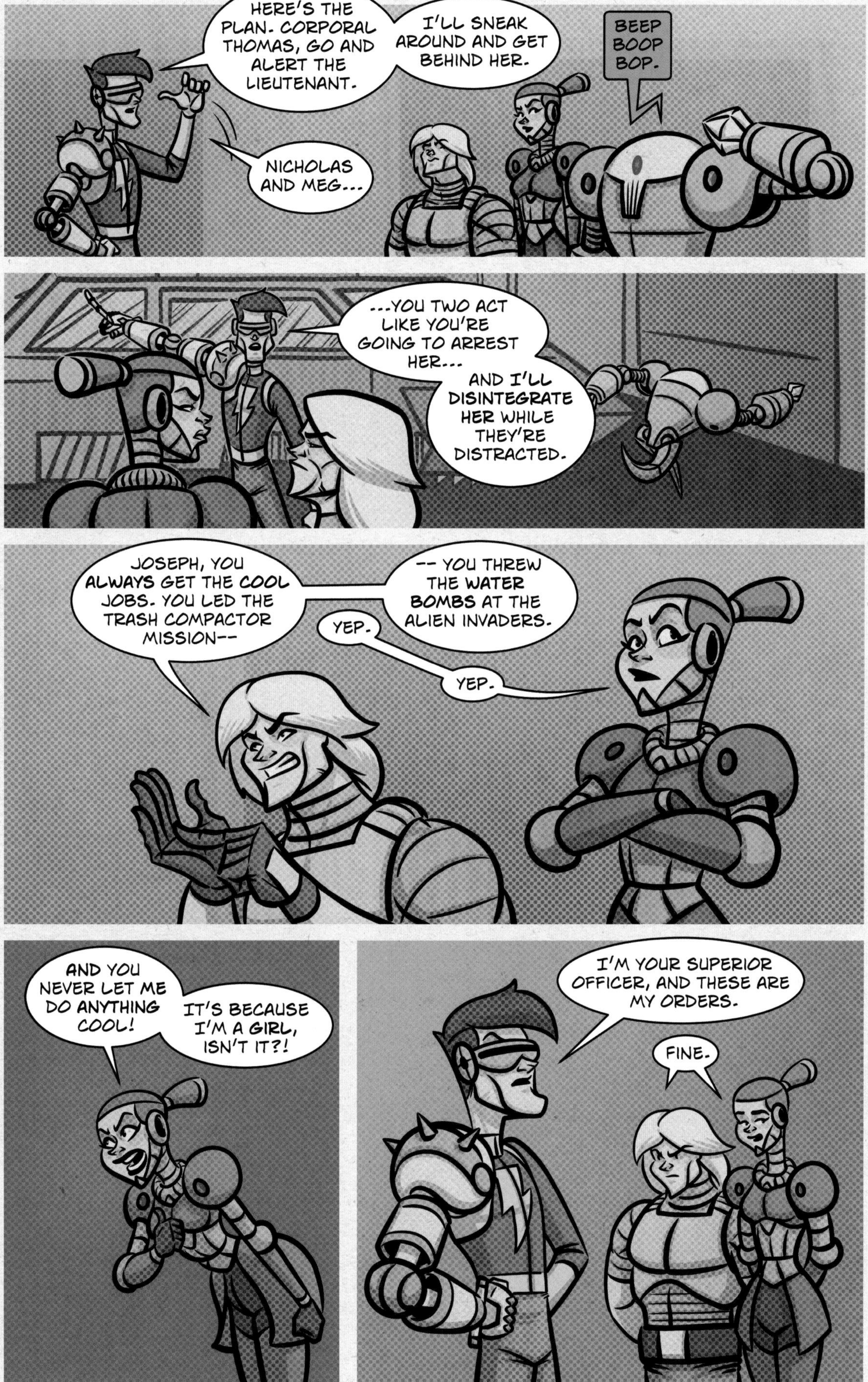
HERE'S THE PLAN. CORPORAL THOMAS, GO AND ALERT THE LIEUTENANT.
I'LL SNEAK AROUND AND GET BEHIND HER.
BEEP BOOP BOP.
NICHOLAS AND MEG...
...YOU TWO ACT LIKE YOU'RE GOING TO ARREST HER...
AND I'LL DISINTEGRATE HER WHILE THEY'RE DISTRACTED.
JOSEPH, YOU ALWAYS GET THE COOL JOBS. YOU LED THE TRASH COMPACTOR MISSION--
-- YOU THREW THE WATER BOMBS AT THE ALIEN INVADERS.
YEP.
YEP.
AND YOU NEVER LET ME DO ANYTHING COOL!
IT'S BECAUSE I'M A GIRL, ISN'T IT?!
I'M YOUR SUPERIOR OFFICER, AND THESE ARE MY ORDERS.
FINE.

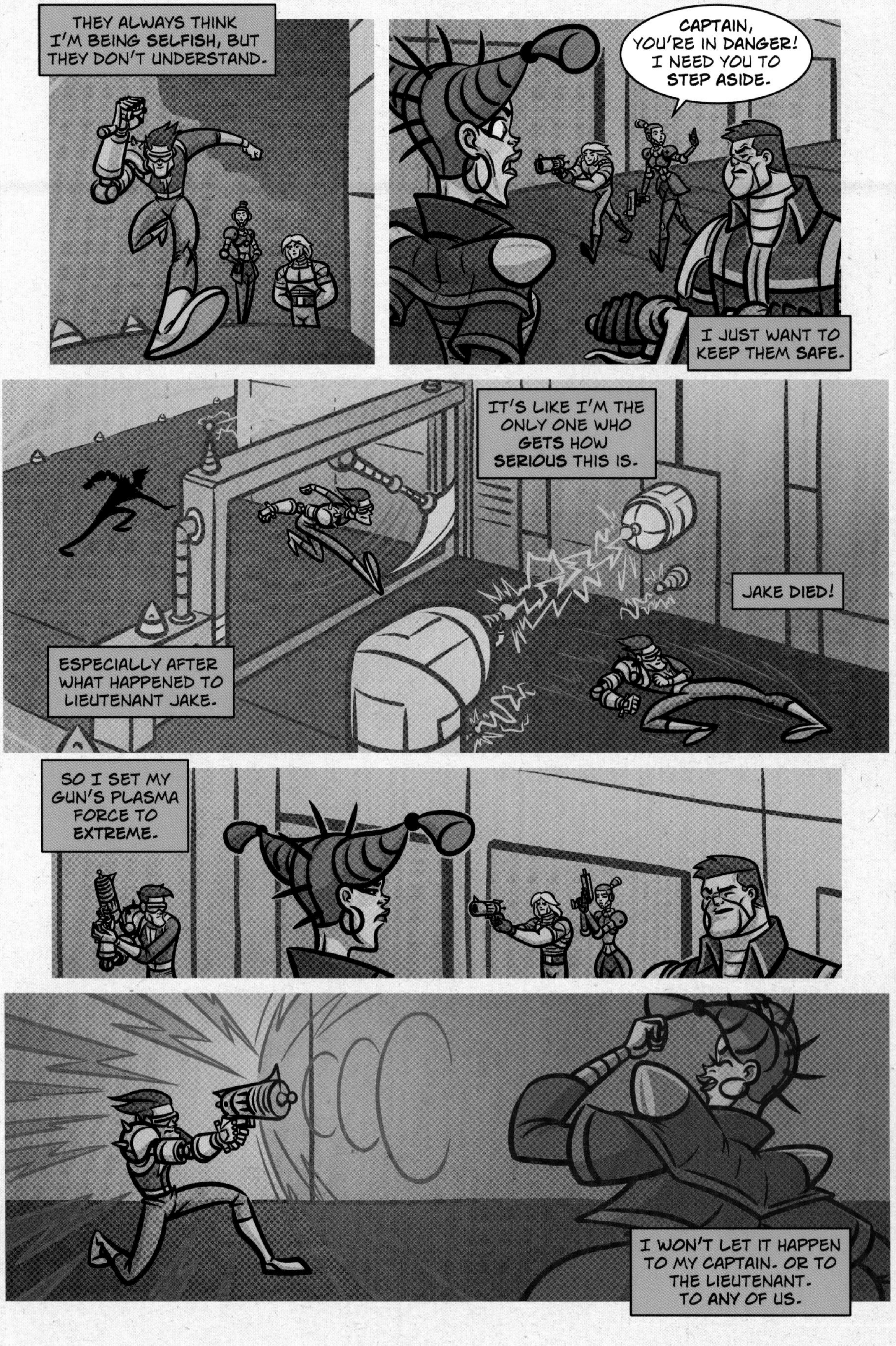
THEY ALWAYS THINK I'M BEING SELFISH, BUT THEY DON'T UNDERSTAND.
CAPTAIN, YOU'RE IN DANGER! I NEED YOU TO STEP ASIDE.
I JUST WANT TO KEEP THEM SAFE.
IT'S LIKE I'M THE ONLY ONE WHO GETS HOW SERIOUS THIS IS.
JAKE DIED!
ESPECIALLY AFTER WHAT HAPPENED TO LIEUTENANT JAKE.
SO I SET MY GUN'S PLASMA FORCE TO EXTREME.
I WON'T LET IT HAPPEN TO MY CAPTAIN. OR TO THE LIEUTENANT. TO ANY OF US.

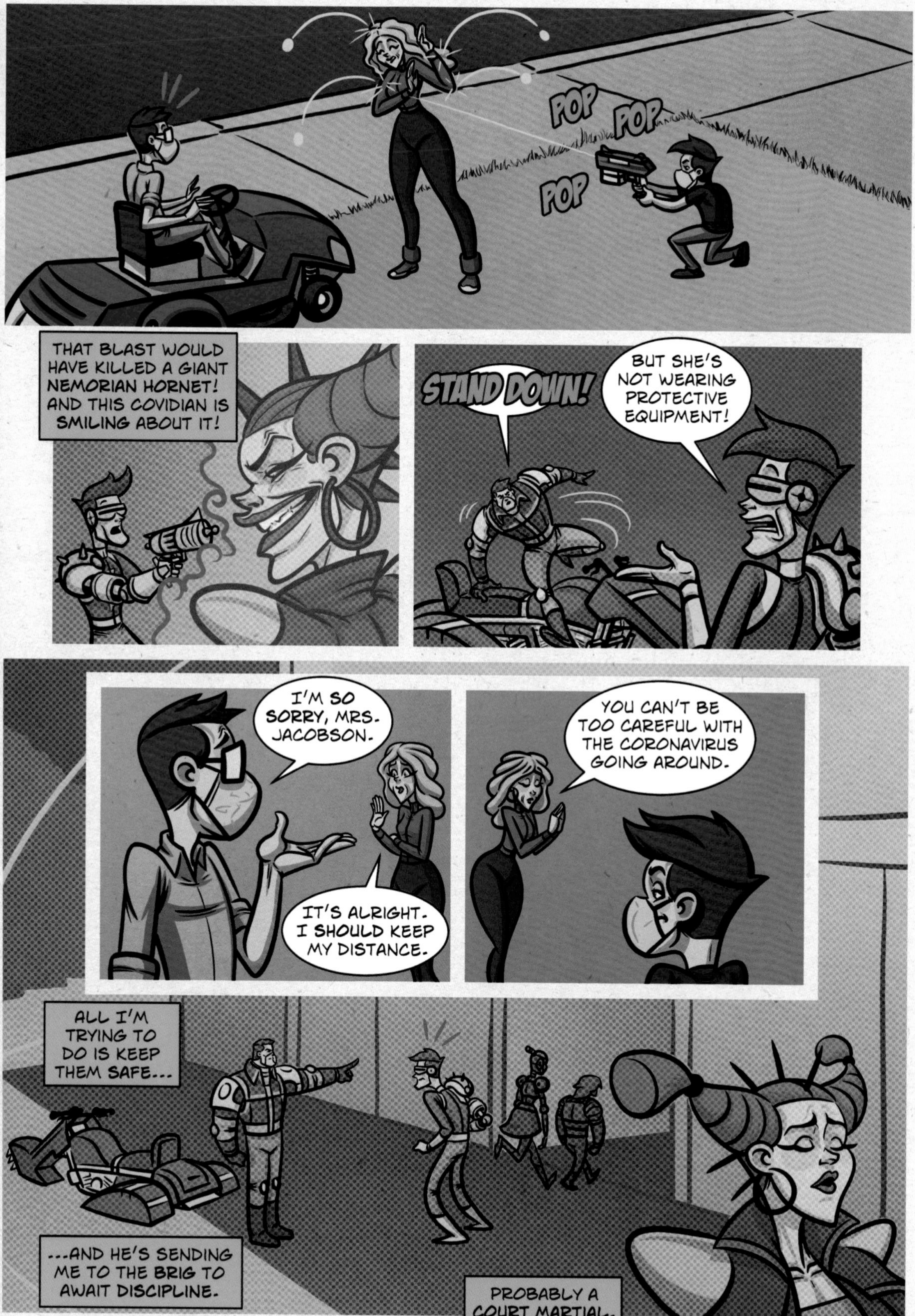
POP
POP
POP
THAT BLAST WOULD HAVE KILLED A GIANT NEMORIAN HORNET! AND THIS COVIDIAN IS SMILING ABOUT IT!
STAND DOWN!
BUT SHE'S NOT WEARING PROTECTIVE EQUIPMENT!
I'M SO SORRY, MRS. JACOBSON.
IT'S ALRIGHT. I SHOULD KEEP MY DISTANCE.
YOU CAN'T BE TOO CAREFUL WITH THE CORONAVIRUS GOING AROUND.
ALL I'M TRYING TO DO IS KEEP THEM SAFE...
...AND HE'S SENDING ME TO THE BRIG TO AWAIT DISCIPLINE.
PROBABLY A COURT MARTIAL.

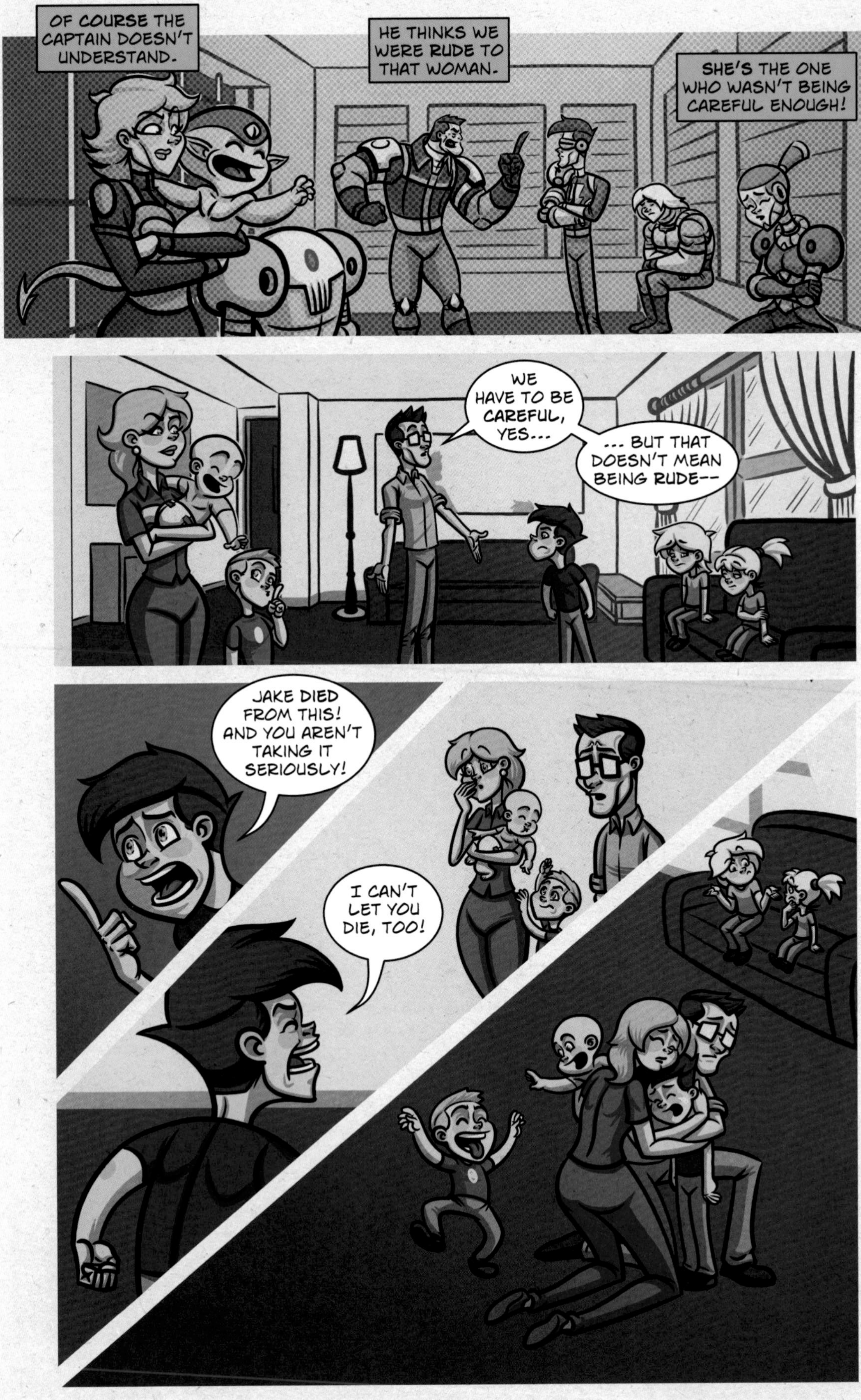
OF COURSE THE CAPTAIN DOESN'T UNDERSTAND.
HE THINKS WE WERE RUDE TO THAT WOMAN.
SHE'S THE ONE WHO WASN'T BEING CAREFUL ENOUGH!
WE HAVE TO BE CAREFUL, YES...
...BUT THAT DOESN'T MEAN BEING RUDE--
JAKE DIED FROM THIS! AND YOU AREN'T TAKING IT SERIOUSLY!
I CAN'T LET YOU DIE, TOO!

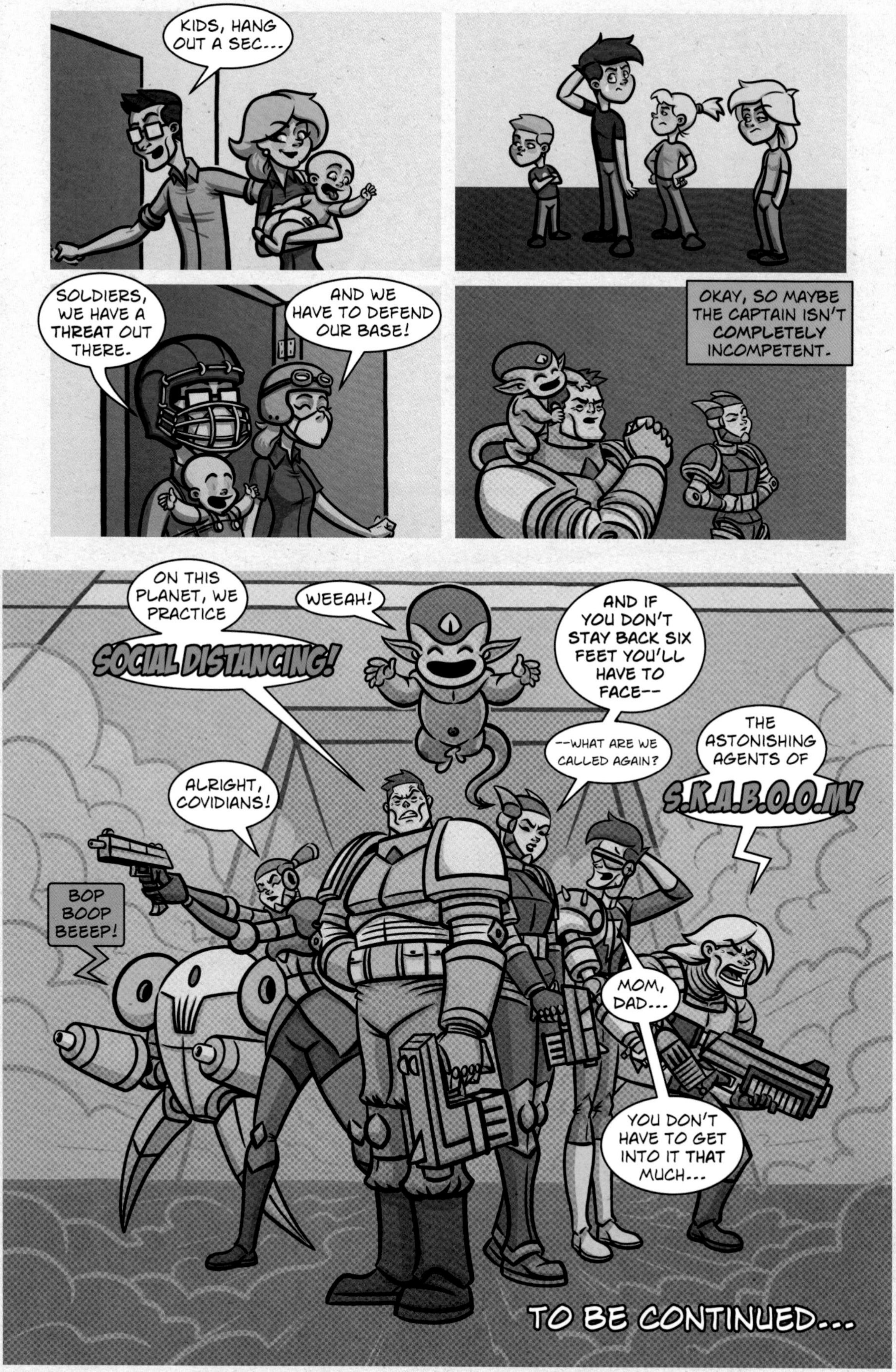
KIDS, HANG OUT A SEC...
SOLDIERS, WE HAVE A THREAT OUT THERE.
AND WE HAVE TO DEFEND OUR BASE!
OKAY, SO MAYBE THE CAPTAIN ISN'T COMPLETELY INCOMPETENT.
ON THIS PLANET, WE PRACTICE SOCIAL DISTANCING!
WEEEAH!
AND IF YOU DON'T STAY BACK SIX FEET YOU'LL HAVE TO FACE--
--WHAT ARE WE CALLED AGAIN?
THE ASTONISHING AGENTS OF S.K.A.B.O.O.M!
ALRIGHT, COVIDIANS!
BOP BOOP BEEEP!
MOM, DAD...
YOU DON'T HAVE TO GET INTO IT THAT MUCH...
TO BE CONTINUED...

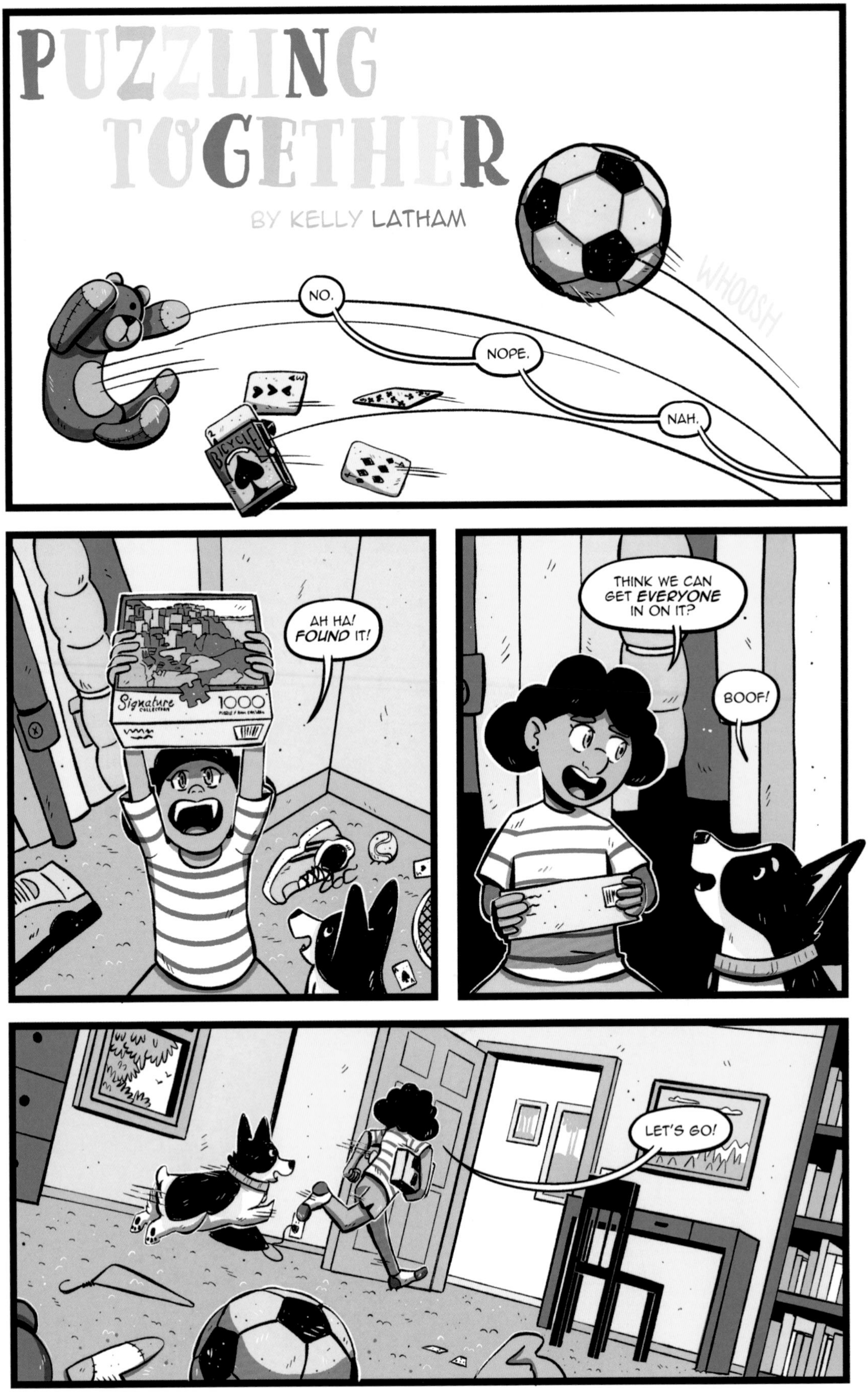
PUZZLING TOGETHER
BY KELLY LATHAM
NO.
NOPE.
NAH.
WHOOSH
BICYCLE
AH HA! FOUND IT!
Signature
1000
THINK WE CAN GET EVERYONE IN ON IT?
BOOF!
LET'S GO!

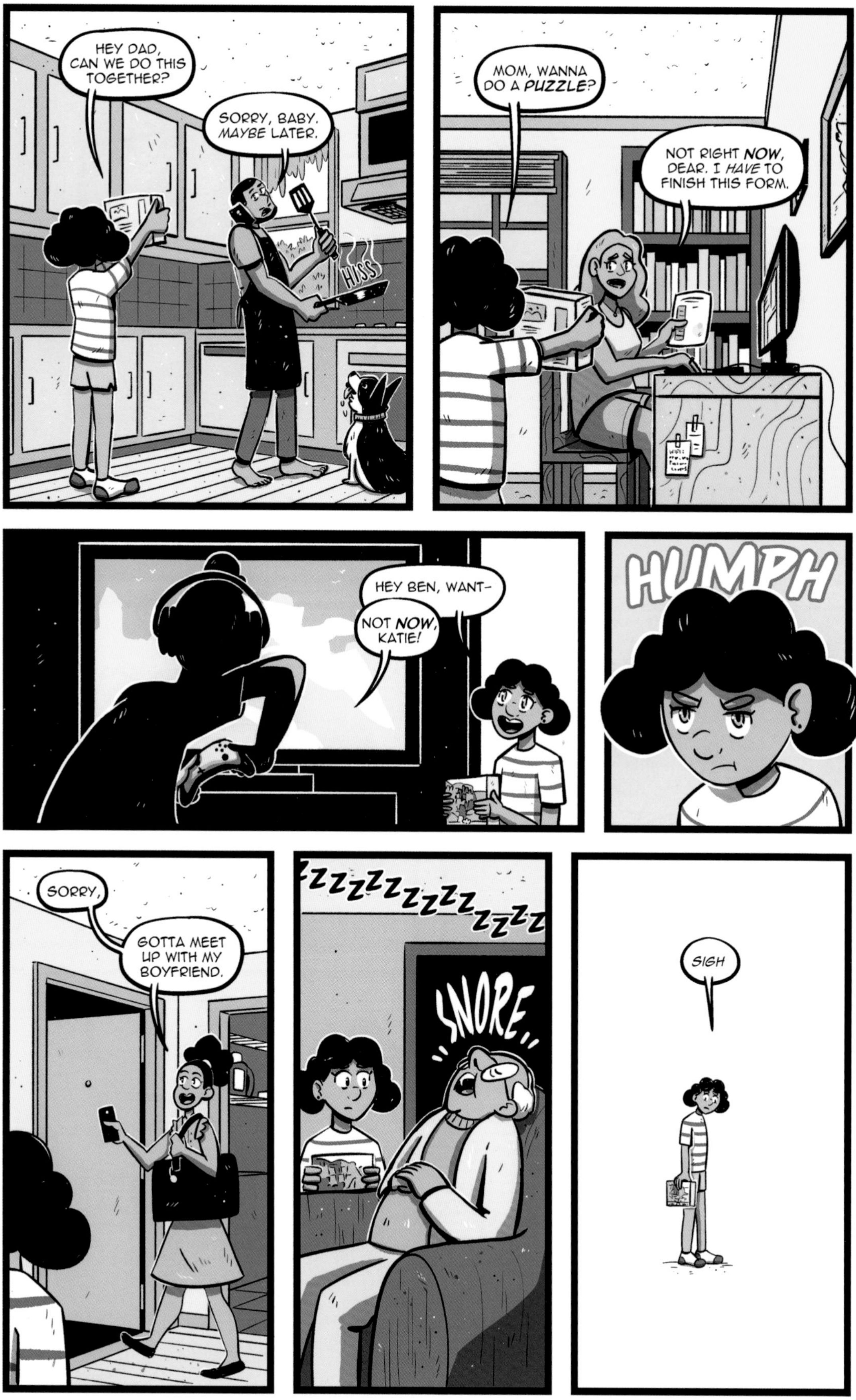
HEY DAD, CAN WE DO THIS TOGETHER?
SORRY, BABY. MAYBE LATER.
HISS
MOM, WANNA DO A PUZZLE?
NOT RIGHT NOW, DEAR. I HAVE TO FINISH THIS FORM.
HEY BEN, WANT-
NOT NOW, KATIE!
HUMPH
SORRY,
GOTTA MEET UP WITH MY BOYFRIEND.
ZZZZZZZZZZZZZZ
SNORE
SIGH

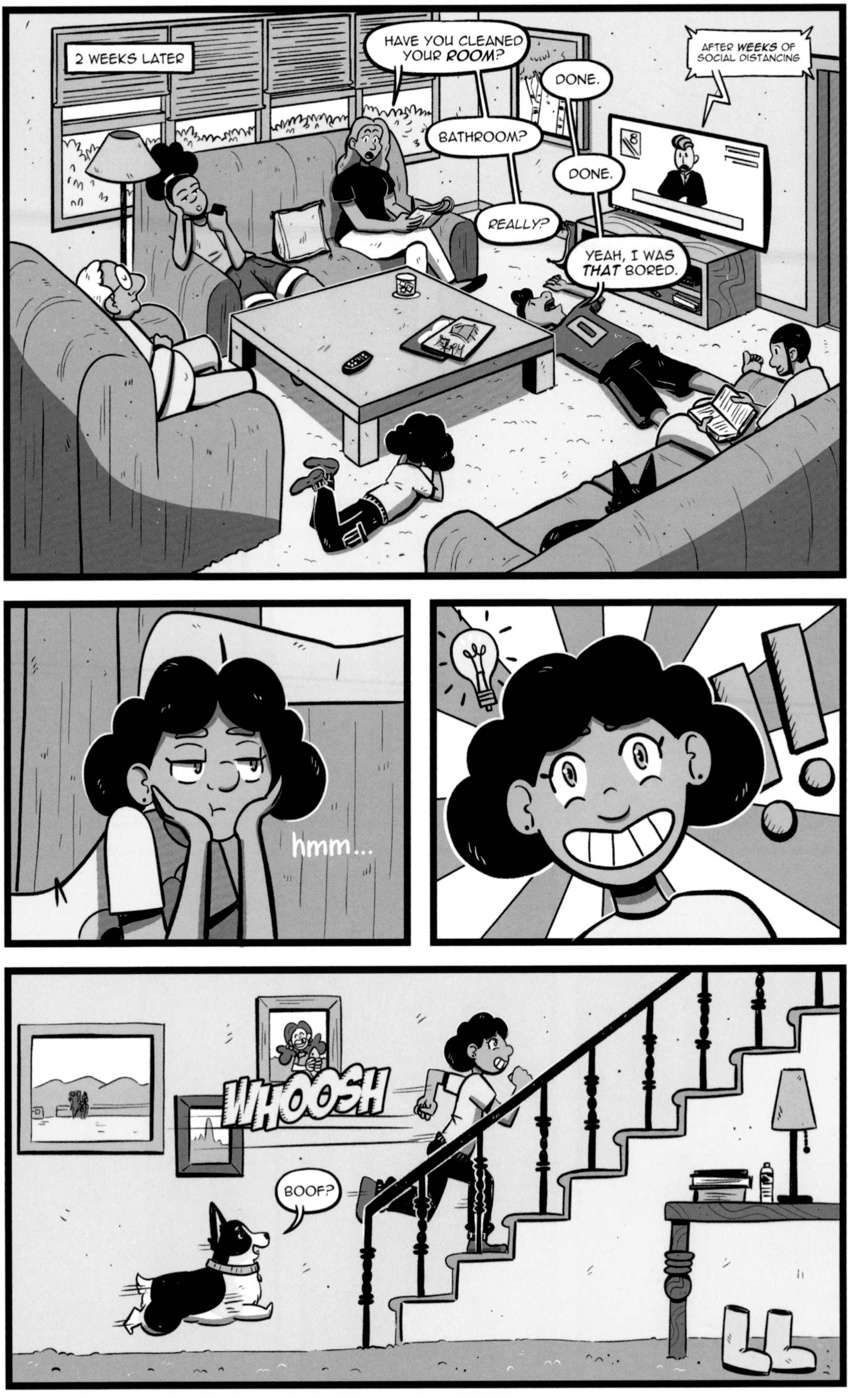
2 WEEKS LATER
HAVE YOU CLEANED YOUR ROOM?
DONE.
BATHROOM?
DONE.
REALLY?
YEAH, I WAS THAT BORED.
AFTER WEEKS OF SOCIAL DISTANCING
hmm...
WHOOSH
BOOF?

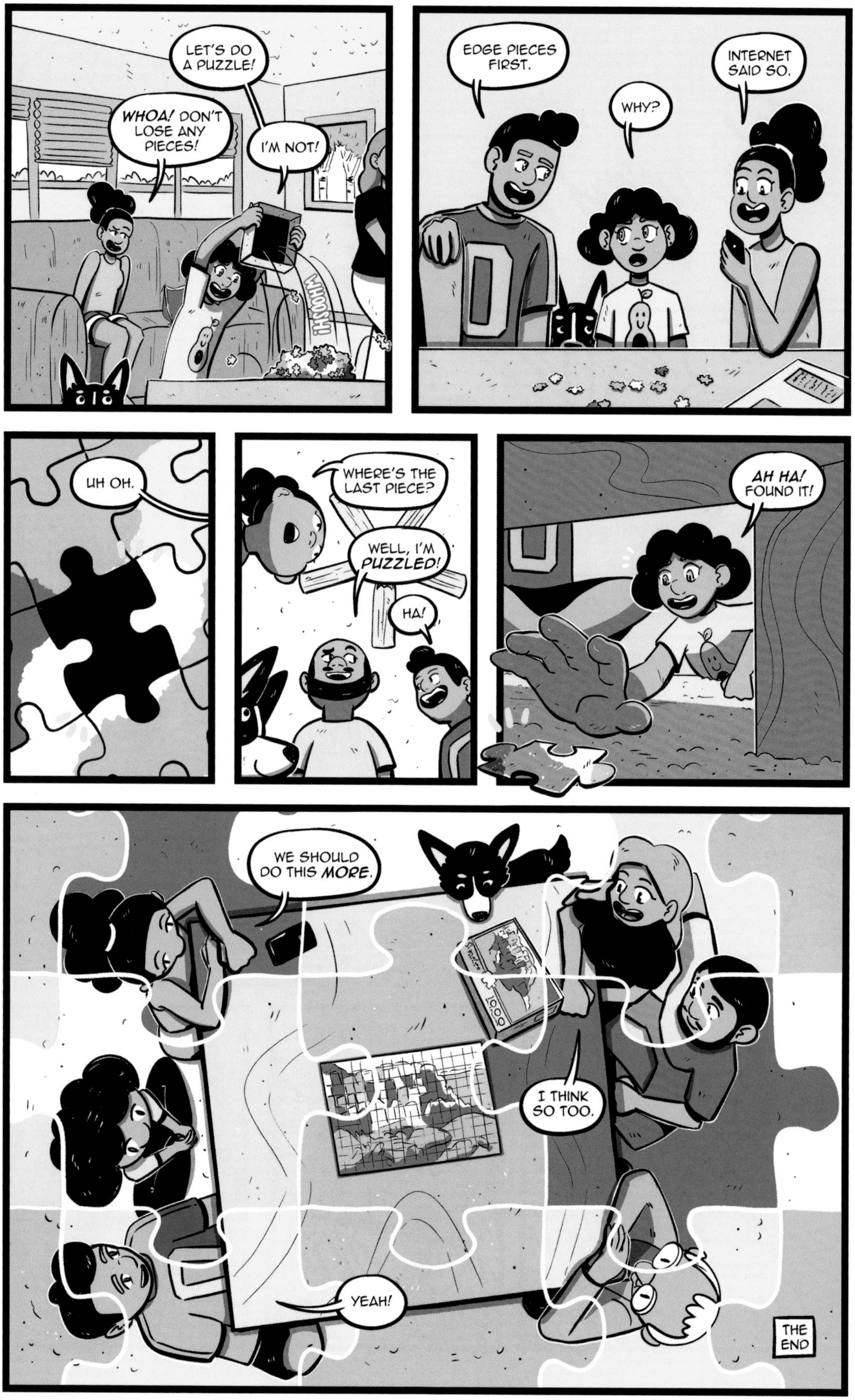

LET'S DO A PUZZLE!
WHOA! DON'T LOSE ANY PIECES!
I'M NOT!
WHOOSH!
EDGE PIECES FIRST.
WHY?
INTERNET SAID SO.
UH OH.
WHERE'S THE LAST PIECE?
WELL, I'M PUZZLED!
HA!
AH HA! FOUND IT!
WE SHOULD DO THIS MORE.
I THINK SO TOO.
YEAH!
THE END

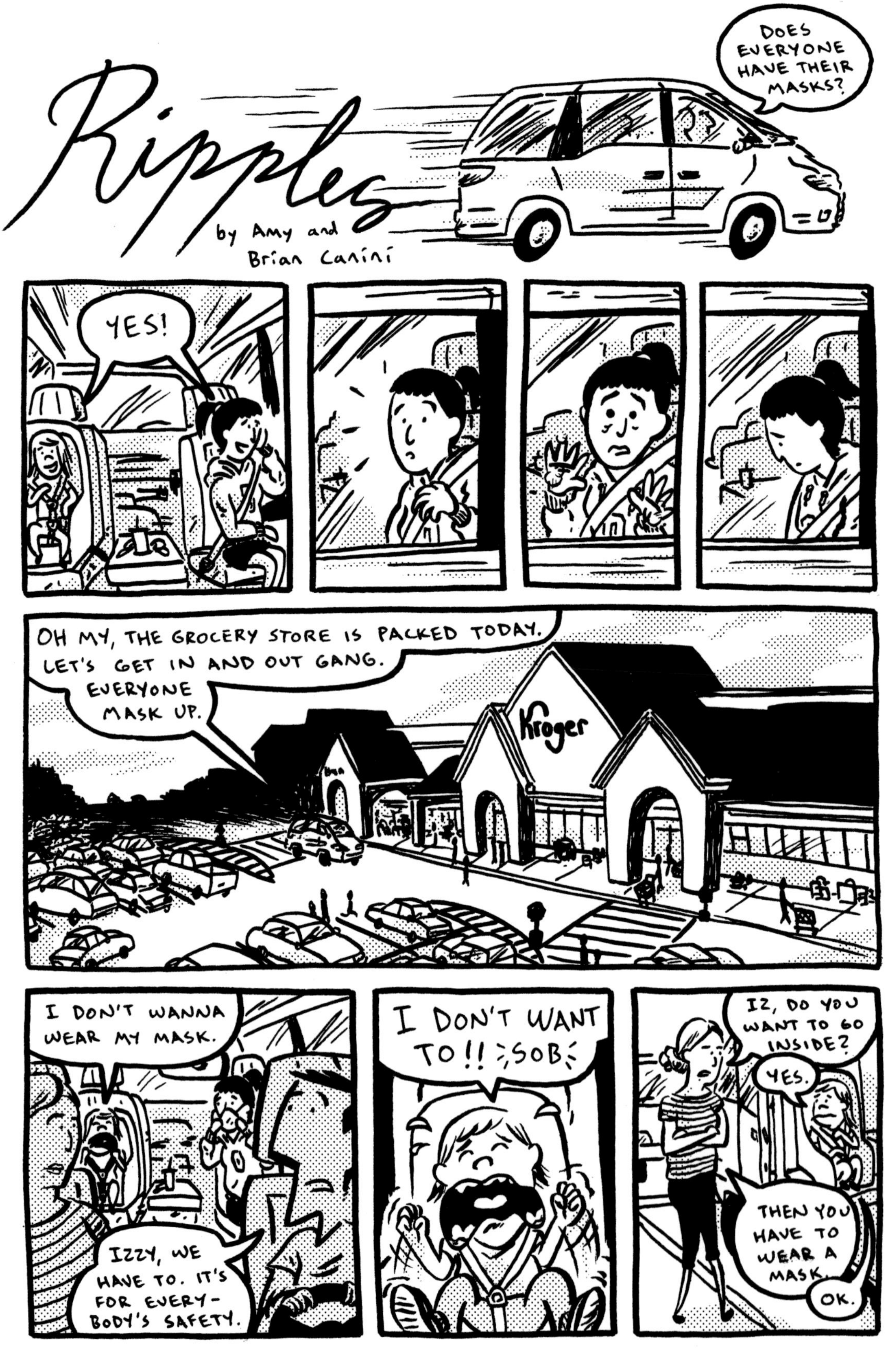
Ripples
by Amy and Brian Canini
DOES EVERYONE HAVE THEIR MASKS?
YES!
OH MY, THE GROCERY STORE IS PACKED TODAY. LET'S GET IN AND OUT GANG. EVERYONE MASK UP.
Kroger
I DON'T WANNA WEAR MY MASK.
IZZY, WE HAVE TO. IT'S FOR EVERY-BODY'S SAFETY.
I DON'T WANT TO!! SOB
IZ, DO YOU WANT TO GO INSIDE?
YES.
THEN YOU HAVE TO WEAR A MASK.
OK.

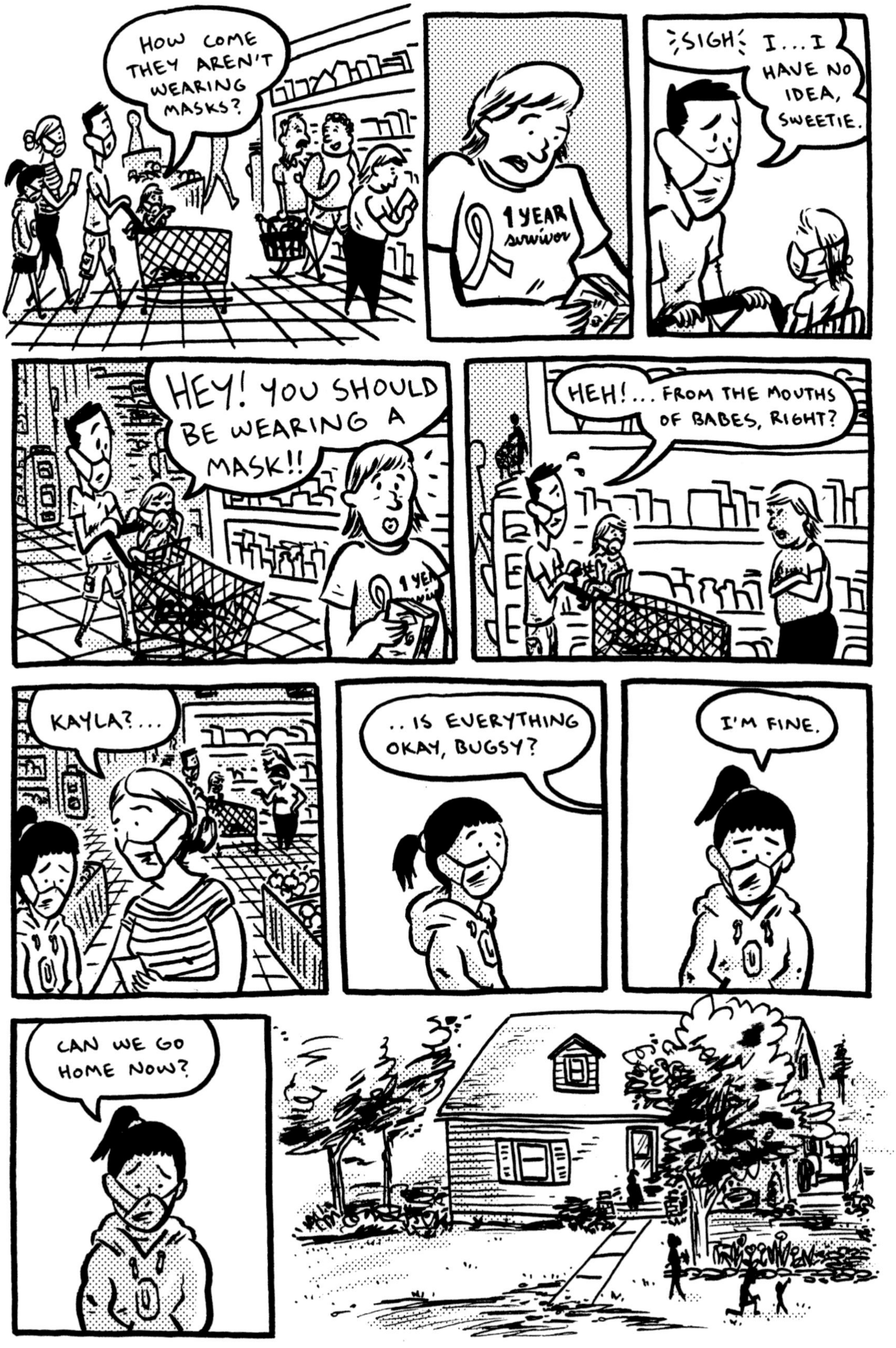
HOW COME THEY AREN'T WEARING MASKS?
1 YEAR survivor
SIGH I...I HAVE NO IDEA, SWEETIE.
HEY! YOU SHOULD BE WEARING A MASK!!
HEH!... FROM THE MOUTHS OF BABES, RIGHT?
KAYLA?...
..IS EVERYTHING OKAY, BUGSY?
I'M FINE.
CAN WE GO HOME NOW?

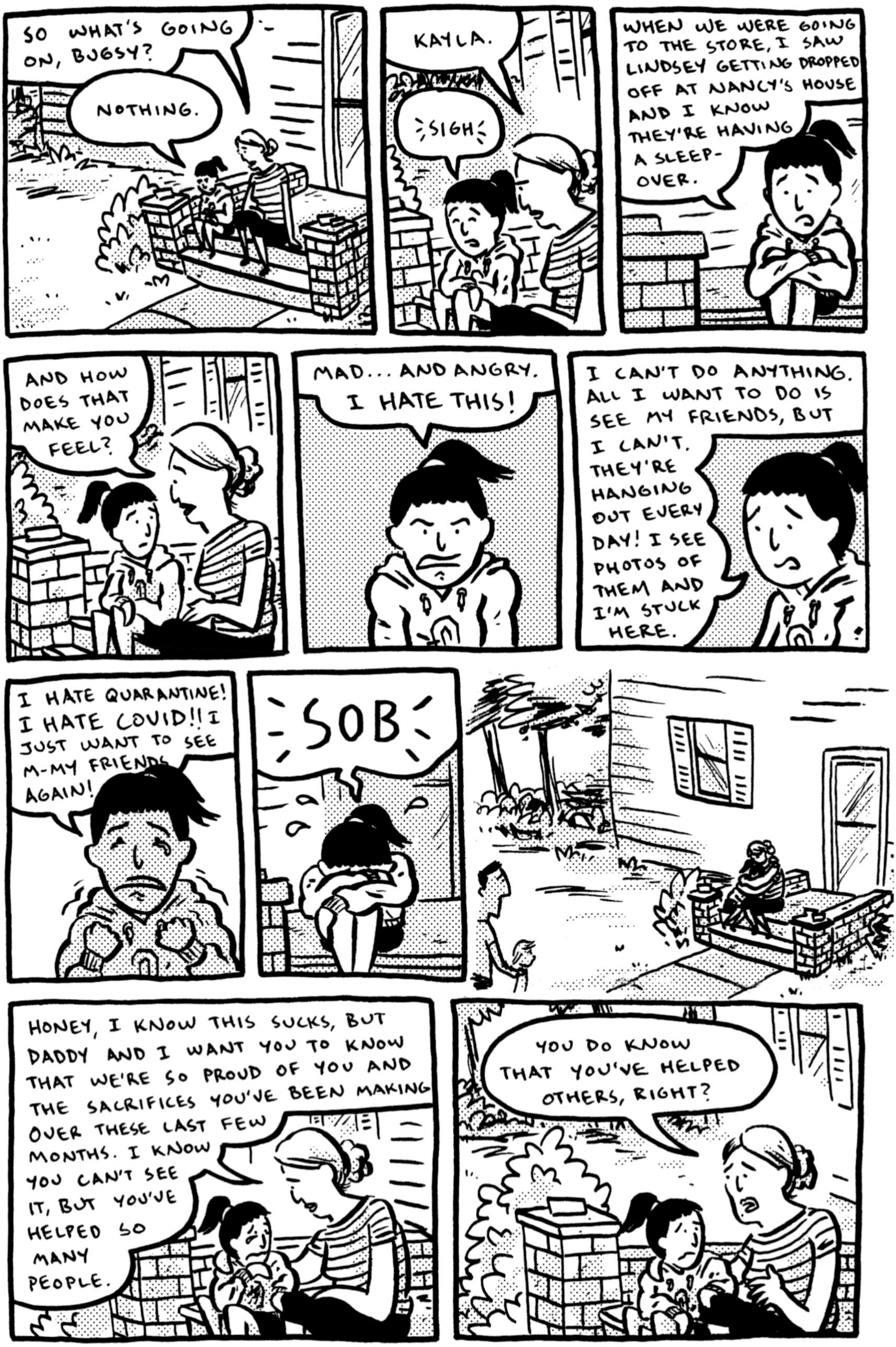
SO WHAT'S GOING ON, BUGSY?
NOTHING.
KAYLA.
SIGH
WHEN WE WERE GOING TO THE STORE, I SAW LINDSEY GETTING DROPPED OFF AT NANCY'S HOUSE AND I KNOW THEY'RE HAVING A SLEEP-OVER.
AND HOW DOES THAT MAKE YOU FEEL?
MAD... AND ANGRY. I HATE THIS!
I CAN'T DO ANYTHING. ALL I WANT TO DO IS SEE MY FRIENDS, BUT I CAN'T. THEY'RE HANGING OUT EVERY DAY! I SEE PHOTOS OF THEM AND I'M STUCK HERE.
I HATE QUARANTINE! I HATE COVID!! I JUST WANT TO SEE M-MY FRIENDS AGAIN!
SOB
HONEY, I KNOW THIS SUCKS, BUT DADDY AND I WANT YOU TO KNOW THAT WE'RE SO PROUD OF YOU AND THE SACRIFICES YOU'VE BEEN MAKING OVER THESE LAST FEW MONTHS. I KNOW YOU CAN'T SEE IT, BUT YOU'VE HELPED SO MANY PEOPLE.
YOU DO KNOW THAT YOU'VE HELPED OTHERS, RIGHT?

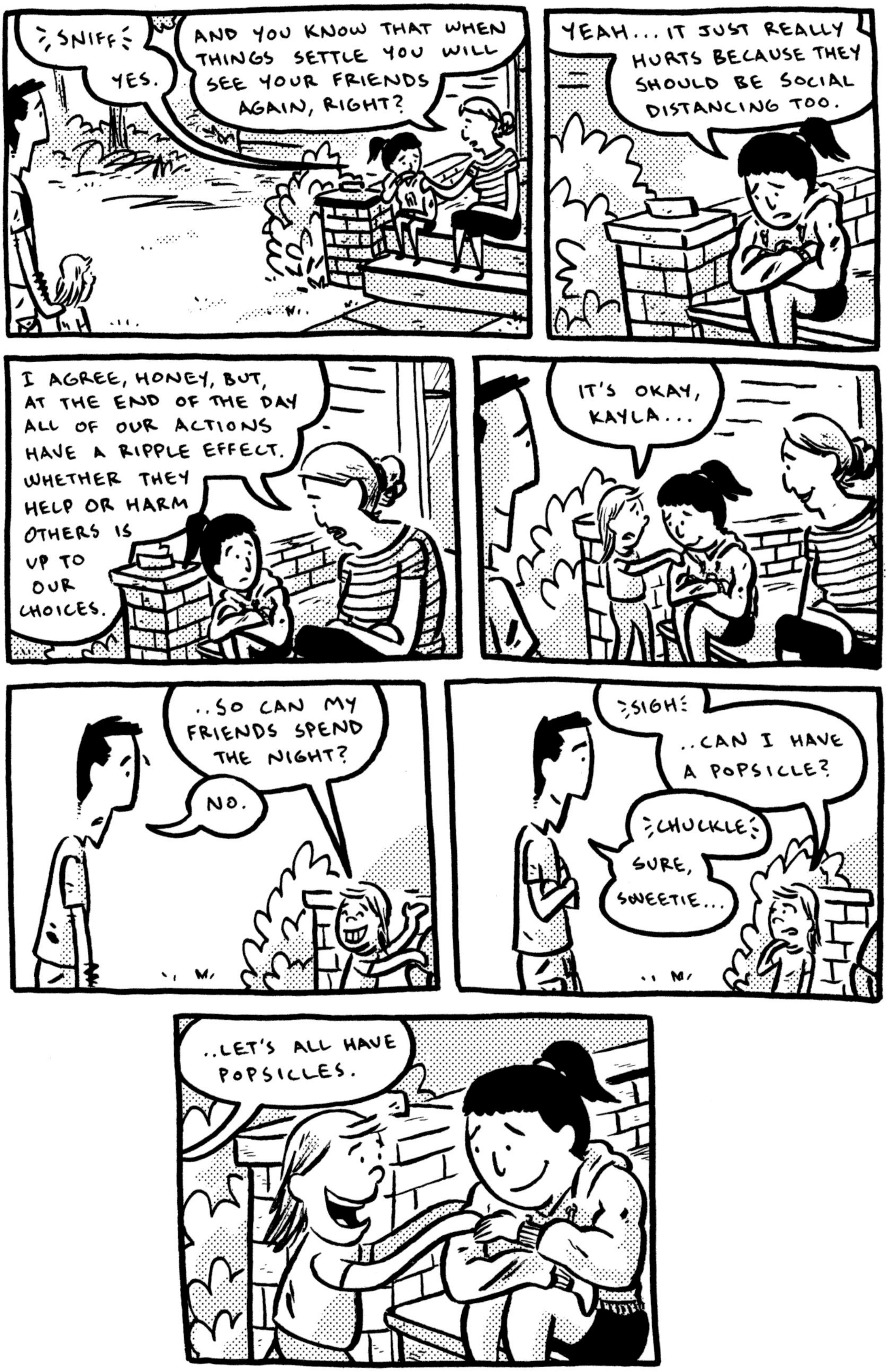
SNIFF
YES.
AND YOU KNOW THAT WHEN THINGS SETTLE YOU WILL SEE YOUR FRIENDS AGAIN, RIGHT?
YEAH... IT JUST REALLY HURTS BECAUSE THEY SHOULD BE SOCIAL DISTANCING TOO.
I AGREE, HONEY, BUT, AT THE END OF THE DAY ALL OF OUR ACTIONS HAVE A RIPPLE EFFECT. WHETHER THEY HELP OR HARM OTHERS IS UP TO OUR CHOICES.
IT'S OKAY, KAYLA...
..SO CAN MY FRIENDS SPEND THE NIGHT?
NO.
SIGH
..CAN I HAVE A POPSICLE?
CHUCKLE
SURE, SWEETIE...
..LET'S ALL HAVE POPSICLES.

LIVE·LOVE·EAT

By Scott J. Jones

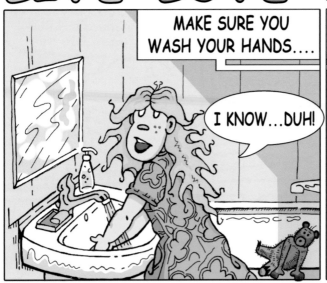

MAKE SURE YOU WASH YOUR HANDS....

I KNOW...DUH!

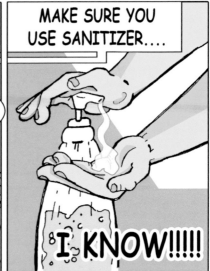

MAKE SURE YOU USE SANITIZER....

I KNOW!!!!!

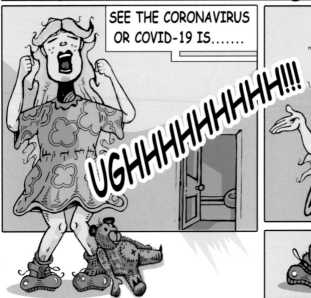

SEE THE CORONAVIRUS OR COVID-19 IS.......

UGHHHHHHHHH!!!!

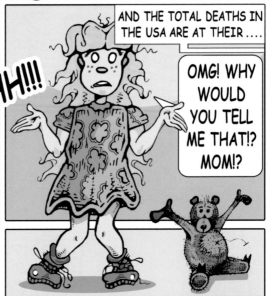

AND THE TOTAL DEATHS IN THE USA ARE AT THEIR ....

OMG! WHY WOULD YOU TELL ME THAT!? MOM!?

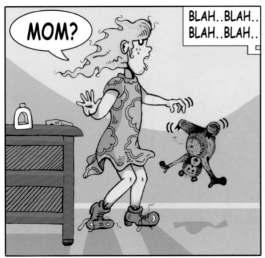

MOM?

BLAH..BLAH.. BLAH..BLAH..

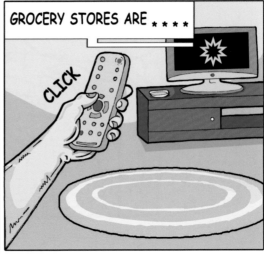

GROCERY STORES ARE ....

CLICK

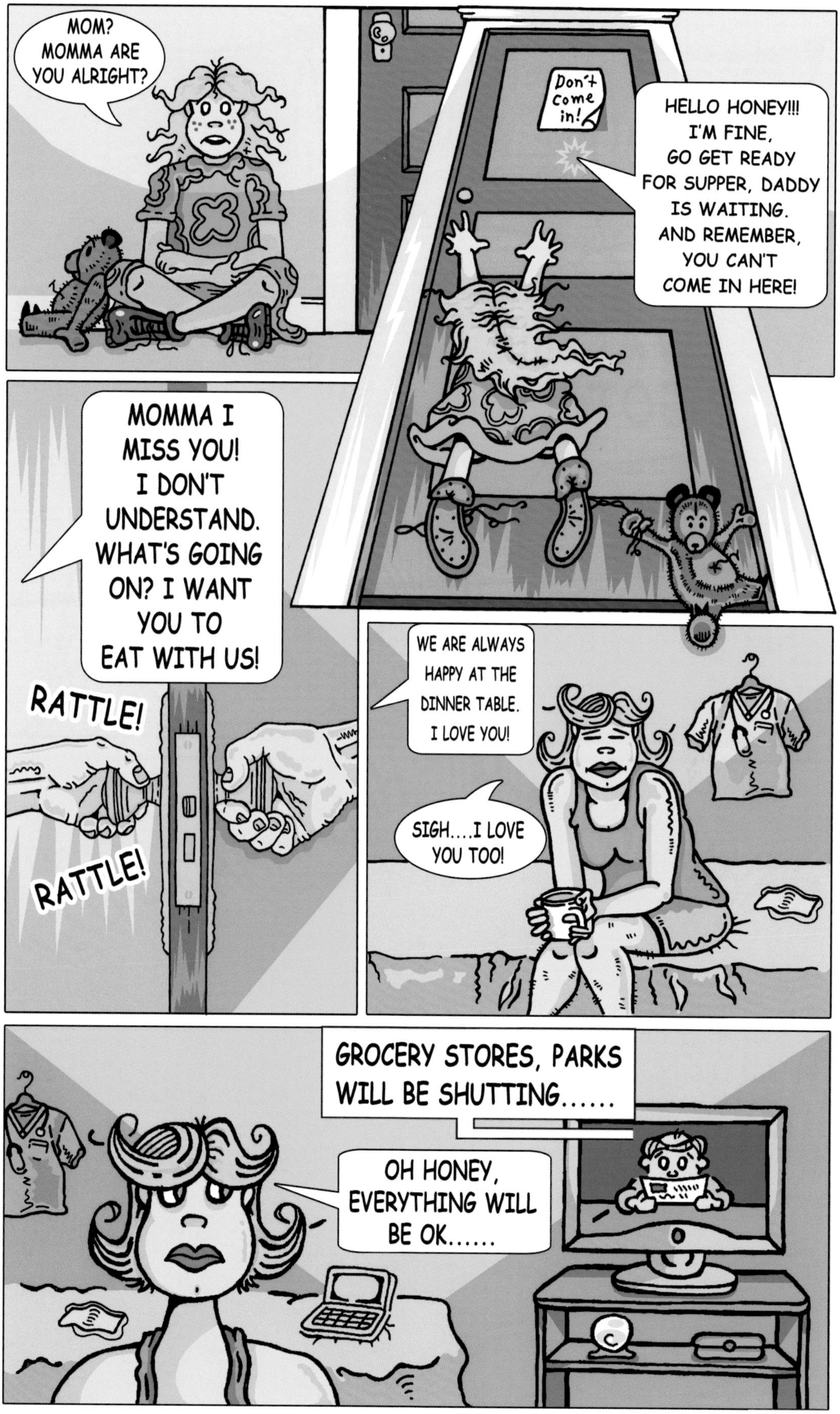
MOM? MOMMA ARE YOU ALRIGHT?
Don't come in!
HELLO HONEY!!! I'M FINE, GO GET READY FOR SUPPER, DADDY IS WAITING. AND REMEMBER, YOU CAN'T COME IN HERE!
MOMMA I MISS YOU! I DON'T UNDERSTAND. WHAT'S GOING ON? I WANT YOU TO EAT WITH US!
RATTLE!
RATTLE!
WE ARE ALWAYS HAPPY AT THE DINNER TABLE. I LOVE YOU!
SIGH....I LOVE YOU TOO!
GROCERY STORES, PARKS WILL BE SHUTTING......
OH HONEY, EVERYTHING WILL BE OK......

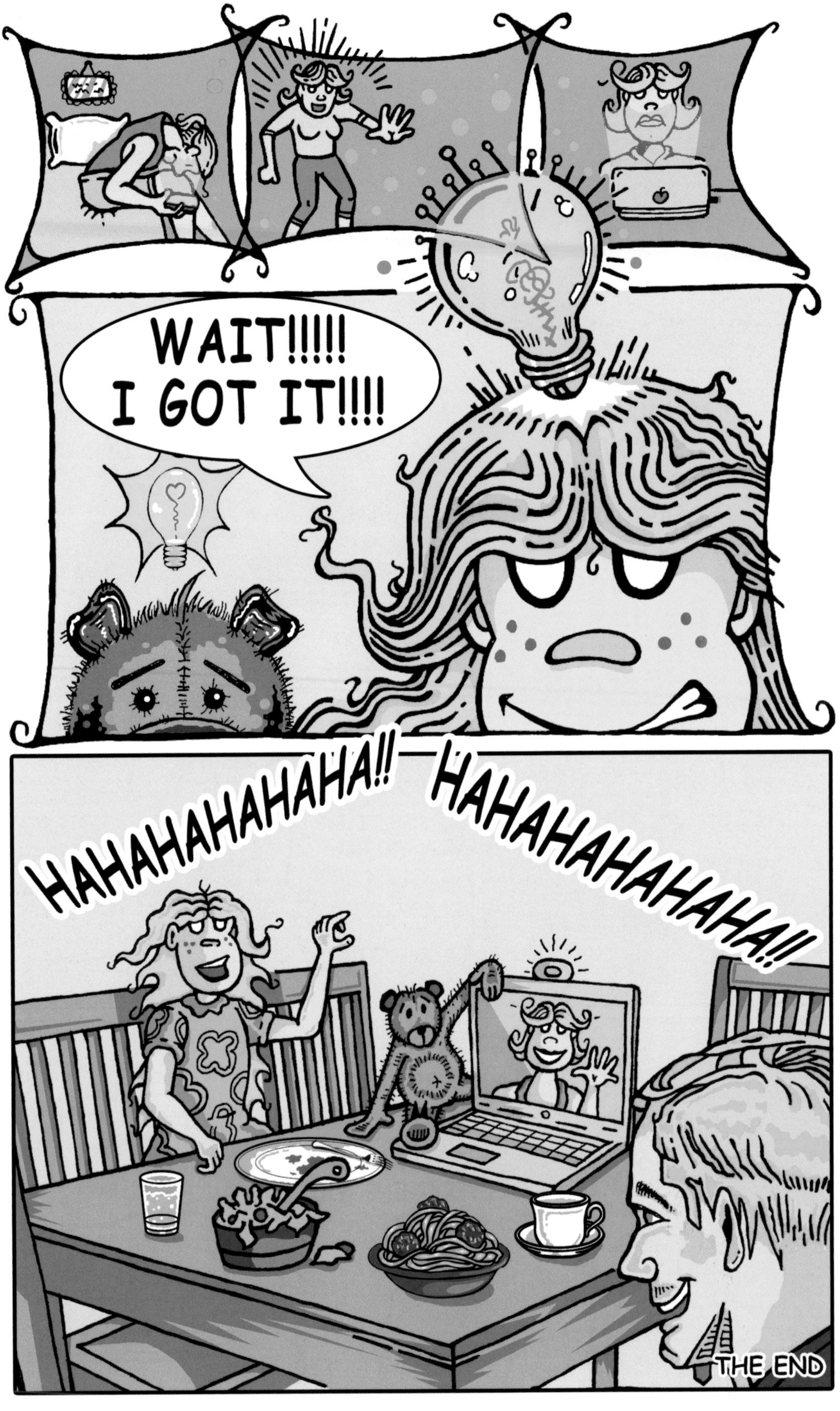
WAIT!!!!!
I GOT IT!!!!
HAHAHAHAHAHA!!
HAHAHAHAHAHAHA!!
THE END

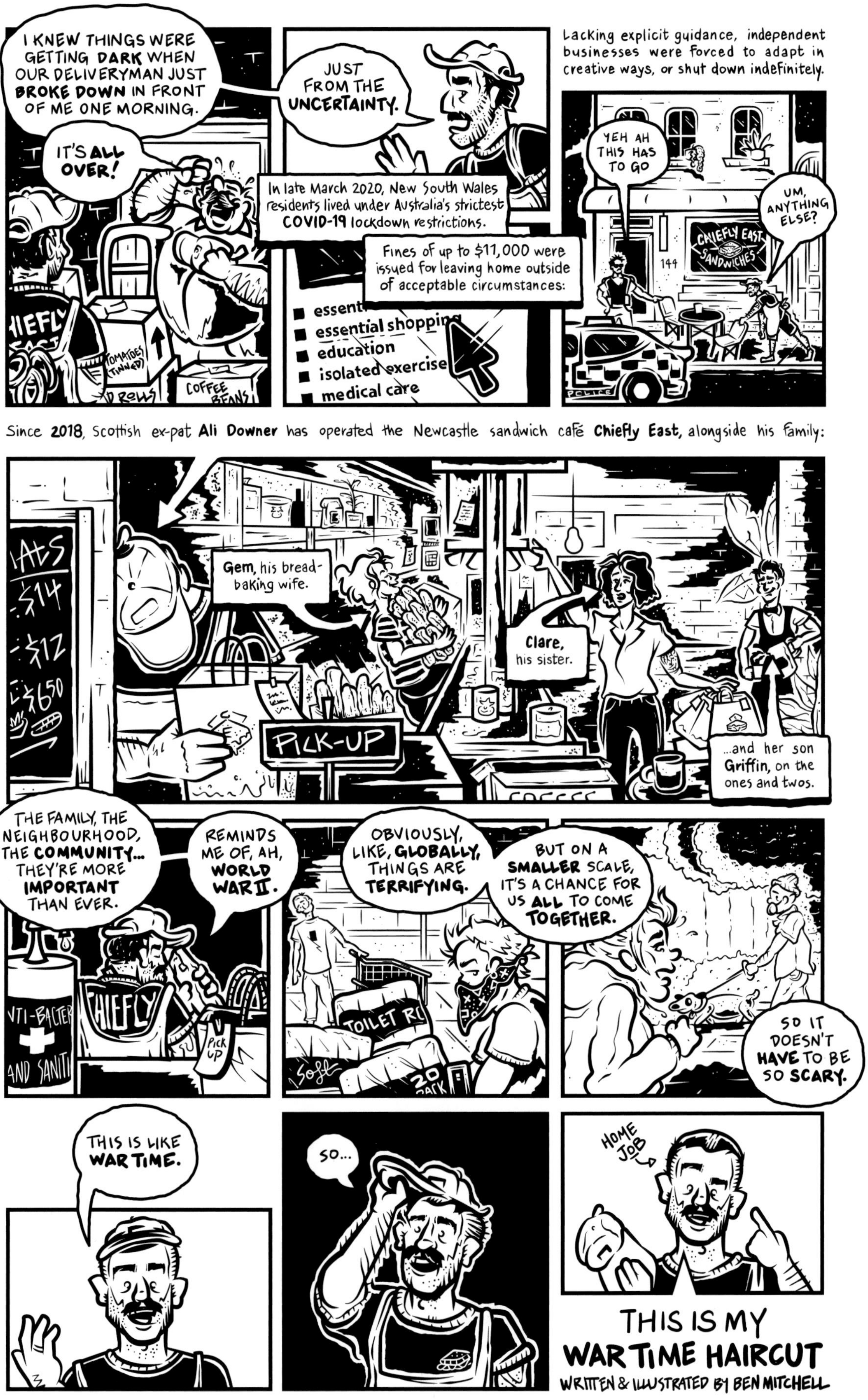

I KNEW THINGS WERE GETTING DARK WHEN OUR DELIVERYMAN JUST BROKE DOWN IN FRONT OF ME ONE MORNING.
IT'S ALL OVER!
CHIEFLY EAST
TOMATOES TINNED
COFFEE BEANS
JUST FROM THE UNCERTAINTY.
In late March 2020, New South Wales residents lived under Australia's strictest COVID-19 lockdown restrictions.
Fines of up to $11,000 were issued for leaving home outside of acceptable circumstances:
essenti
essential shopping
education
isolated exercise
medical care
Lacking explicit guidance, independent businesses were forced to adapt in creative ways, or shut down indefinitely.
YEH AH THIS HAS TO GO
UM, ANYTHING ELSE?
CHIEFLY EAST SANDWICHES
144
POLICE
Since 2018, Scottish ex-pat Ali Downer has operated the Newcastle sandwich café Chiefly East, alongside his family:
Gem, his bread-baking wife.
Clare, his sister.
...and her son Griffin, on the ones and twos.
PICK-UP
THE FAMILY, THE NEIGHBOURHOOD, THE COMMUNITY... THEY'RE MORE IMPORTANT THAN EVER.
REMINDS ME OF, AH, WORLD WAR II.
CHIEFLY
PICK UP
NTI-BACTER
AND SANITI
OBVIOUSLY, LIKE, GLOBALLY, THINGS ARE TERRIFYING.
BUT ON A SMALLER SCALE, IT'S A CHANCE FOR US ALL TO COME TOGETHER.
TOILET R
20 PACK
SO IT DOESN'T HAVE TO BE SO SCARY.
THIS IS LIKE WAR TIME.
SO...
HOME JOB
THIS IS MY
WAR TIME HAIRCUT
WRITTEN & ILLUSTRATED BY BEN MITCHELL

Ali's family moved in 2014 from **Glasgow,** where they ran a café out of an old schoolhouse building.

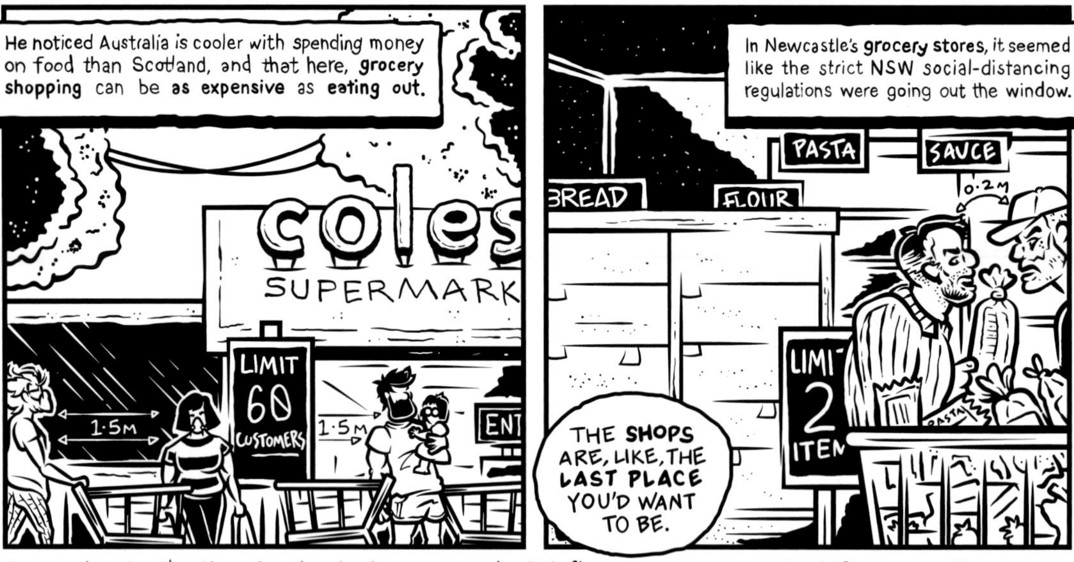
He noticed Australia is cooler with spending money on food than Scotland, and that here, **grocery shopping** can be **as expensive** as **eating out.**
coles
SUPERMARK
LIMIT 60 CUSTOMERS
1·5M
1·5M
ENT
In Newcastle's **grocery stores,** it seemed like the strict NSW social-distancing regulations were going out the window.
PASTA
SAUCE
BREAD
FLOUR
0·2M
LIMIT 2 ITEM
THE **SHOPS** ARE, LIKE, THE **LAST PLACE** YOU'D WANT TO BE.

By early April, the family had converted **Chiefly East** to a **makeshift community grocer.**

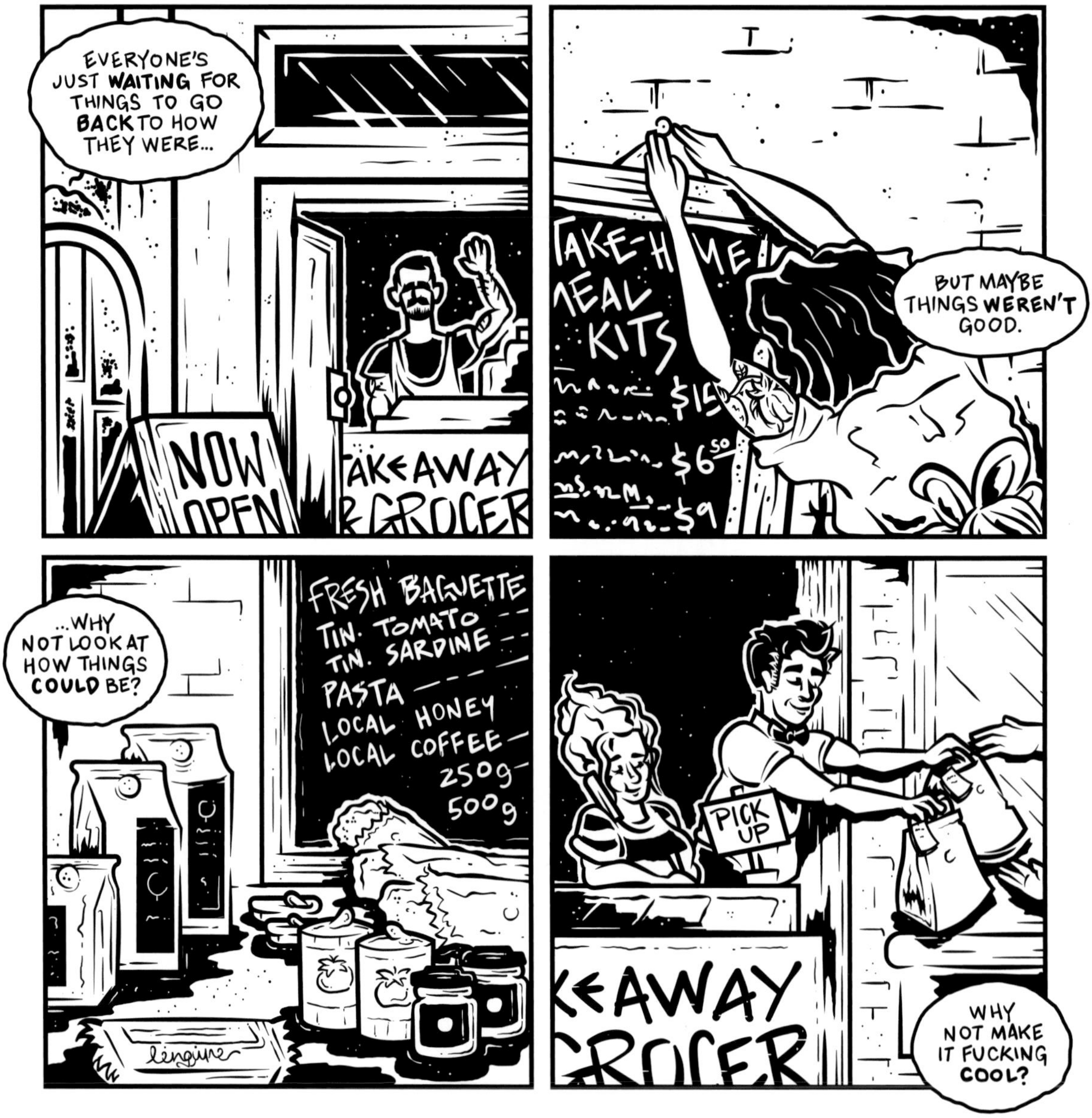
EVERYONE'S JUST **WAITING** FOR THINGS TO GO **BACK** TO HOW THEY WERE...
NOW OPEN
AKEAWAY GROCER
AKE-HOME MEAL KITS
$15
$6.50
$9
BUT MAYBE THINGS **WEREN'T** GOOD.
...WHY NOT LOOK AT HOW THINGS **COULD** BE?
FRESH BAGUETTE
TIN. TOMATO
TIN. SARDINE
PASTA
LOCAL HONEY
LOCAL COFFEE
250g
500g
PICK UP
KEAWAY GROCER
WHY NOT MAKE IT FUCKING **COOL?**

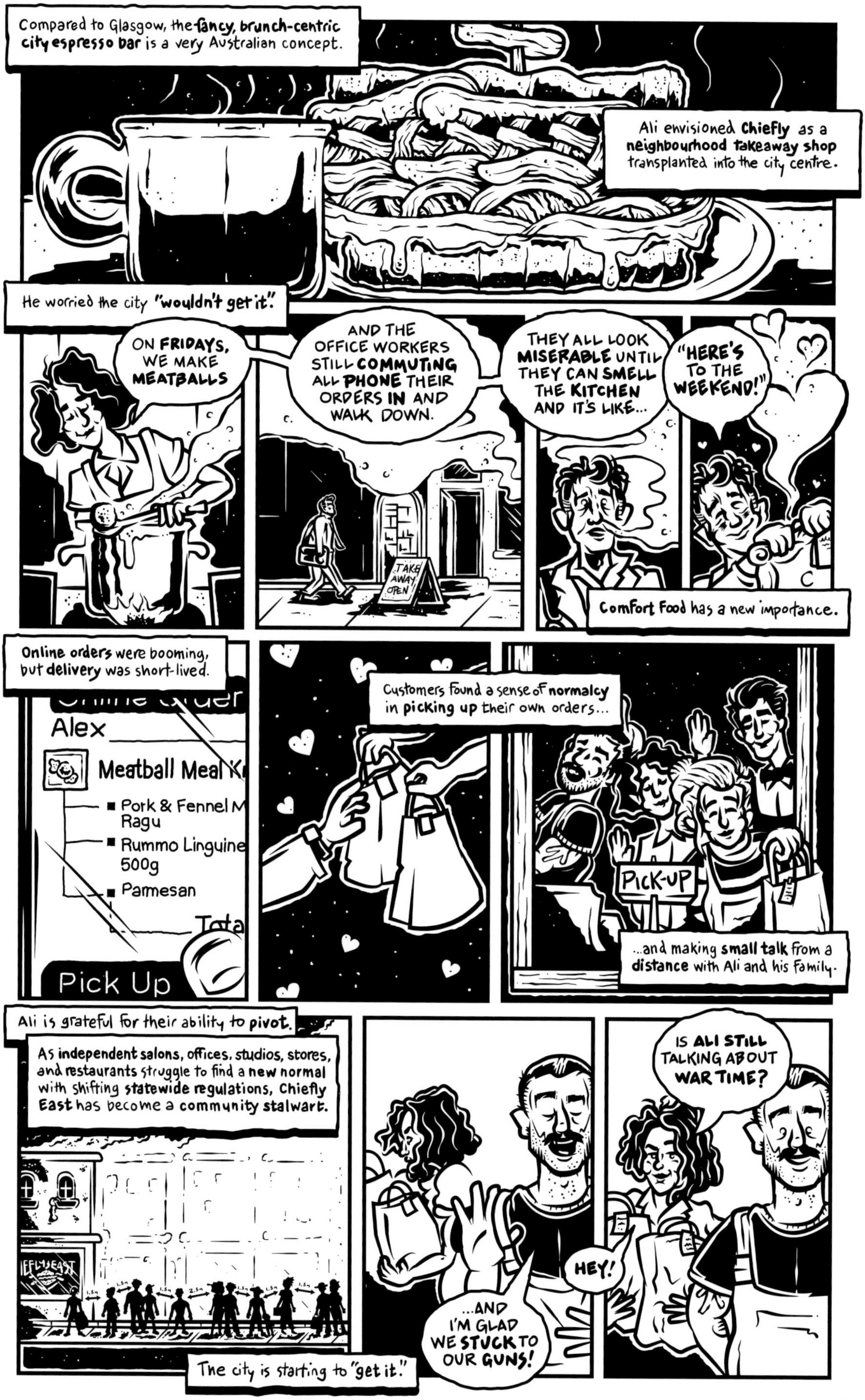

Compared to Glasgow, the fancy, brunch-centric city espresso bar is a very Australian concept.
Ali envisioned Chiefly as a neighbourhood takeaway shop transplanted into the city centre.
He worried the city "wouldn't get it."
ON FRIDAYS, WE MAKE MEATBALLS
AND THE OFFICE WORKERS STILL COMMUTING ALL PHONE THEIR ORDERS IN AND WALK DOWN.
TAKE AWAY OPEN
THEY ALL LOOK MISERABLE UNTIL THEY CAN SMELL THE KITCHEN AND IT'S LIKE...
"HERE'S TO THE WEEKEND!"
Comfort Food has a new importance.
Online orders were booming, but delivery was short-lived.
Alex
Meatball Meal Ki
Pork & Fennel M
Ragu
Rummo Linguine
500g
Parmesan
Tota
Pick Up
Customers found a sense of normalcy in picking up their own orders...
PICK-UP
...and making small talk from a distance with Ali and his family.
Ali is grateful for their ability to pivot.
As independent salons, offices, studios, stores, and restaurants struggle to find a new normal with shifting statewide regulations, Chiefly East has become a community stalwart.
The city is starting to "get it."
HEY!
...AND I'M GLAD WE STUCK TO OUR GUNS!
IS ALI STILL TALKING ABOUT WAR TIME?

BRAID ROUND CHALLAH
IN SIX SIMPLE STEPS
1.
2.
4.
5.
6.
Which step are you on?
....?!?!

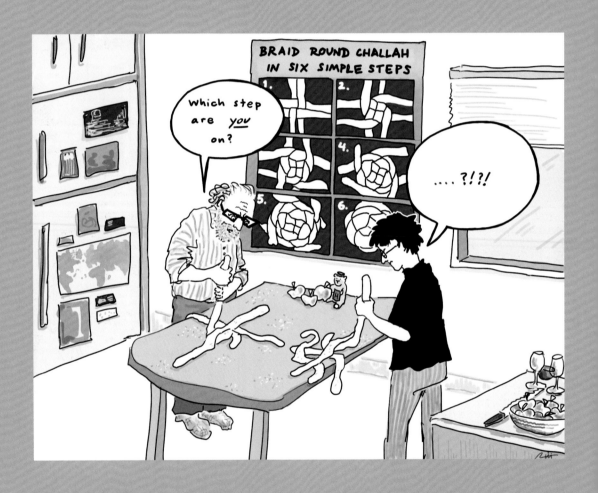

APRIL 11 – 15, 2020 BY ROB KIRBY

SATURDAY 4/11/20

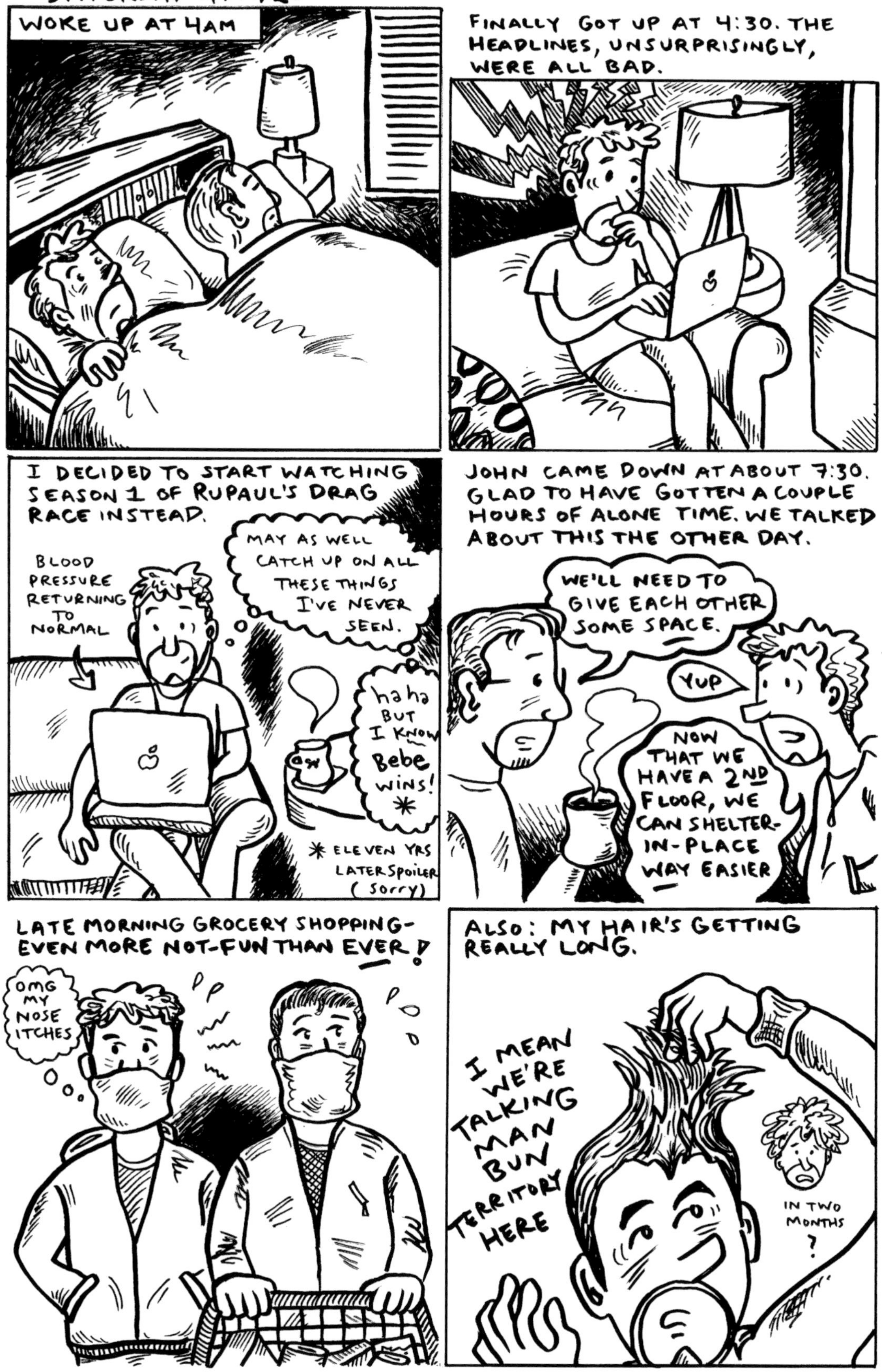
WOKE UP AT 4AM
FINALLY GOT UP AT 4:30. THE HEADLINES, UNSURPRISINGLY, WERE ALL BAD.
I DECIDED TO START WATCHING SEASON 1 OF RUPAUL'S DRAG RACE INSTEAD.
BLOOD PRESSURE RETURNING TO NORMAL
MAY AS WELL CATCH UP ON ALL THESE THINGS I'VE NEVER SEEN.
haha BUT I KNOW Bebe WINS! *
* ELEVEN YRS LATER SPOILER (SORRY)
JOHN CAME DOWN AT ABOUT 7:30. GLAD TO HAVE GOTTEN A COUPLE HOURS OF ALONE TIME. WE TALKED ABOUT THIS THE OTHER DAY.
WE'LL NEED TO GIVE EACH OTHER SOME SPACE.
YUP
NOW THAT WE HAVE A 2ND FLOOR, WE CAN SHELTER-IN-PLACE WAY EASIER
LATE MORNING GROCERY SHOPPING – EVEN MORE NOT-FUN THAN EVER!
OMG MY NOSE ITCHES
ALSO: MY HAIR'S GETTING REALLY LONG.
I MEAN WE'RE TALKING MAN BUN TERRITORY HERE
IN TWO MONTHS ?

SUNDAY 4/12/20

IT'S A COLD AND SNOWY EASTER SUNDAY AND I'M GLAD.

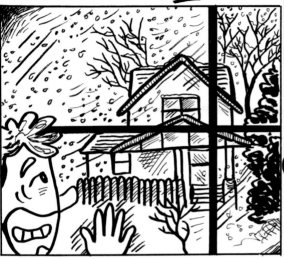

IF MOST OF US HAVE TO BE INSIDE 95% OF THE TIME ANYWAY, WHY NOT MAKE IT WORTHWHILE, BE ALL COZY?

maybe it was worth moving here after all

GAS FIREPLACE →

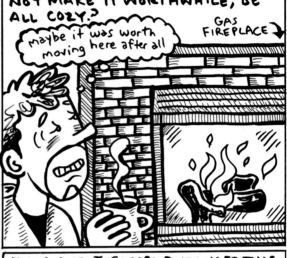

AN OLD FRIEND OF MINE TOLD ME THAT WHEN SHE LIVED IN LA SHE WAS ALWAYS A LITTLE DEPRESSED. SHE FINALLY REALIZED IT WAS BECAUSE IT WAS ALWAYS SUNNY THERE AND SHE NEVER GOT TO ENJOY A MOODY DAY.

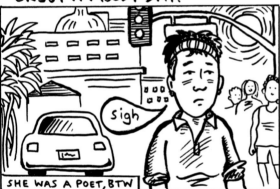

sigh

SHE WAS A POET, BTW

JOHN AND I SOCIAL DISTANCED THIS AFTERNOON — FROM EACH OTHER.

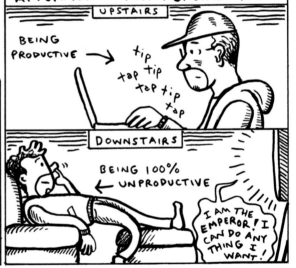

UPSTAIRS

BEING PRODUCTIVE →

tip tap tip tap tip tap

DOWNSTAIRS

BEING 100% ← UNPRODUCTIVE

I AM THE EMPEROR! I CAN DO ANY THING I WANT!

WE HAD BEEN TOGETHER ALMOST 24/7 FOR THE PAST TWO SLIGHTLY HELLISH WEEKS OF MOVING.*

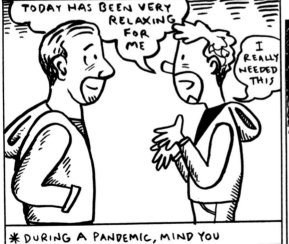

TODAY HAS BEEN VERY RELAXING FOR ME

I REALLY NEEDED THIS

* DURING A PANDEMIC, MIND YOU

The US Now Has the Most Reported Coronavirus Deaths of Any Country

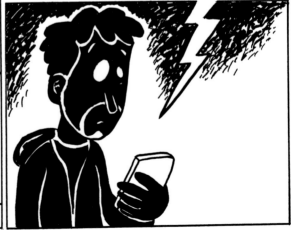

MONDAY 4/13/20

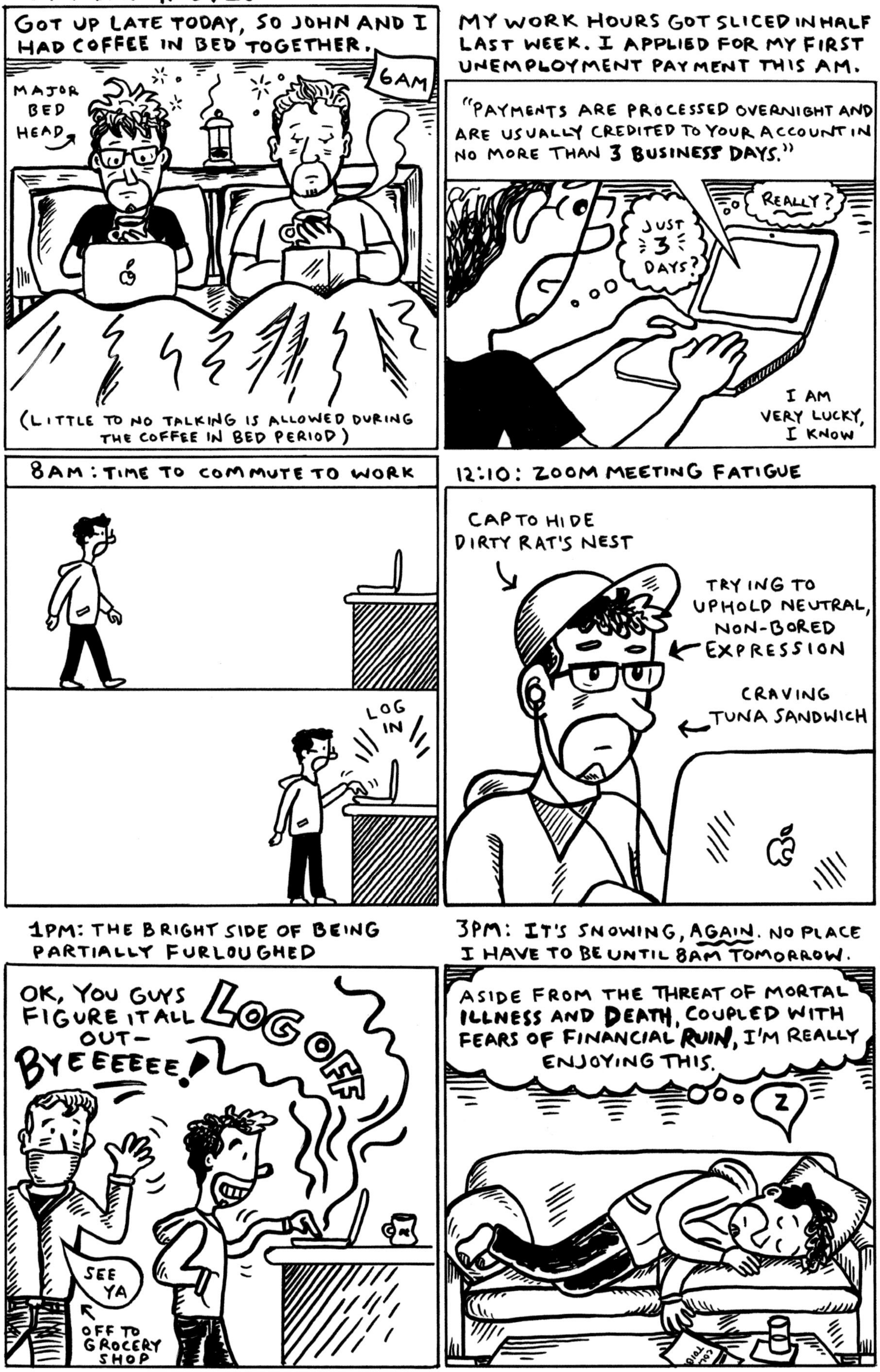
GOT UP LATE TODAY, SO JOHN AND I HAD COFFEE IN BED TOGETHER.
6AM
MAJOR BED HEAD
(LITTLE TO NO TALKING IS ALLOWED DURING THE COFFEE IN BED PERIOD)
MY WORK HOURS GOT SLICED IN HALF LAST WEEK. I APPLIED FOR MY FIRST UNEMPLOYMENT PAYMENT THIS AM.
"PAYMENTS ARE PROCESSED OVERNIGHT AND ARE USUALLY CREDITED TO YOUR ACCOUNT IN NO MORE THAN 3 BUSINESS DAYS."
JUST 3 DAYS?
REALLY?
I AM VERY LUCKY, I KNOW
8AM: TIME TO COMMUTE TO WORK
LOG IN
12:10: ZOOM MEETING FATIGUE
CAP TO HIDE DIRTY RAT'S NEST
TRYING TO UPHOLD NEUTRAL, NON-BORED EXPRESSION
CRAVING TUNA SANDWICH
1PM: THE BRIGHT SIDE OF BEING PARTIALLY FURLOUGHED
OK, YOU GUYS FIGURE IT ALL OUT— BYEEEEEE!
LOG OFF
SEE YA
OFF TO GROCERY SHOP
3PM: IT'S SNOWING, AGAIN. NO PLACE I HAVE TO BE UNTIL 8AM TOMORROW.
ASIDE FROM THE THREAT OF MORTAL ILLNESS AND DEATH, COUPLED WITH FEARS OF FINANCIAL RUIN, I'M REALLY ENJOYING THIS.
Z

TUESDAY 4/14/20

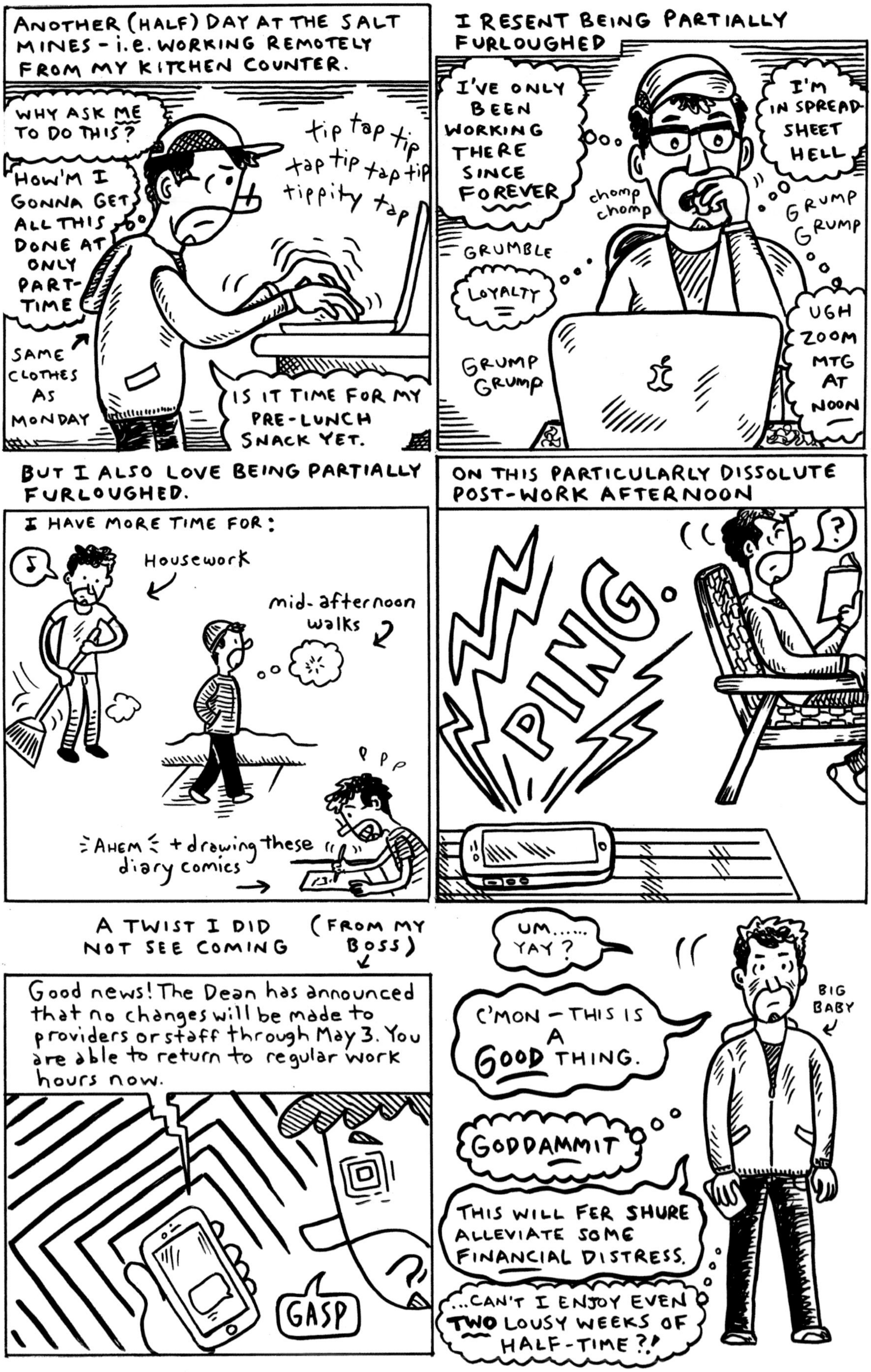

ANOTHER (HALF) DAY AT THE SALT MINES - i.e. WORKING REMOTELY FROM MY KITCHEN COUNTER.
WHY ASK ME TO DO THIS?
HOW'M I GONNA GET ALL THIS DONE AT ONLY PART-TIME
tip tap tip tap tip tap tip tippity tap
SAME CLOTHES AS MONDAY
IS IT TIME FOR MY PRE-LUNCH SNACK YET.
I RESENT BEING PARTIALLY FURLOUGHED
I'VE ONLY BEEN WORKING THERE SINCE FOREVER
chomp chomp
I'M IN SPREADSHEET HELL
GRUMP GRUMP
GRUMBLE
LOYALTY
GRUMP GRUMP
UGH ZOOM MTG AT NOON
BUT I ALSO LOVE BEING PARTIALLY FURLOUGHED.
I HAVE MORE TIME FOR:
Housework
mid-afternoon walks
AHEM + drawing these diary comics
ON THIS PARTICULARLY DISSOLUTE POST-WORK AFTERNOON
PING.
?
A TWIST I DID NOT SEE COMING
(FROM MY BOSS)
Good news! The Dean has announced that no changes will be made to providers or staff through May 3. You are able to return to regular work hours now.
GASP
UM...... YAY?
C'MON - THIS IS A GOOD THING.
BIG BABY
GODDAMMIT
THIS WILL FER SHURE ALLEVIATE SOME FINANCIAL DISTRESS.
...CAN'T I ENJOY EVEN TWO LOUSY WEEKS OF HALF-TIME?!

WEDNESDAY 4/15/20

5AM: THE MORNING PEE BEFORE THE MORNING COFFEE

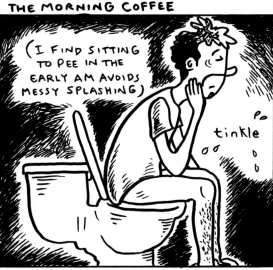

(I FIND SITTING TO PEE IN THE EARLY AM AVOIDS MESSY SPLASHING)

tinkle

I'VE HAD THIS LITTLE CLOCK SINCE FOREVER. I STUCK IT IN THIS LITTLE SECOND BATHROOM WHEN WE MOVED IN A COUPLE OF WEEKS AGO.

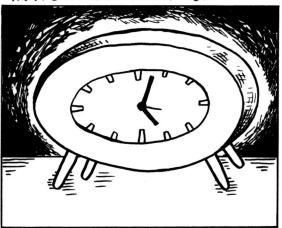

WE HAVE TO KEEP IT AWAY FROM ANYWHERE PEOPLE SLEEP BECAUSE THE TICKING SOUND IT MAKES CAN BOTHER PEOPLE.

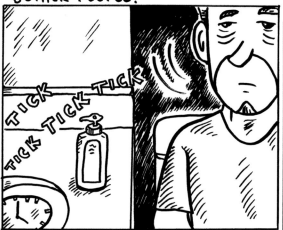

TICK TICK TICK

IN THE OTHERWISE SILENT DARK-NESS THAT SOUND SOMEHOW TRIGGERED AN AWFUL DESOLATION IN ME... IT SEEMED TO BORE ITS WAY STRAIGHT TO MY CORE.

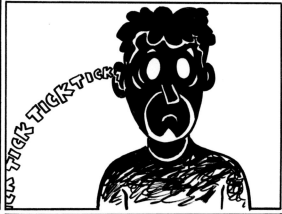

TICK TICK TICK TICK

ONCE AGAIN I STARTED THINKING ABOUT THINGS I **REALLY** DIDN'T WANT TO THINK ABOUT.

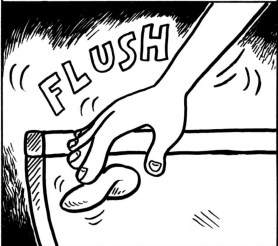

((FLUSH))

THIRTY MINUTES LATER: NOT SURE IF MY ABILITY TO RECOVER QUICKLY FROM EXISTENTIAL DESPAIR IS MY SUPER POWER OR MY KRYPTONITE.

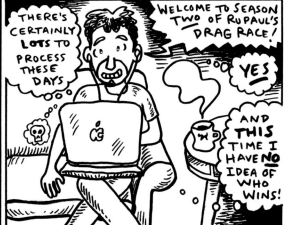

THERE'S CERTAINLY **LOTS** TO PROCESS THESE DAYS

WELCOME TO SEASON TWO OF RUPAUL'S DRAG RACE!

YES

AND **THIS** TIME I HAVE **NO** IDEA OF WHO WINS!

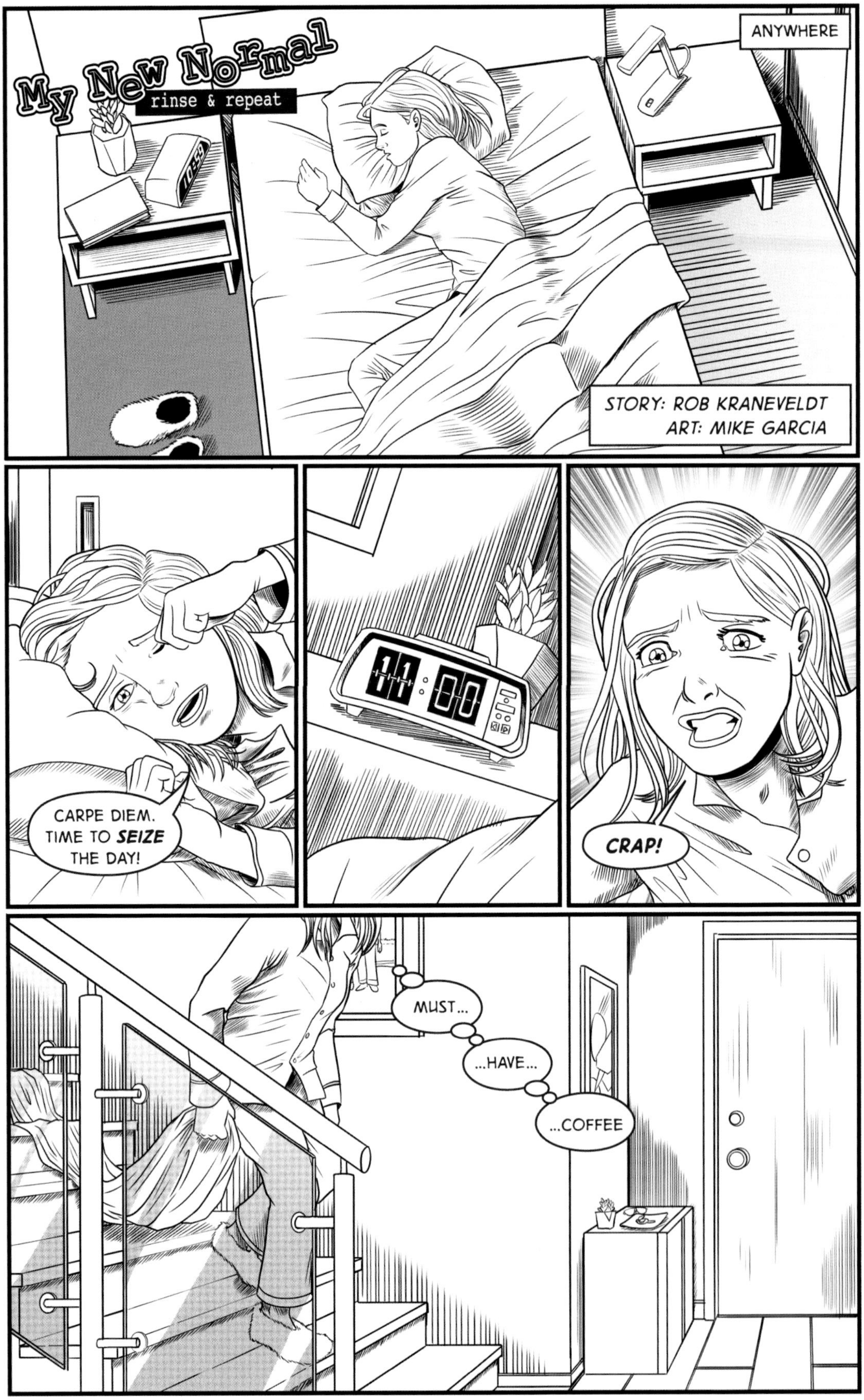
My New Normal
rinse & repeat
ANYWHERE
10:59
STORY: ROB KRANEVELDT
ART: MIKE GARCIA
CARPE DIEM. TIME TO SEIZE THE DAY!
11:00
CRAP!
MUST...
...HAVE...
...COFFEE

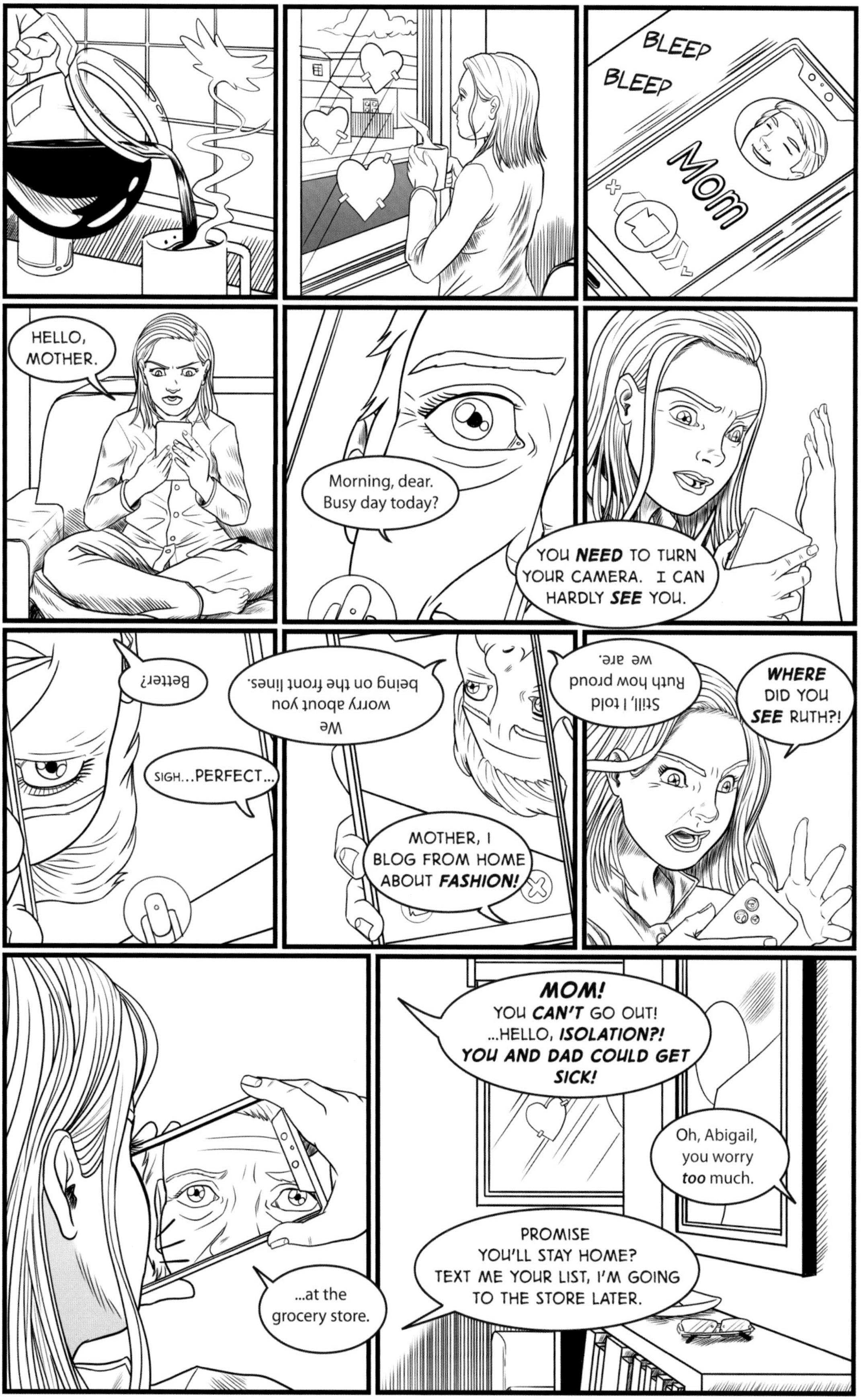
BLEEP
BLEEP
Mom
HELLO, MOTHER.
Morning, dear. Busy day today?
YOU **NEED** TO TURN YOUR CAMERA. I CAN HARDLY **SEE** YOU.
Better?
SIGH...PERFECT...
We worry about you being on the front lines.
MOTHER, I BLOG FROM HOME ABOUT **FASHION!**
Still, I told Ruth how proud we are.
WHERE DID YOU **SEE** RUTH?!
...at the grocery store.
MOM! YOU **CAN'T** GO OUT! ...HELLO, **ISOLATION?! YOU AND DAD COULD GET SICK!**
Oh, Abigail, you worry ***too*** much.
PROMISE YOU'LL STAY HOME? TEXT ME YOUR LIST, I'M GOING TO THE STORE LATER.

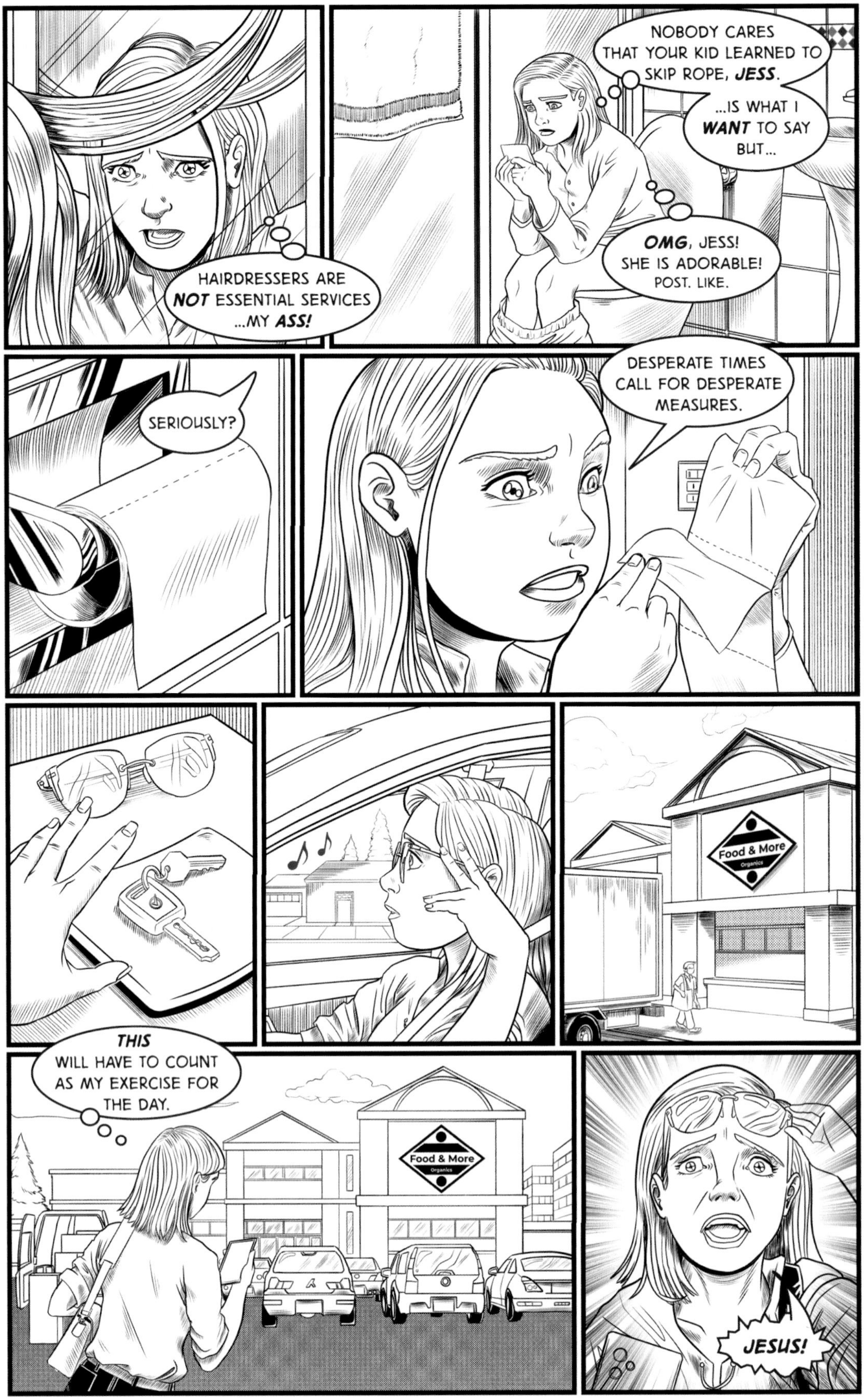
HAIRDRESSERS ARE NOT ESSENTIAL SERVICES ...MY ASS!
NOBODY CARES THAT YOUR KID LEARNED TO SKIP ROPE, JESS.
...IS WHAT I WANT TO SAY BUT...
OMG, JESS! SHE IS ADORABLE! POST. LIKE.
SERIOUSLY?
DESPERATE TIMES CALL FOR DESPERATE MEASURES.
Food & More Organics
THIS WILL HAVE TO COUNT AS MY EXERCISE FOR THE DAY.
Food & More Organics
JESUS!

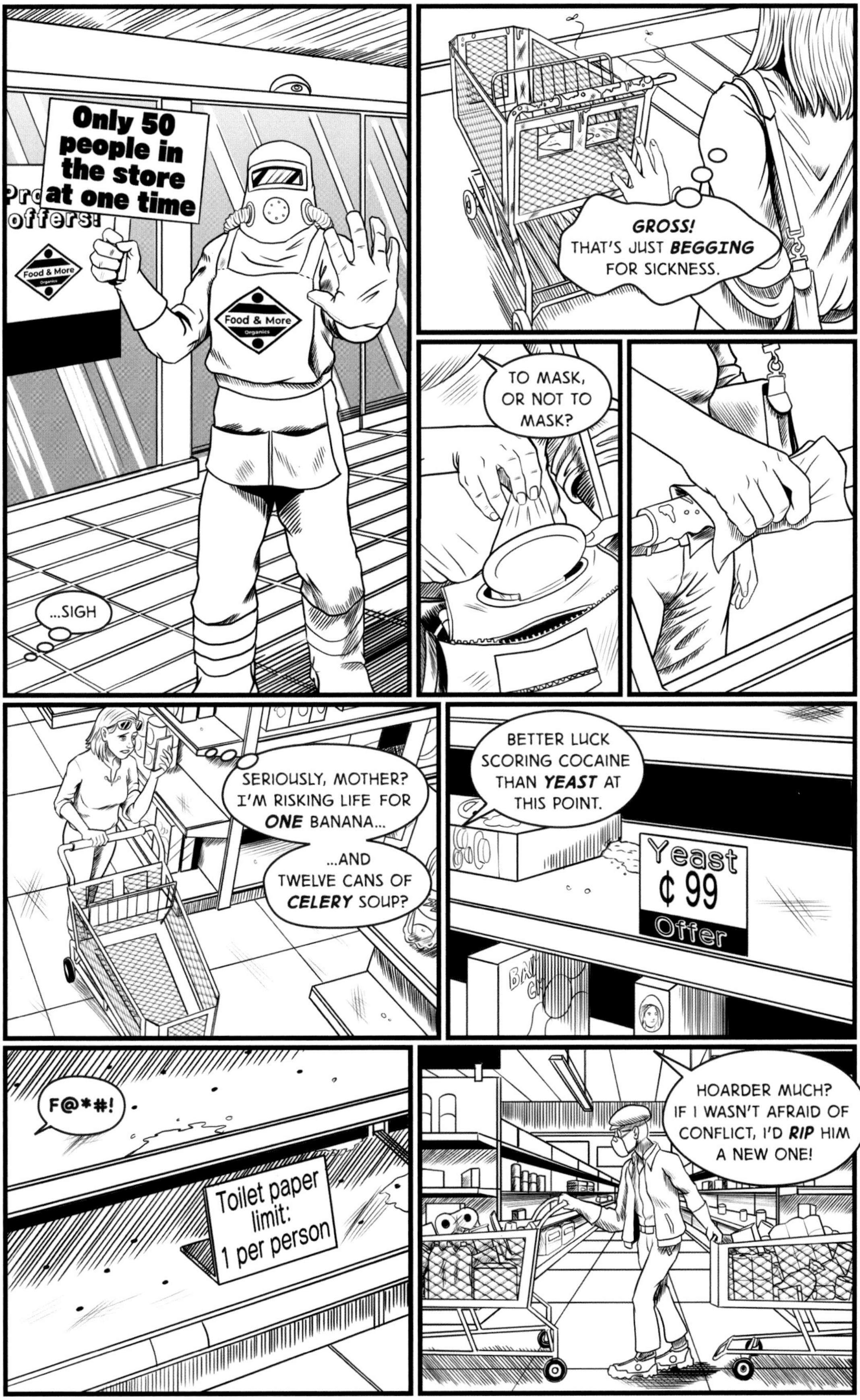
Only 50 people in the store at one time
Pro offers!
Food & More Organics
Food & More Organics
...SIGH
GROSS! THAT'S JUST BEGGING FOR SICKNESS.
TO MASK, OR NOT TO MASK?
SERIOUSLY, MOTHER? I'M RISKING LIFE FOR ONE BANANA...
...AND TWELVE CANS OF CELERY SOUP?
BETTER LUCK SCORING COCAINE THAN YEAST AT THIS POINT.
Yeast ¢ 99 Offer
F@*#!
Toilet paper limit: 1 per person
HOARDER MUCH? IF I WASN'T AFRAID OF CONFLICT, I'D RIP HIM A NEW ONE!

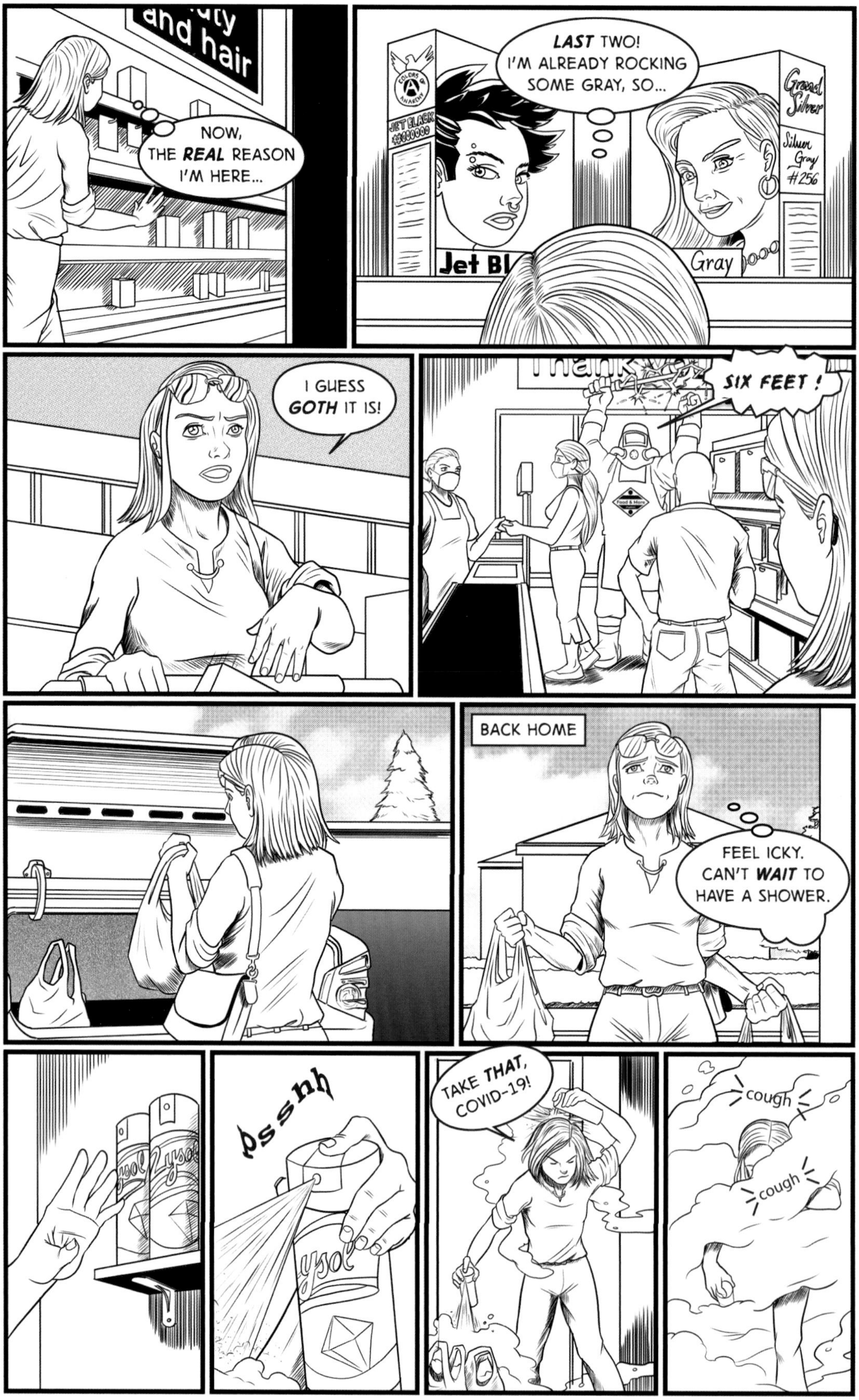
and hair
NOW, THE REAL REASON I'M HERE...
LAST TWO! I'M ALREADY ROCKING SOME GRAY, SO...
JET BLACK #000000
Jet Bl
Grand Silver
Silver Gray #256
Gray
I GUESS GOTH IT IS!
SIX FEET!
BACK HOME
FEEL ICKY. CAN'T WAIT TO HAVE A SHOWER.
pssshh
TAKE THAT, COVID-19!
cough
cough

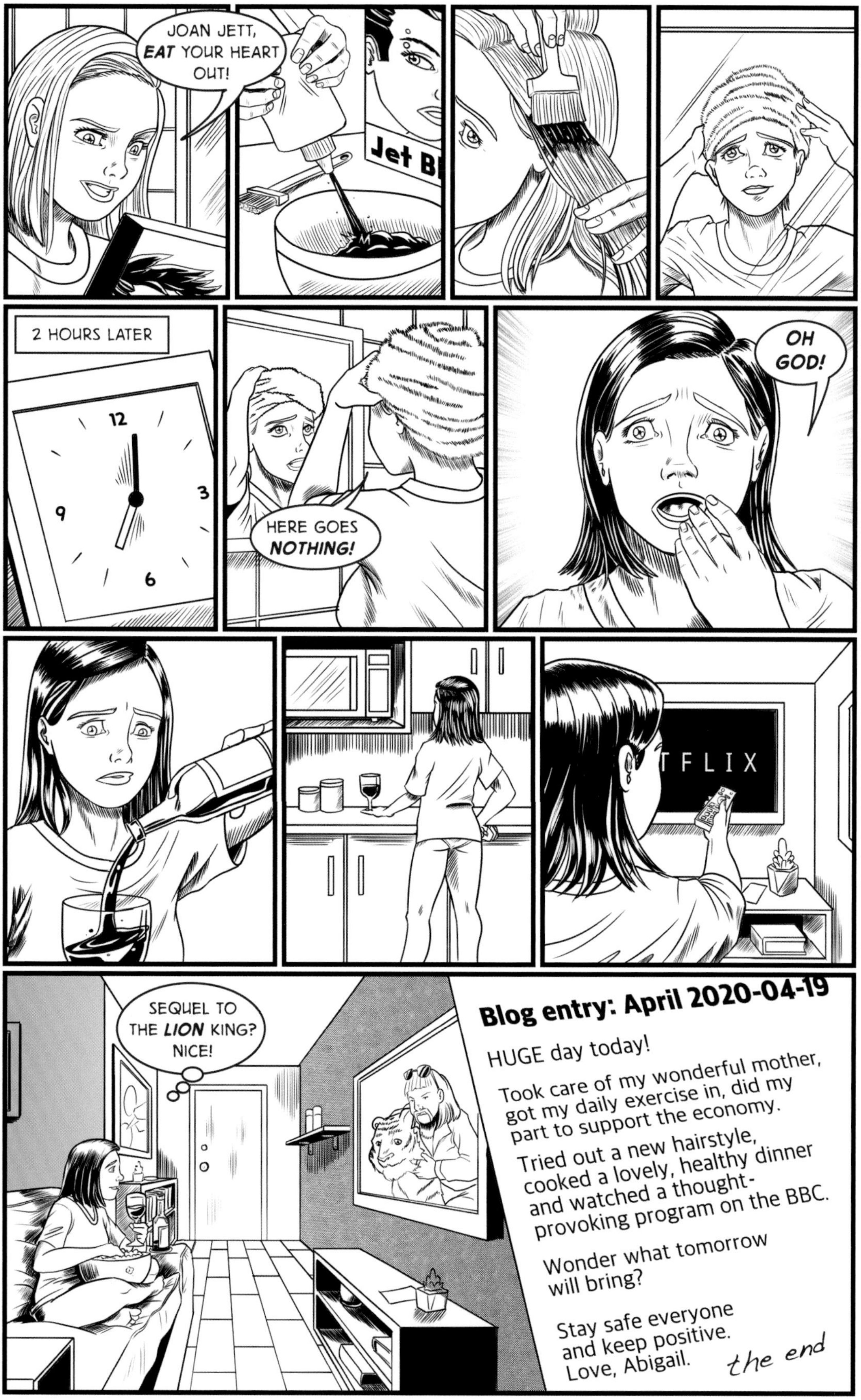
JOAN JETT, EAT YOUR HEART OUT!
Jet Bl
2 HOURS LATER
12
3
6
9
HERE GOES NOTHING!
OH GOD!
TFLIX
SEQUEL TO THE LION KING? NICE!
Blog entry: April 2020-04-19
HUGE day today!
Took care of my wonderful mother, got my daily exercise in, did my part to support the economy.
Tried out a new hairstyle, cooked a lovely, healthy dinner and watched a thought-provoking program on the BBC.
Wonder what tomorrow will bring?
Stay safe everyone and keep positive.
Love, Abigail.
the end

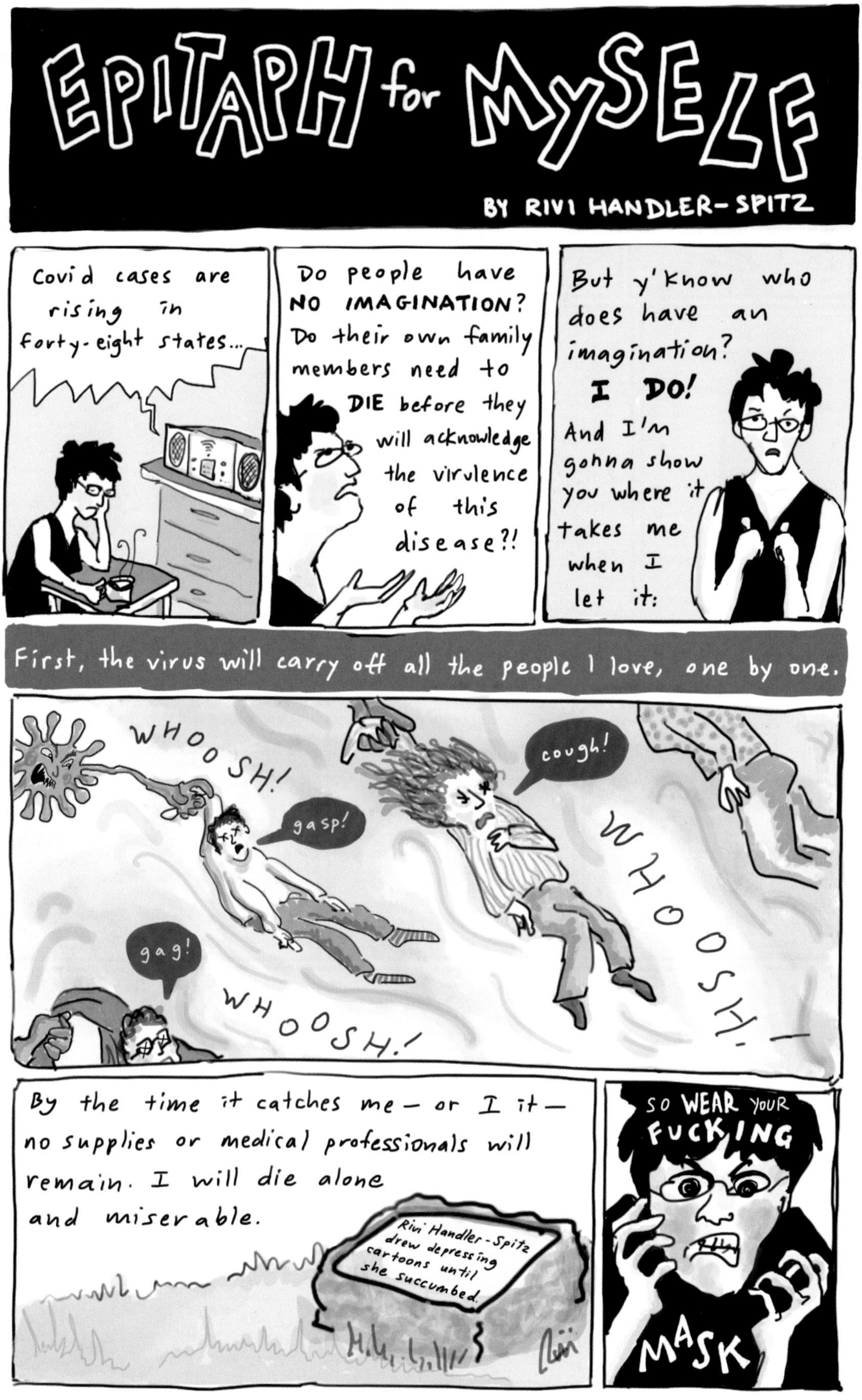
EPITAPH for MYSELF
BY RIVI HANDLER-SPITZ
Covid cases are rising in forty-eight states...
Do people have NO IMAGINATION? Do their own family members need to DIE before they will acknowledge the virulence of this disease?!
But y'know who does have an imagination? I DO! And I'm gonna show you where it takes me when I let it:
First, the virus will carry off all the people I love, one by one.
WHOOSH!
gasp!
cough!
WHOOSH!
gag!
WHOOSH!
By the time it catches me—or I it—no supplies or medical professionals will remain. I will die alone and miserable.
Rivi Handler-Spitz drew depressing cartoons until she succumbed.
Rivi
SO WEAR YOUR FUCKING MASK

The Dance of DEATH

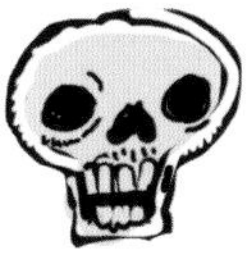

BY PETER DUNLAP-SHOHL

A lesson from the pandemic: Humankind is inextricably linked in both space and time. Dance of Death allegories were a popular meme of the Middle Ages, where Death is depicted as the great equalizer, taking both princes and peasants. Death walked everywhere and came for anyone at any time. A *memento mori*, the Dance of Death reminds us we are here for a short time, and gone for eternity.

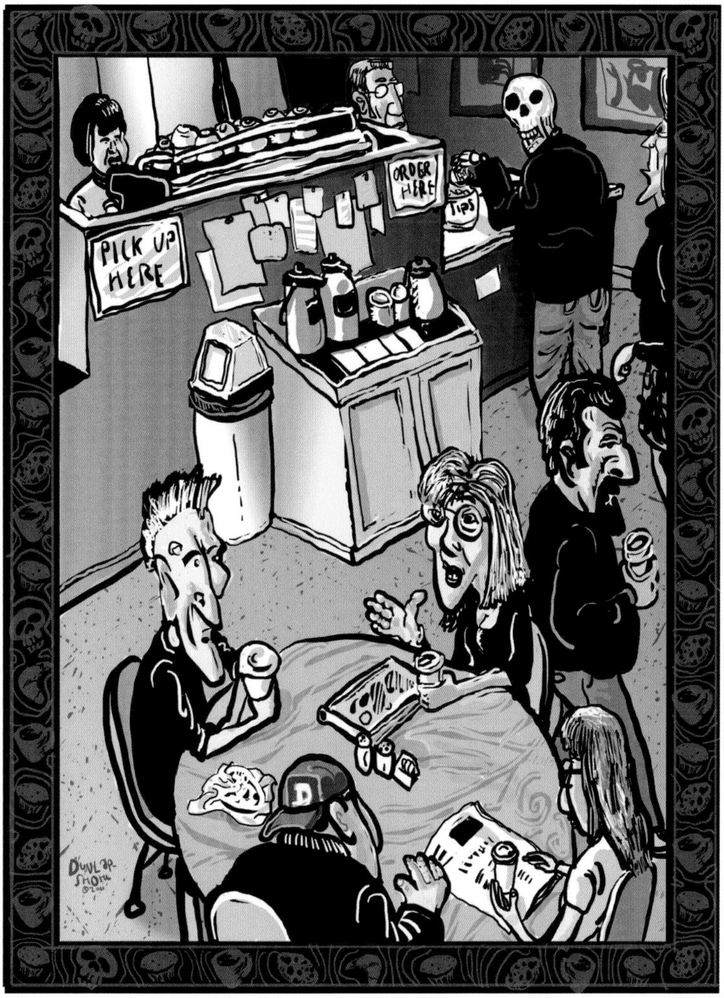
ORDER HERE
TIPS
PICK UP HERE
DUNLAP-SHOHL

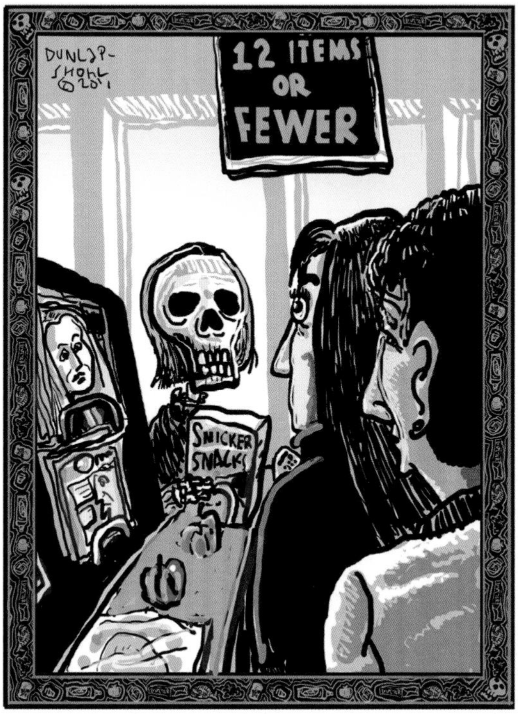
DUNLAP-SHOHL
12 ITEMS OR FEWER
SNICKER SNACKS

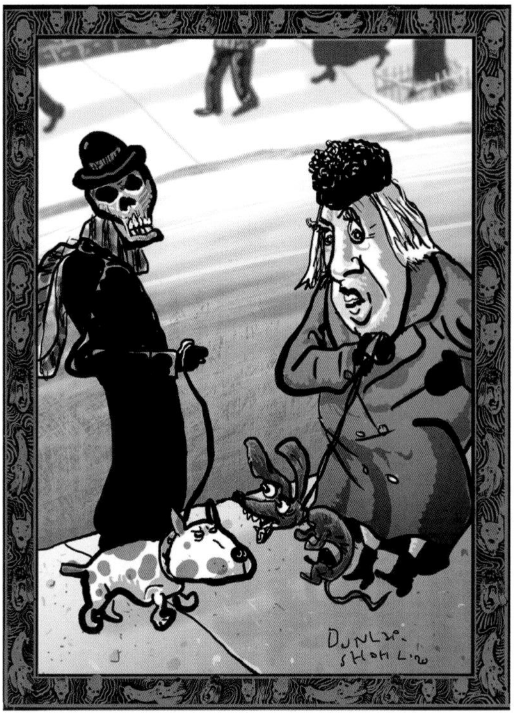
DUNLAP-SHOHL

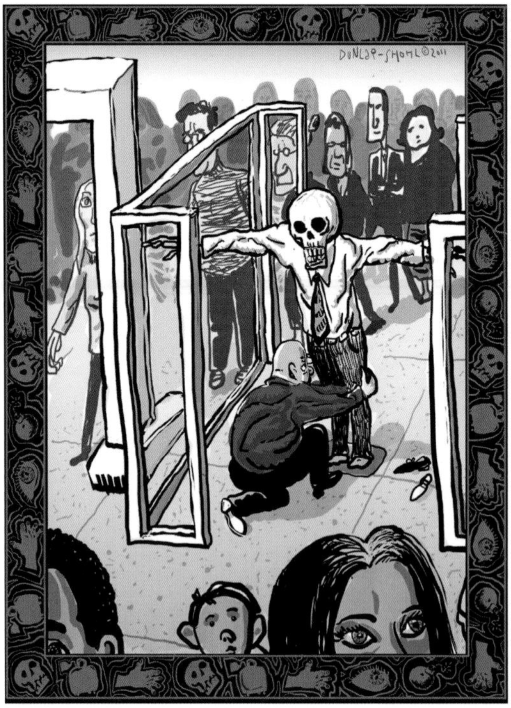
DUNLAP-SHOHL©2011

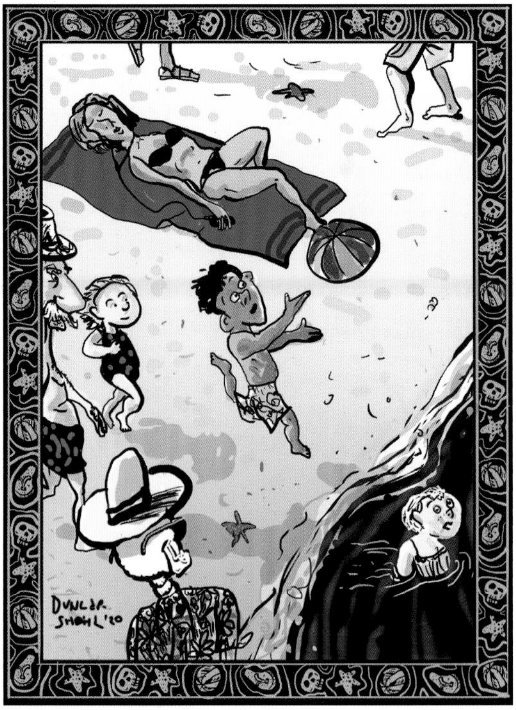
DUNLAP-SHOHL'20

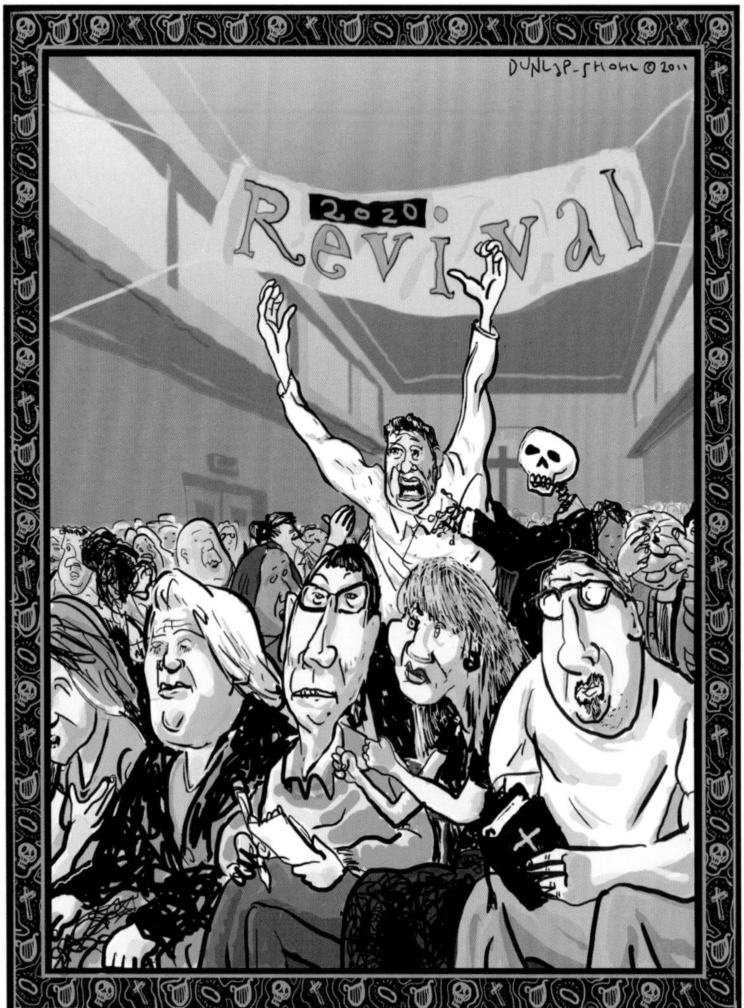
DUNLAP-SHOHL©2011
2020
Revival

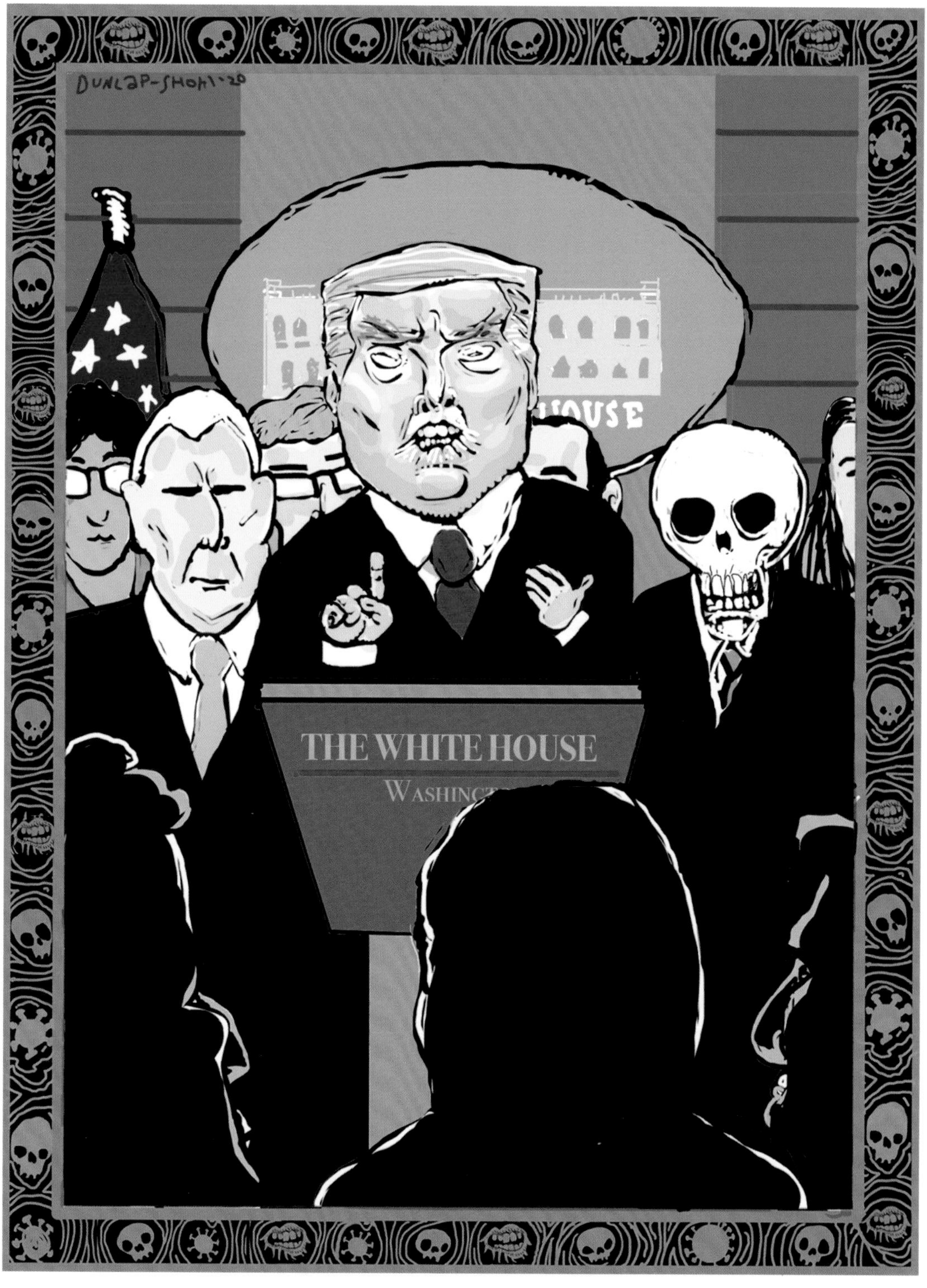
DUNLAP-SHOHL '20
THE WHITE HOUSE

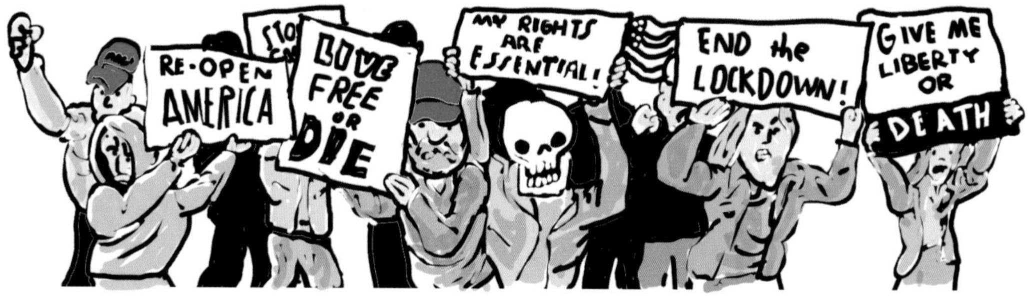
RE-OPEN AMERICA
LIVE FREE OR DIE
MY RIGHTS ARE ESSENTIAL!
END the LOCKDOWN!
GIVE ME LIBERTY OR DEATH

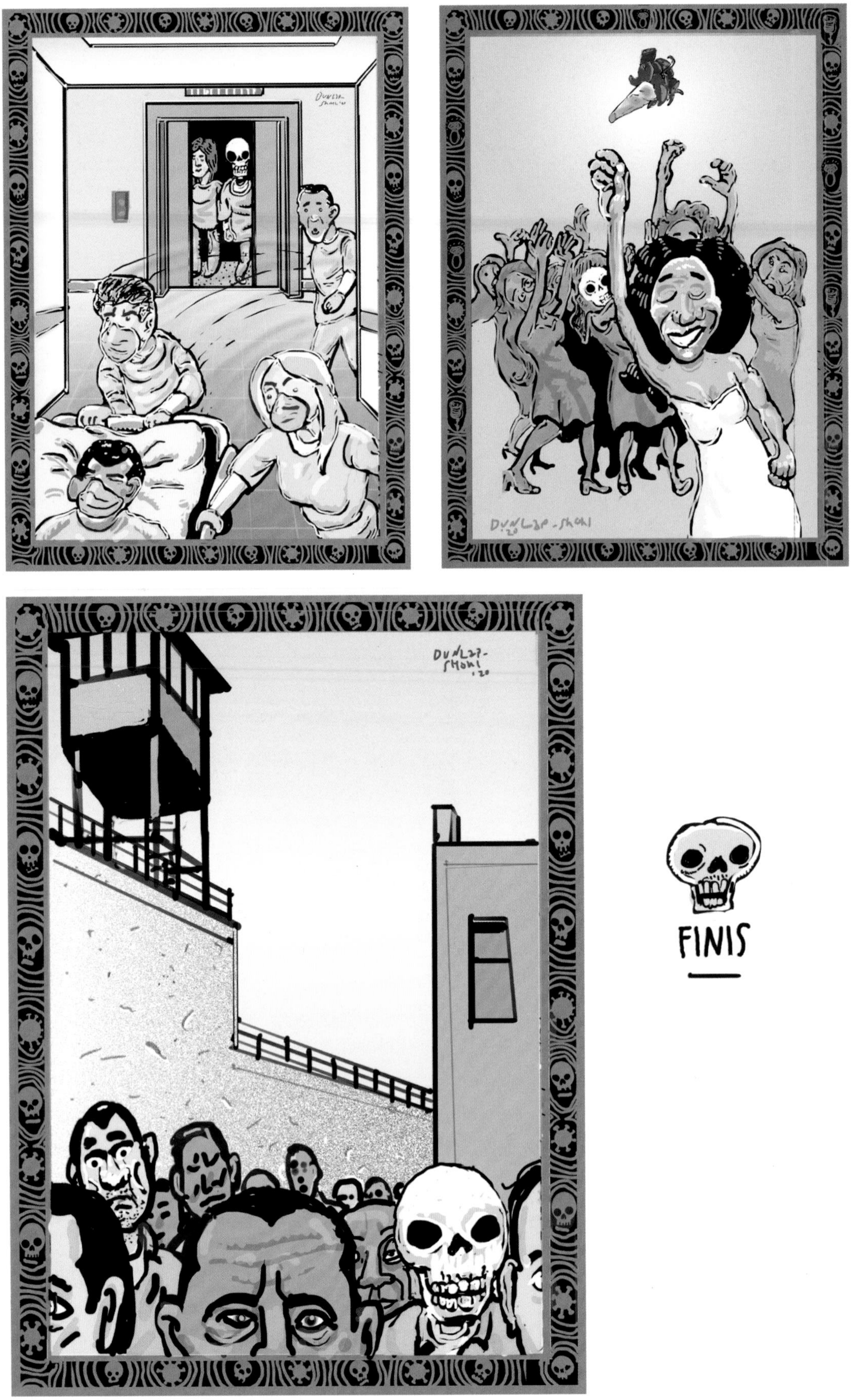
FINIS

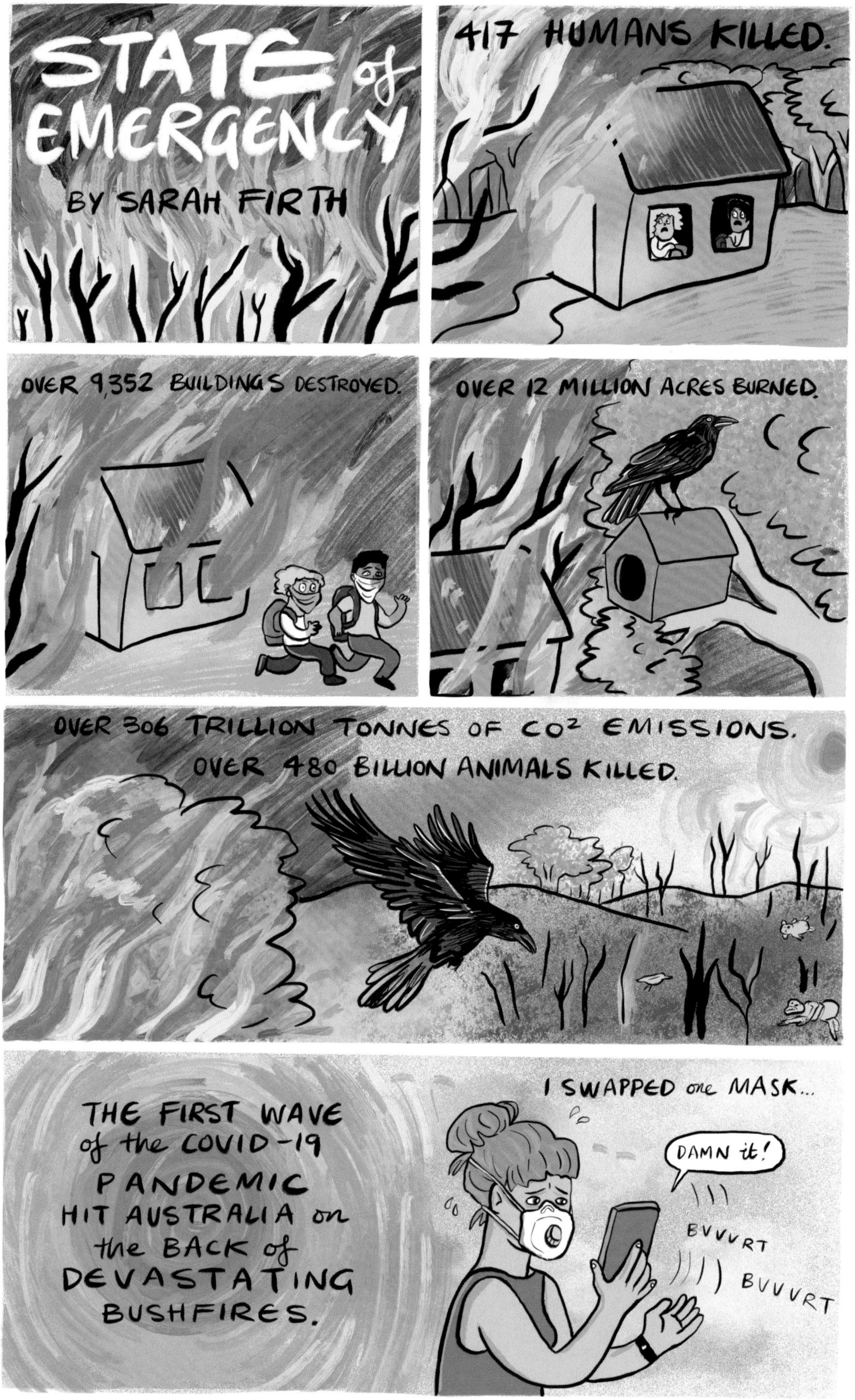
STATE of EMERGENCY
BY SARAH FIRTH
417 HUMANS KILLED.
OVER 9,352 BUILDINGS DESTROYED.
OVER 12 MILLION ACRES BURNED.
OVER 306 TRILLION TONNES OF CO^2 EMISSIONS.
OVER 480 BILLION ANIMALS KILLED.
THE FIRST WAVE of the COVID-19 PANDEMIC HIT AUSTRALIA on the BACK of DEVASTATING BUSHFIRES.
I SWAPPED one MASK...
DAMN it!
BVVVRT
BVVVRT

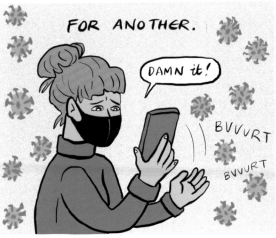

FOR ANOTHER.

DAMN it!

BVVURT

BVVURT

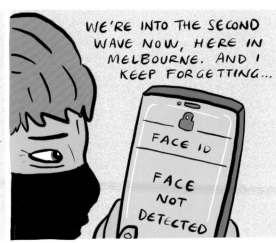

WE'RE INTO THE SECOND WAVE NOW, HERE IN MELBOURNE. AND I KEEP FORGETTING...

FACE ID

FACE NOT DETECTED

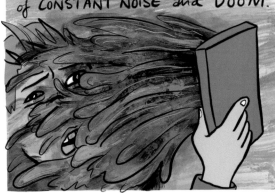

DAMN it!

TAK TAK TAK

PASSCODE

THAT I STILL CAN'T QUICKLY UNLOCK MY PHONE.

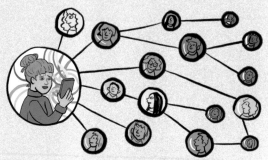

IT'S BEEN SEVEN LONG MONTHS OF ISOLATING. I MISS SO MUCH. FOR NOW, ONLINE IS A LIFELINE.

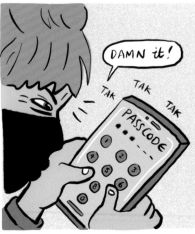

BUT IT'S ALSO A FIREHOSE of CONSTANT NOISE and DOOM.

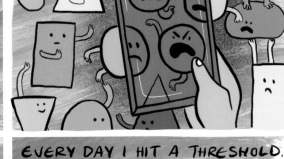

DISTORTING and FRAGMENTING EVENTS and INFORMATION. CUTTING AWAY CONTEXT.

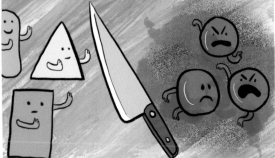

EVERY DAY I HIT A THRESHOLD. AND REMEMBER I CAN ONLY HANDLE SO MUCH.

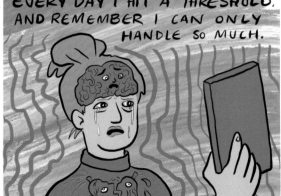

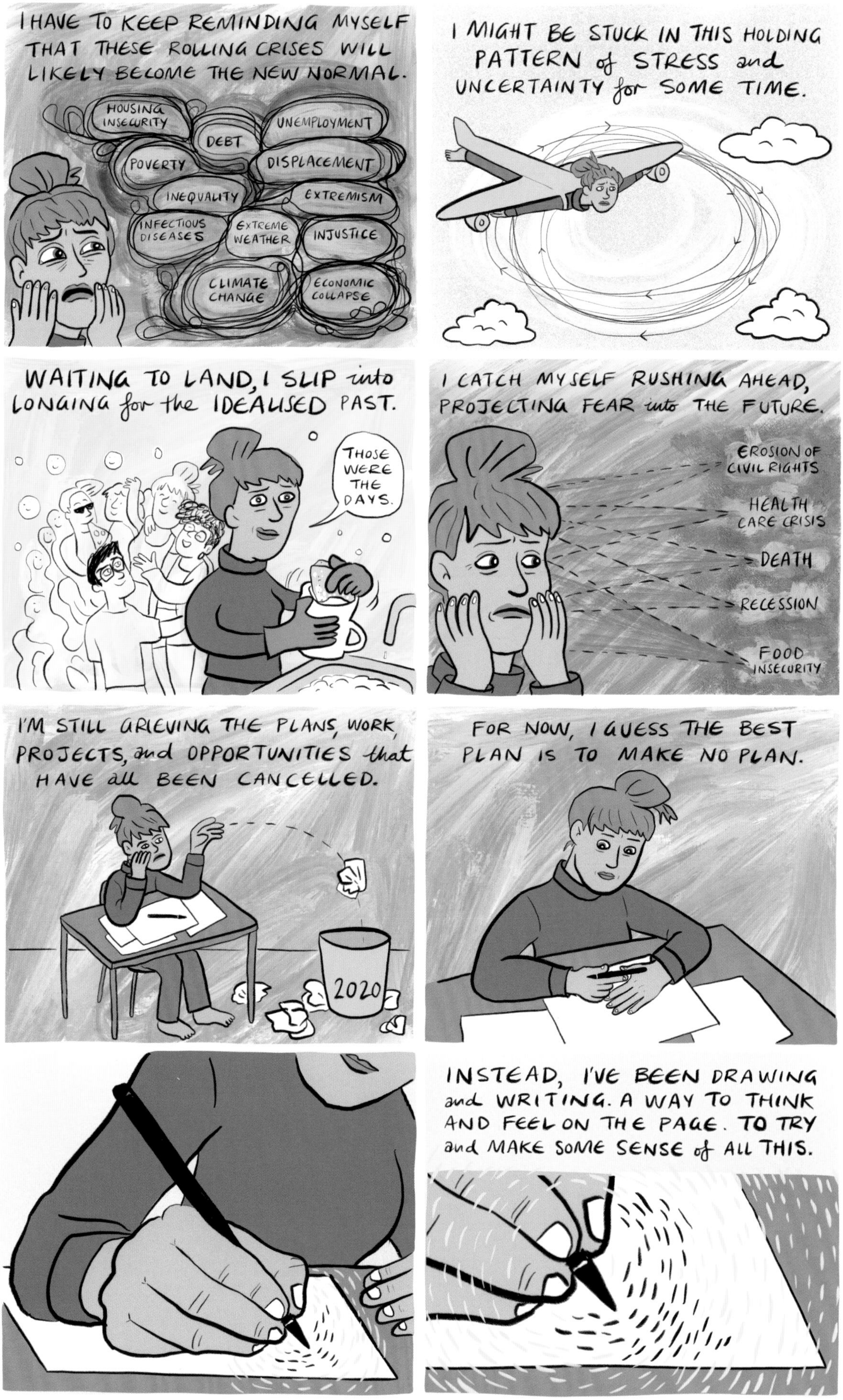
I HAVE TO KEEP REMINDING MYSELF THAT THESE ROLLING CRISES WILL LIKELY BECOME THE NEW NORMAL.
HOUSING INSECURITY
DEBT
UNEMPLOYMENT
POVERTY
DISPLACEMENT
INEQUALITY
EXTREMISM
INFECTIOUS DISEASES
EXTREME WEATHER
INJUSTICE
CLIMATE CHANGE
ECONOMIC COLLAPSE
I MIGHT BE STUCK IN THIS HOLDING PATTERN of STRESS and UNCERTAINTY for SOME TIME.
WAITING TO LAND, I SLIP into LONGING for the IDEALISED PAST.
THOSE WERE THE DAYS.
I CATCH MYSELF RUSHING AHEAD, PROJECTING FEAR into THE FUTURE.
EROSION OF CIVIL RIGHTS
HEALTH CARE CRISIS
DEATH
RECESSION
FOOD INSECURITY
I'M STILL GRIEVING THE PLANS, WORK, PROJECTS, and OPPORTUNITIES that HAVE all BEEN CANCELLED.
2020
FOR NOW, I GUESS THE BEST PLAN IS TO MAKE NO PLAN.
INSTEAD, I'VE BEEN DRAWING and WRITING. A WAY TO THINK AND FEEL ON THE PAGE. TO TRY and MAKE SOME SENSE of ALL THIS.

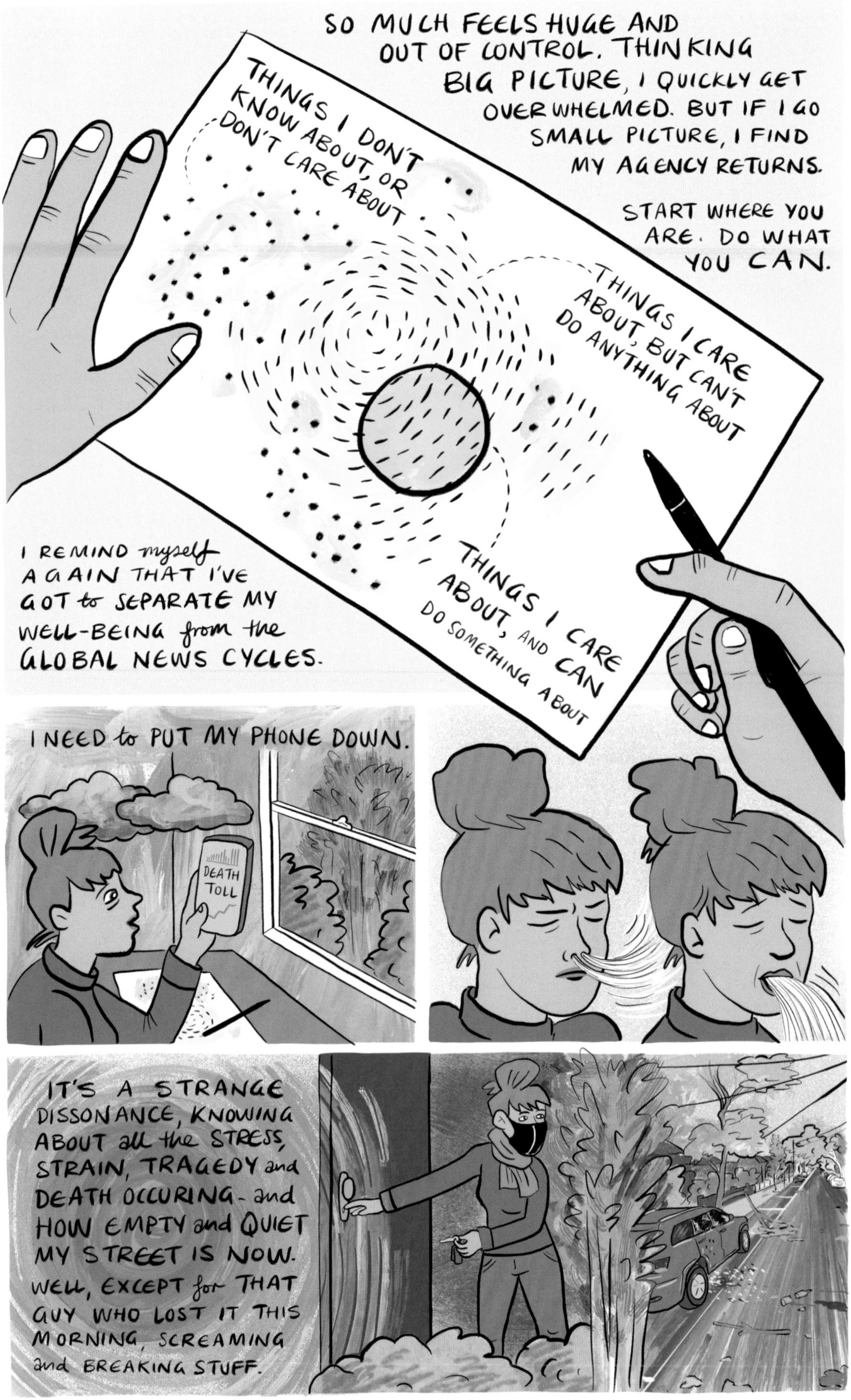
SO MUCH FEELS HUGE AND OUT OF CONTROL. THINKING BIG PICTURE, I QUICKLY GET OVERWHELMED. BUT IF I GO SMALL PICTURE, I FIND MY AGENCY RETURNS.
START WHERE YOU ARE. DO WHAT YOU CAN.
THINGS I DON'T KNOW ABOUT, OR DON'T CARE ABOUT
THINGS I CARE ABOUT, BUT CAN'T DO ANYTHING ABOUT
THINGS I CARE ABOUT, AND CAN DO SOMETHING ABOUT
I REMIND myself AGAIN THAT I'VE GOT to SEPARATE MY WELL-BEING from the GLOBAL NEWS CYCLES.
I NEED to PUT MY PHONE DOWN.
DEATH TOLL
IT'S A STRANGE DISSONANCE, KNOWING ABOUT all the STRESS, STRAIN, TRAGEDY and DEATH OCCURING - and HOW EMPTY and QUIET MY STREET IS NOW. WELL, EXCEPT for THAT GUY WHO LOST IT THIS MORNING, SCREAMING and BREAKING STUFF.

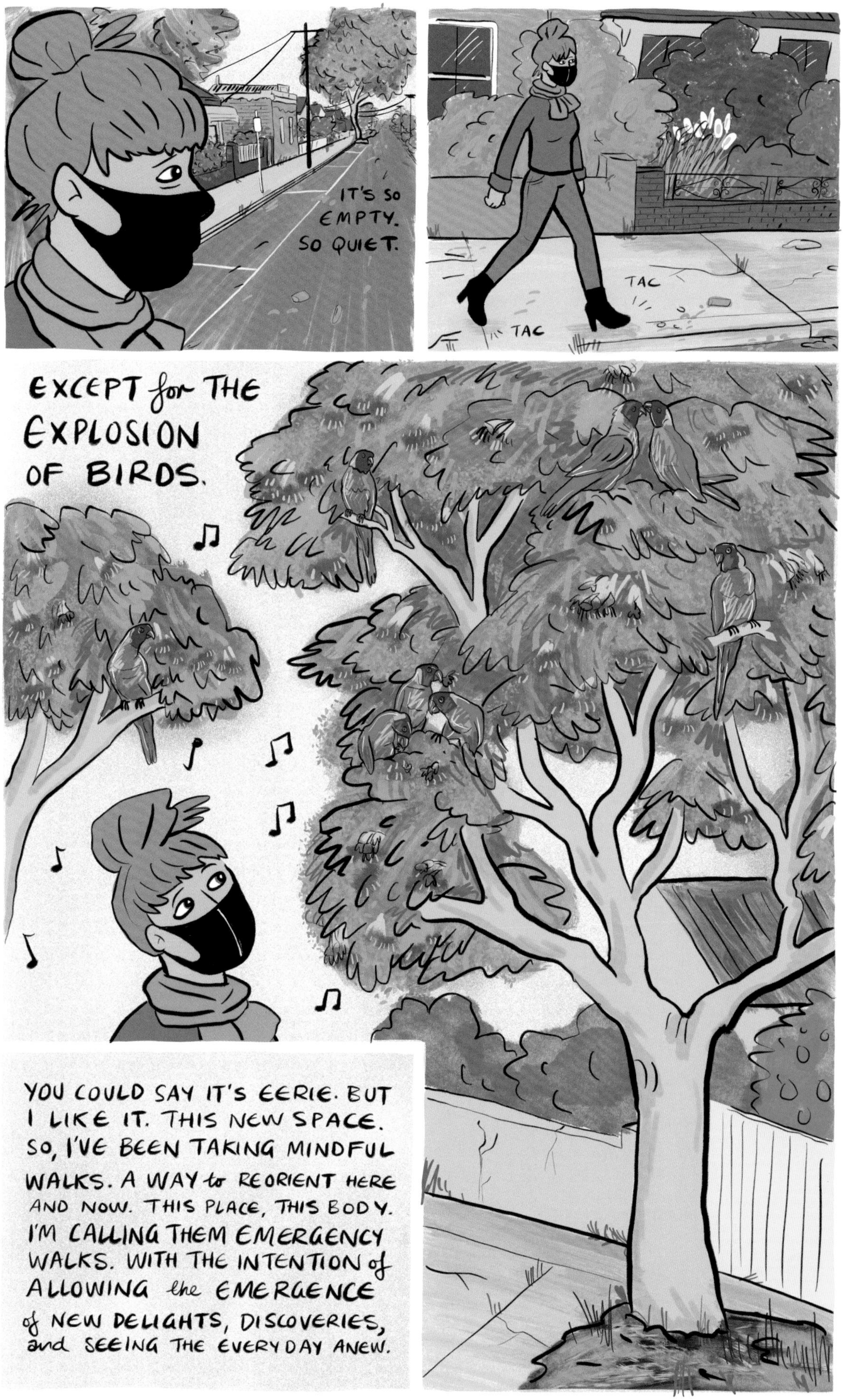
IT'S SO EMPTY. SO QUIET.
TAC
TAC
EXCEPT for THE EXPLOSION OF BIRDS.
YOU COULD SAY IT'S EERIE. BUT I LIKE IT. THIS NEW SPACE. SO, I'VE BEEN TAKING MINDFUL WALKS. A WAY to REORIENT HERE AND NOW. THIS PLACE, THIS BODY. I'M CALLING THEM EMERGENCY WALKS. WITH THE INTENTION of ALLOWING the EMERGENCE of NEW DELIGHTS, DISCOVERIES, and SEEING THE EVERYDAY ANEW.

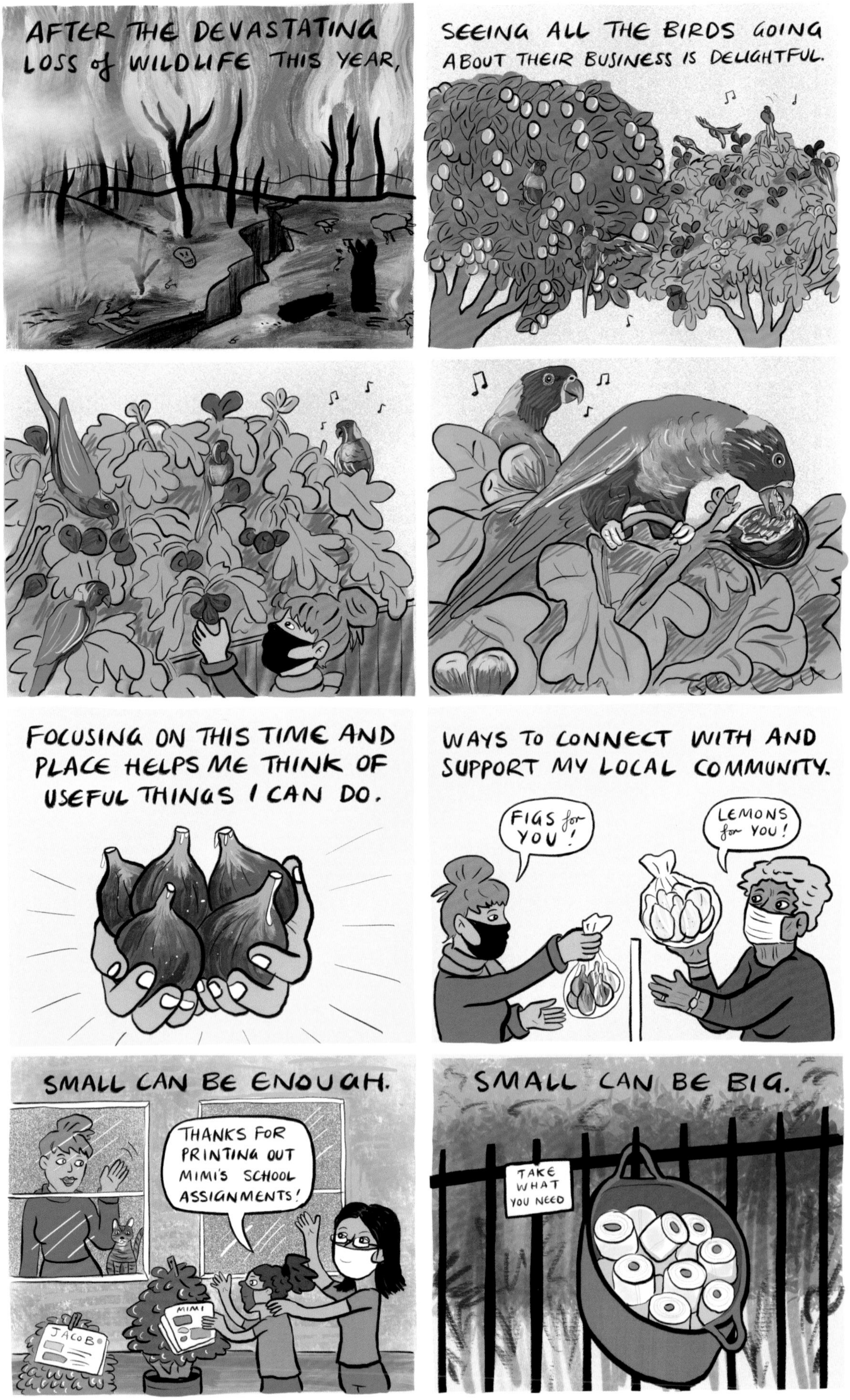
AFTER THE DEVASTATING LOSS of WILDLIFE THIS YEAR,
SEEING ALL THE BIRDS GOING ABOUT THEIR BUSINESS IS DELIGHTFUL.
FOCUSING ON THIS TIME AND PLACE HELPS ME THINK OF USEFUL THINGS I CAN DO.
WAYS TO CONNECT WITH AND SUPPORT MY LOCAL COMMUNITY.
FIGS for YOU!
LEMONS for YOU!
SMALL CAN BE ENOUGH.
THANKS FOR PRINTING OUT MIMI'S SCHOOL ASSIGNMENTS!
JACOB
MIMI
SMALL CAN BE BIG.
TAKE WHAT YOU NEED

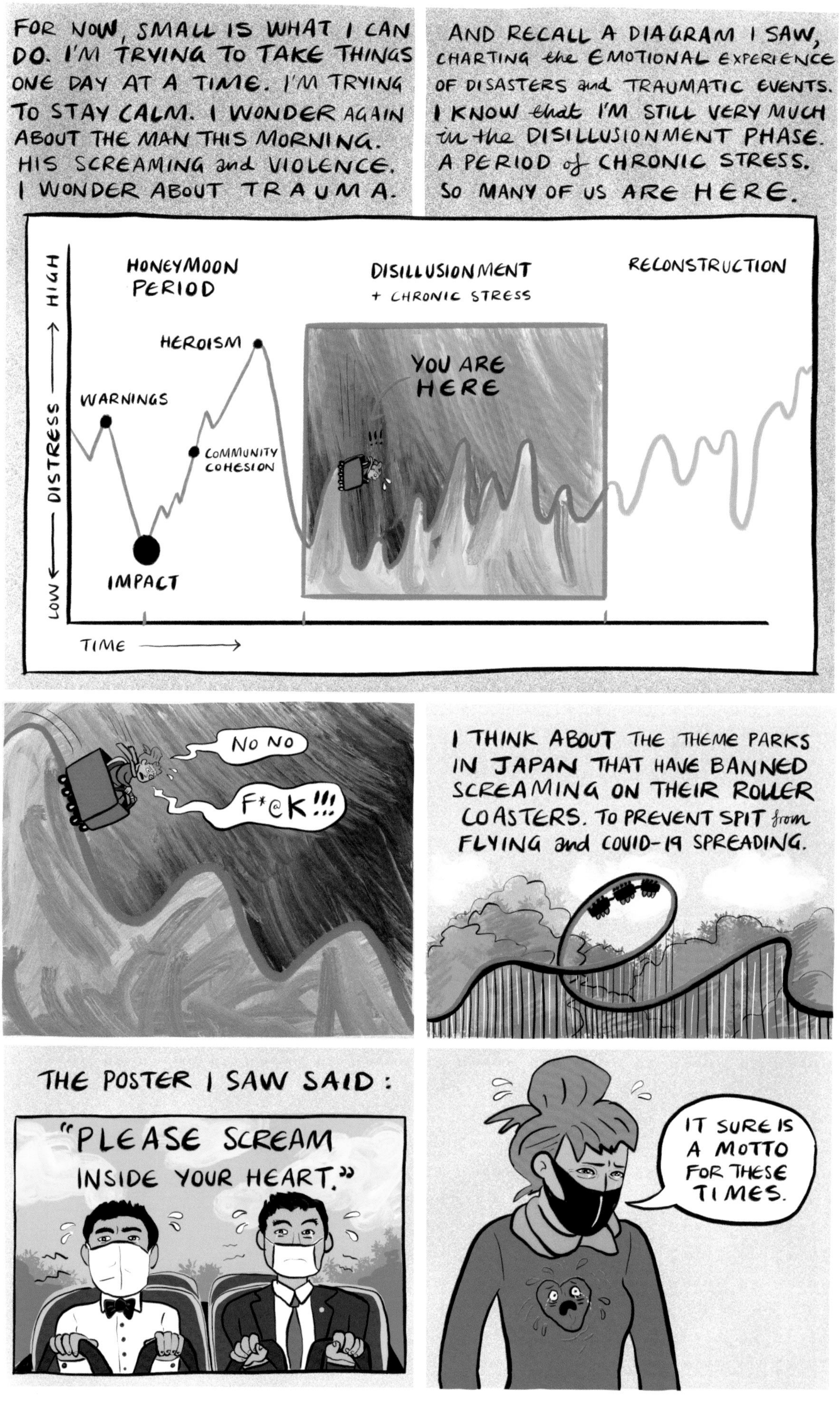

FOR NOW, SMALL IS WHAT I CAN DO. I'M TRYING TO TAKE THINGS ONE DAY AT A TIME. I'M TRYING TO STAY CALM. I WONDER AGAIN ABOUT THE MAN THIS MORNING. HIS SCREAMING and VIOLENCE. I WONDER ABOUT TRAUMA.
AND RECALL A DIAGRAM I SAW, CHARTING the EMOTIONAL EXPERIENCE OF DISASTERS and TRAUMATIC EVENTS. I KNOW that I'M STILL VERY MUCH in the DISILLUSIONMENT PHASE. A PERIOD of CHRONIC STRESS. SO MANY OF US ARE HERE.
HONEYMOON PERIOD
DISILLUSIONMENT + CHRONIC STRESS
RECONSTRUCTION
HEROISM
WARNINGS
COMMUNITY COHESION
IMPACT
YOU ARE HERE
!!!
LOW ← DISTRESS → HIGH
TIME →
No No
F*@K!!!
I THINK ABOUT THE THEME PARKS IN JAPAN THAT HAVE BANNED SCREAMING ON THEIR ROLLER COASTERS. TO PREVENT SPIT from FLYING and COVID-19 SPREADING.
THE POSTER I SAW SAID:
"PLEASE SCREAM INSIDE YOUR HEART."
IT SURE IS A MOTTO FOR THESE TIMES.

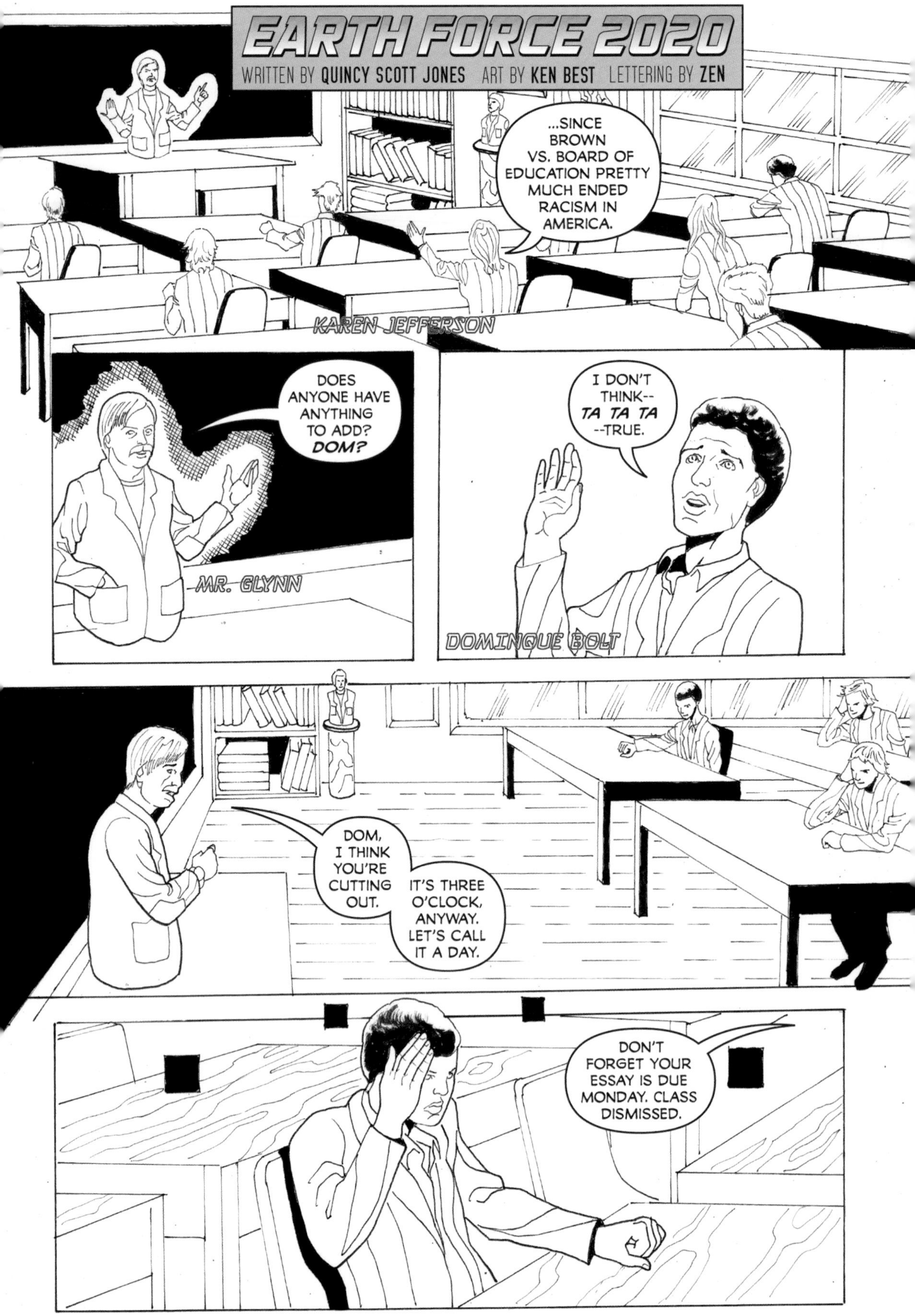
EARTH FORCE 2020
WRITTEN BY QUINCY SCOTT JONES ART BY KEN BEST LETTERING BY ZEN
...SINCE BROWN VS. BOARD OF EDUCATION PRETTY MUCH ENDED RACISM IN AMERICA.
KAREN JEFFERSON
DOES ANYONE HAVE ANYTHING TO ADD? DOM?
MR. GLYNN
I DON'T THINK-- TA TA TA --TRUE.
DOMINQUE BOLT
DOM, I THINK YOU'RE CUTTING OUT.
IT'S THREE O'CLOCK, ANYWAY. LET'S CALL IT A DAY.
DON'T FORGET YOUR ESSAY IS DUE MONDAY. CLASS DISMISSED.

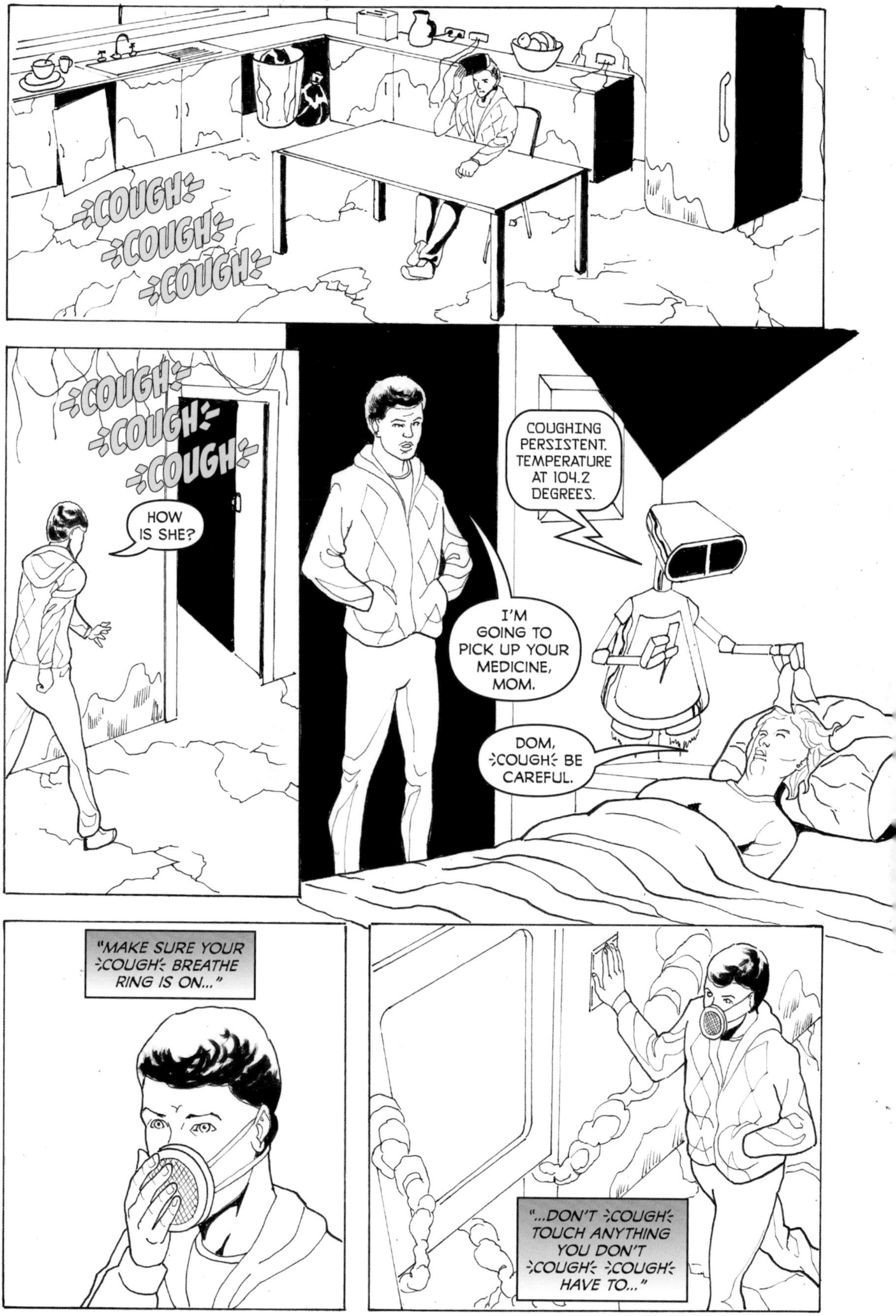
COUGH
COUGH
COUGH
COUGH
COUGH
COUGH
HOW IS SHE?
COUGHING PERSISTENT. TEMPERATURE AT 104.2 DEGREES.
I'M GOING TO PICK UP YOUR MEDICINE, MOM.
DOM, COUGH BE CAREFUL.
"MAKE SURE YOUR COUGH BREATHE RING IS ON..."
"...DON'T COUGH TOUCH ANYTHING YOU DON'T COUGH COUGH HAVE TO..."

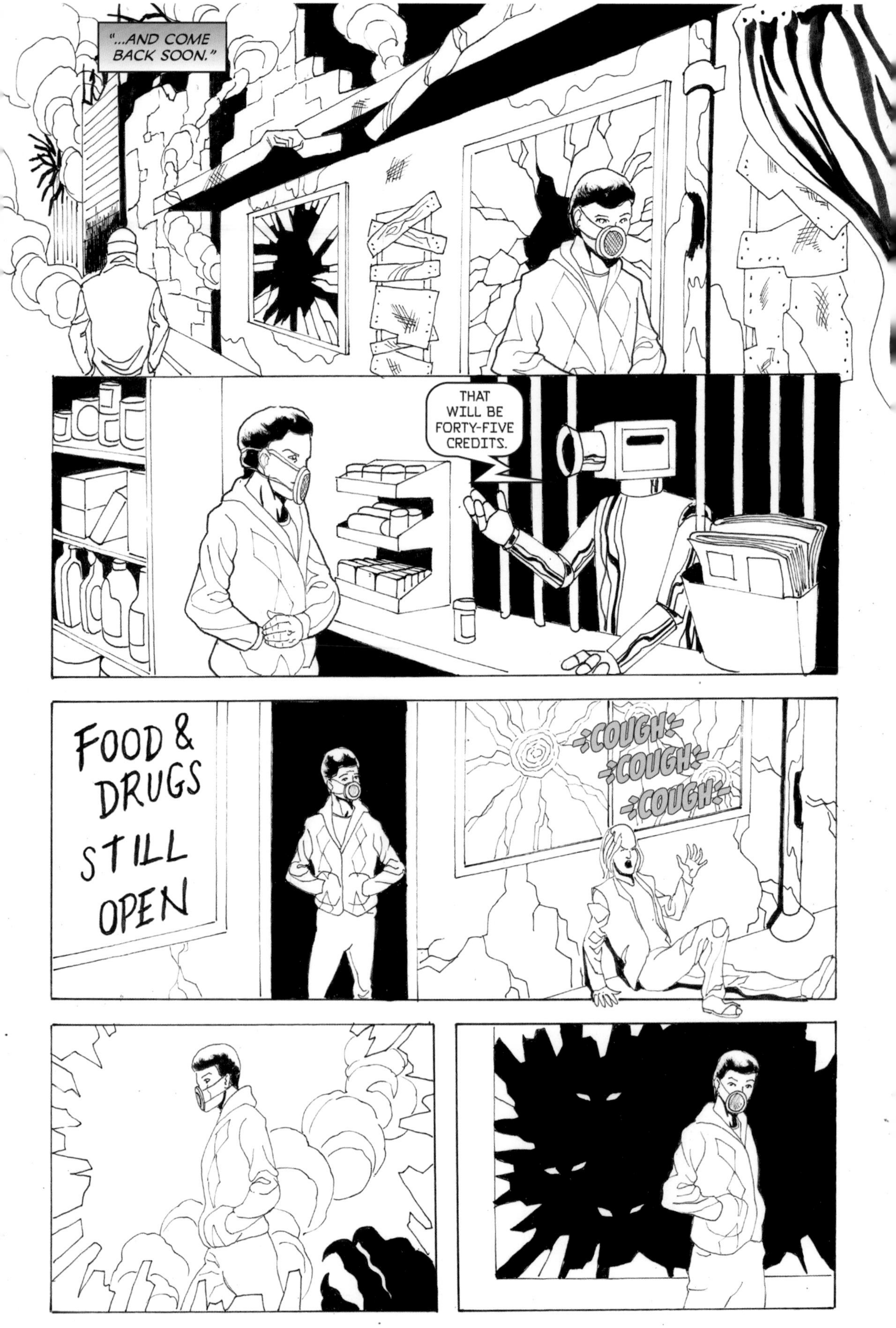
"...AND COME BACK SOON."
THAT WILL BE FORTY-FIVE CREDITS.
FOOD & DRUGS STILL OPEN
COUGH
COUGH
COUGH

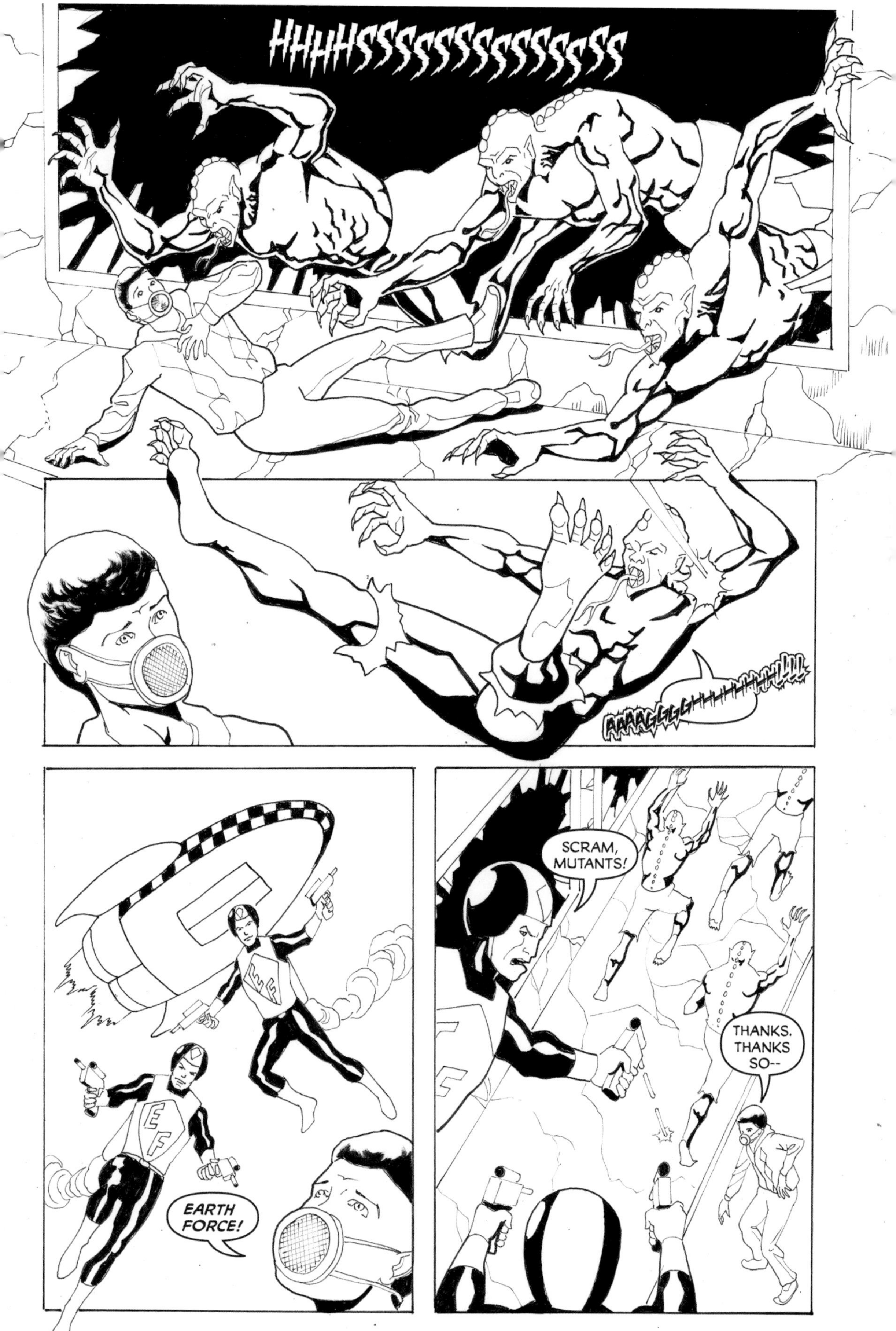
HHHHSSSSSSSSSSSSSS
AAAAAGGGGHHHHHHHHH!!!
EARTH FORCE!
SCRAM, MUTANTS!
THANKS. THANKS SO--

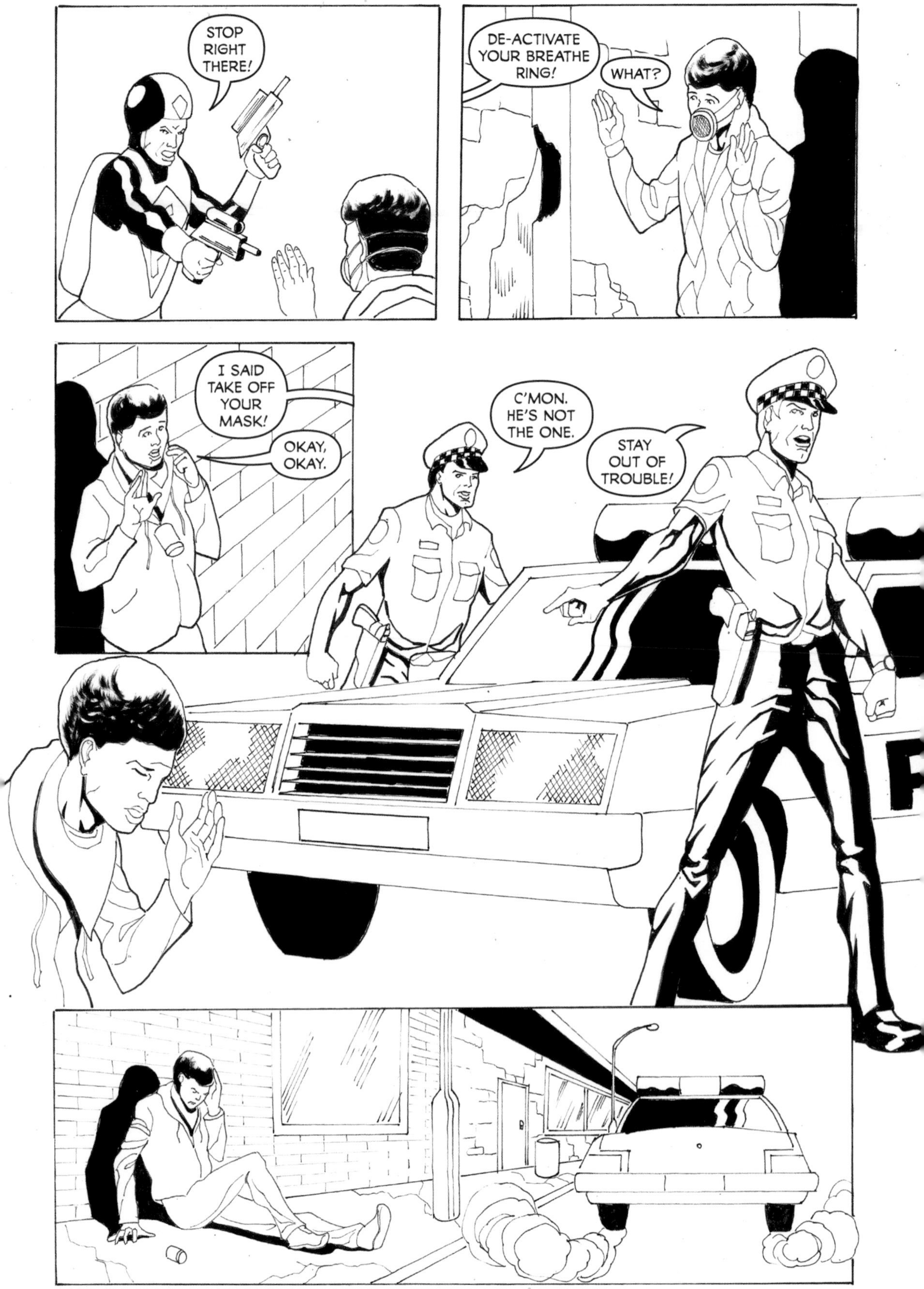
STOP RIGHT THERE!
DE-ACTIVATE YOUR BREATHE RING!
WHAT?
I SAID TAKE OFF YOUR MASK!
OKAY, OKAY.
C'MON. HE'S NOT THE ONE.
STAY OUT OF TROUBLE!

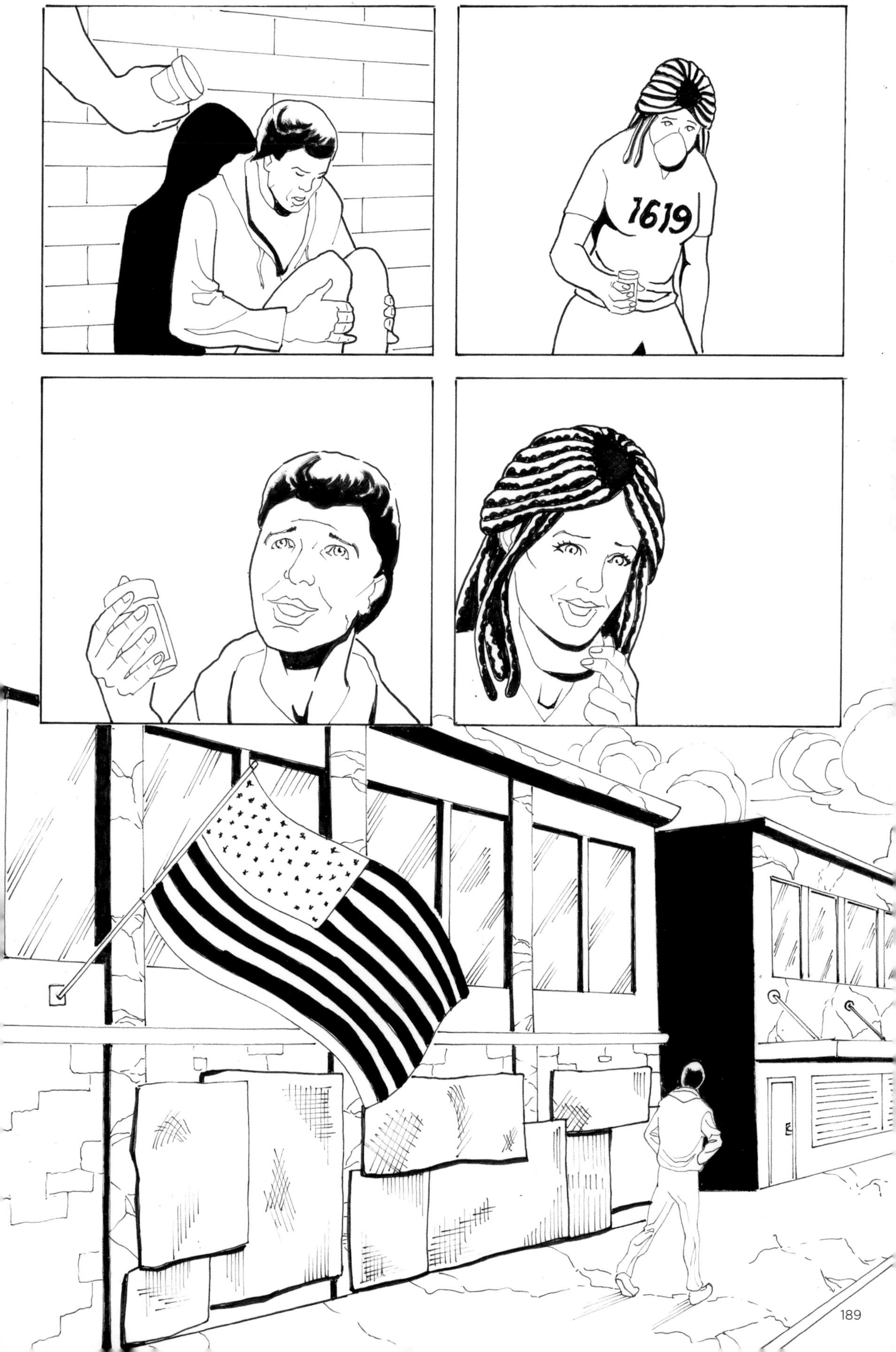
1619

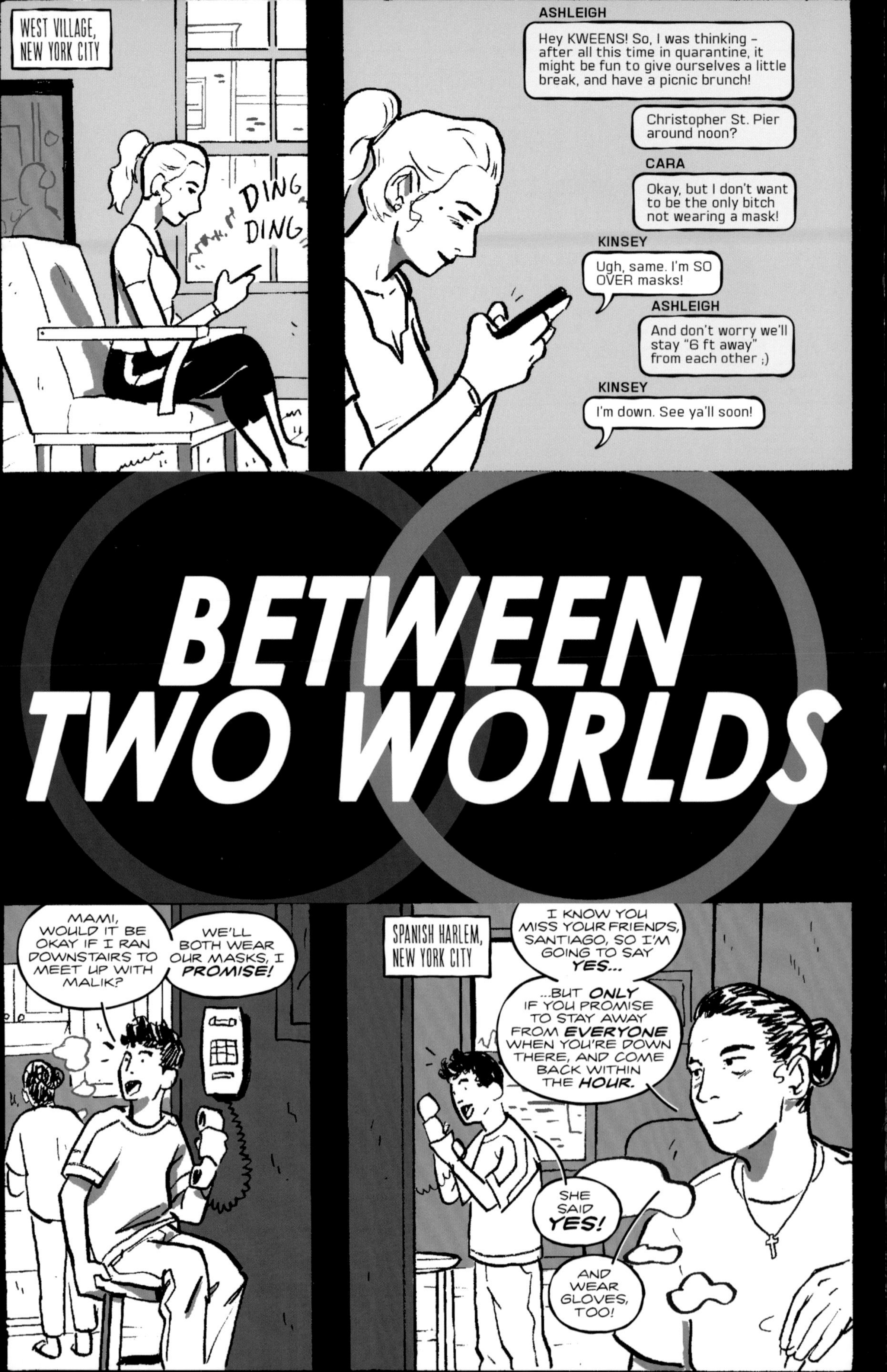
WEST VILLAGE, NEW YORK CITY
DING DING
ASHLEIGH
Hey KWEENS! So, I was thinking – after all this time in quarantine, it might be fun to give ourselves a little break, and have a picnic brunch!
Christopher St. Pier around noon?
CARA
Okay, but I don't want to be the only bitch not wearing a mask!
KINSEY
Ugh, same. I'm SO OVER masks!
ASHLEIGH
And don't worry we'll stay "6 ft away" from each other ;)
KINSEY
I'm down. See ya'll soon!
BETWEEN TWO WORLDS
MAMI, WOULD IT BE OKAY IF I RAN DOWNSTAIRS TO MEET UP WITH MALIK?
WE'LL BOTH WEAR OUR MASKS, I PROMISE!
SPANISH HARLEM, NEW YORK CITY
I KNOW YOU MISS YOUR FRIENDS, SANTIAGO, SO I'M GOING TO SAY YES...
...BUT ONLY IF YOU PROMISE TO STAY AWAY FROM EVERYONE WHEN YOU'RE DOWN THERE, AND COME BACK WITHIN THE HOUR.
SHE SAID YES!
AND WEAR GLOVES, TOO!

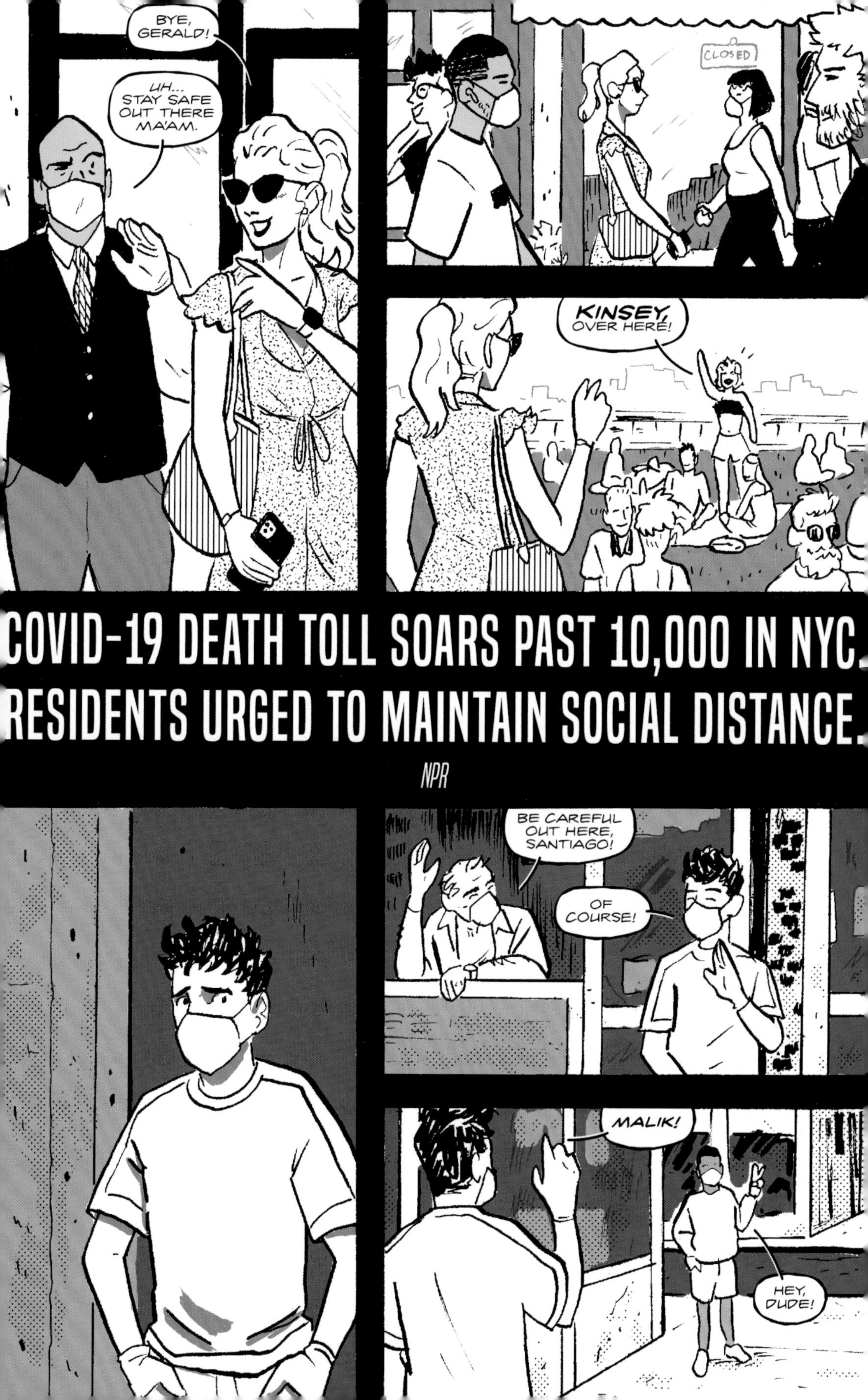
BYE, GERALD!
UH... STAY SAFE OUT THERE MA'AM.
CLOSED
KINSEY, OVER HERE!
COVID-19 DEATH TOLL SOARS PAST 10,000 IN NYC.
RESIDENTS URGED TO MAINTAIN SOCIAL DISTANCE.
NPR
BE CAREFUL OUT HERE, SANTIAGO!
OF COURSE!
MALIK!
HEY, DUDE!

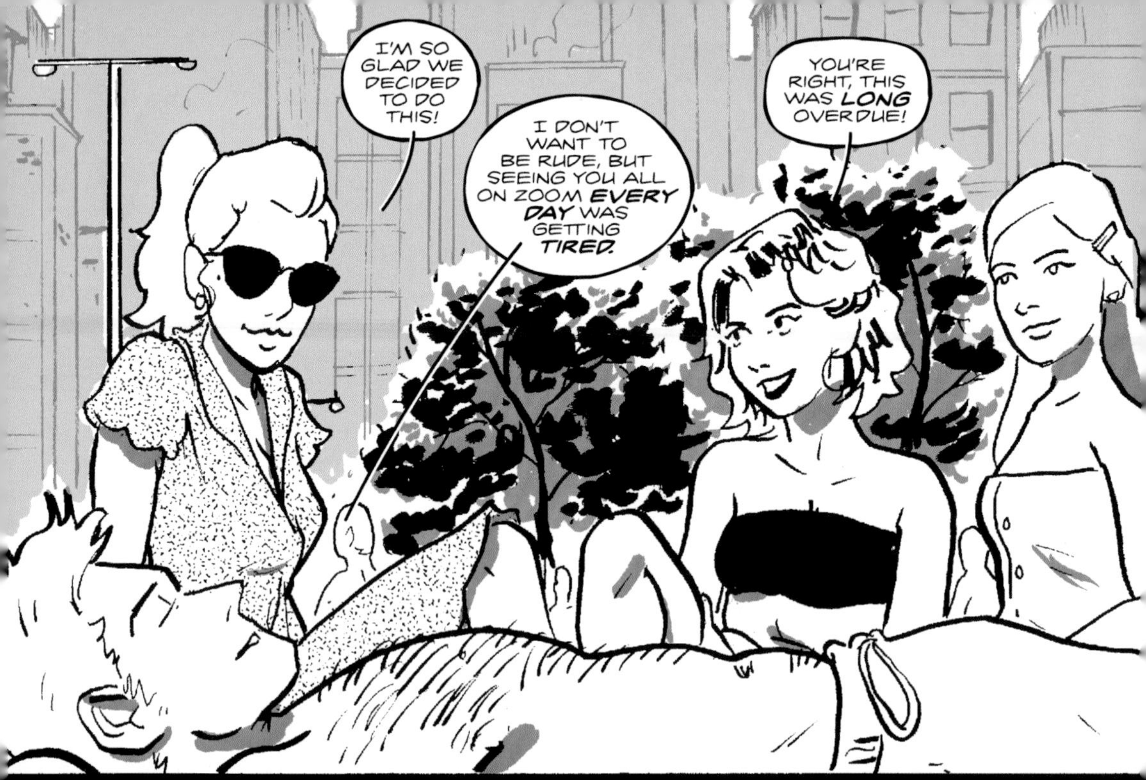
I'M SO GLAD WE DECIDED TO DO THIS!
I DON'T WANT TO BE RUDE, BUT SEEING YOU ALL ON ZOOM EVERY DAY WAS GETTING TIRED.
YOU'RE RIGHT, THIS WAS LONG OVERDUE!

NYC FACES SOCIAL TEST AS NICE WEATHER LURES MANY OUTSIDE

NY1 NEWS

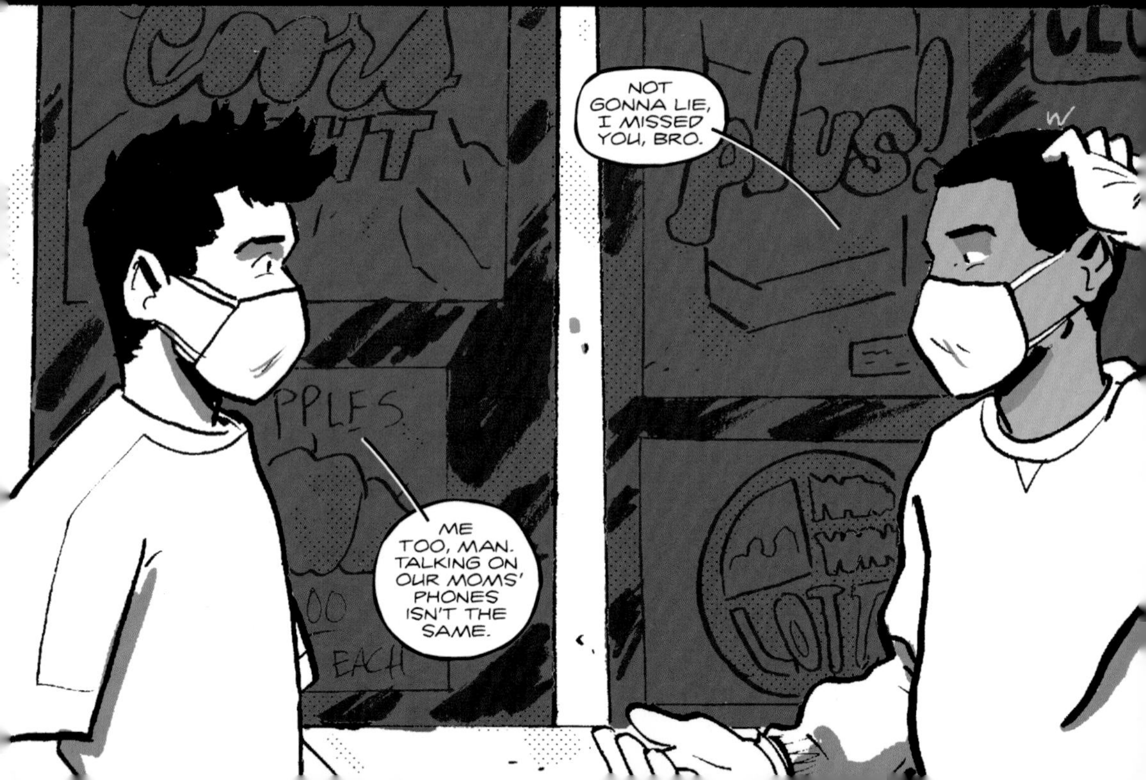
NOT GONNA LIE, I MISSED YOU, BRO.
ME TOO, MAN. TALKING ON OUR MOMS' PHONES ISN'T THE SAME.

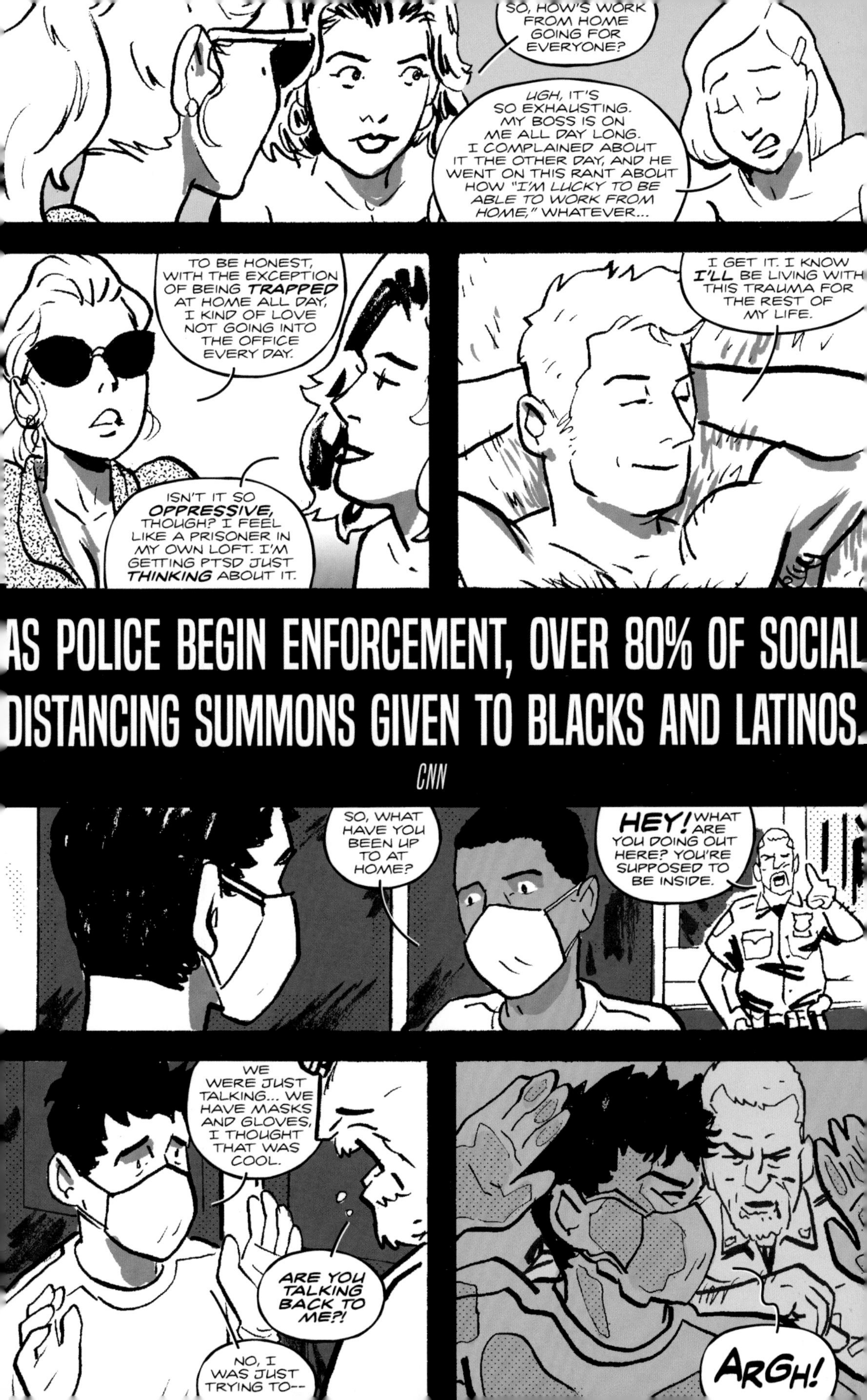
SO, HOW'S WORK FROM HOME GOING FOR EVERYONE?
UGH, IT'S SO EXHAUSTING. MY BOSS IS ON ME ALL DAY LONG. I COMPLAINED ABOUT IT THE OTHER DAY, AND HE WENT ON THIS RANT ABOUT HOW "I'M LUCKY TO BE ABLE TO WORK FROM HOME," WHATEVER...
TO BE HONEST, WITH THE EXCEPTION OF BEING TRAPPED AT HOME ALL DAY, I KIND OF LOVE NOT GOING INTO THE OFFICE EVERY DAY.
ISN'T IT SO OPPRESSIVE, THOUGH? I FEEL LIKE A PRISONER IN MY OWN LOFT. I'M GETTING PTSD JUST THINKING ABOUT IT.
I GET IT. I KNOW I'LL BE LIVING WITH THIS TRAUMA FOR THE REST OF MY LIFE.
AS POLICE BEGIN ENFORCEMENT, OVER 80% OF SOCIAL DISTANCING SUMMONS GIVEN TO BLACKS AND LATINOS.
CNN
SO, WHAT HAVE YOU BEEN UP TO AT HOME?
HEY! WHAT ARE YOU DOING OUT HERE? YOU'RE SUPPOSED TO BE INSIDE.
WE WERE JUST TALKING... WE HAVE MASKS AND GLOVES, I THOUGHT THAT WAS COOL.
ARE YOU TALKING BACK TO ME?!
NO, I WAS JUST TRYING TO--
ARGH!

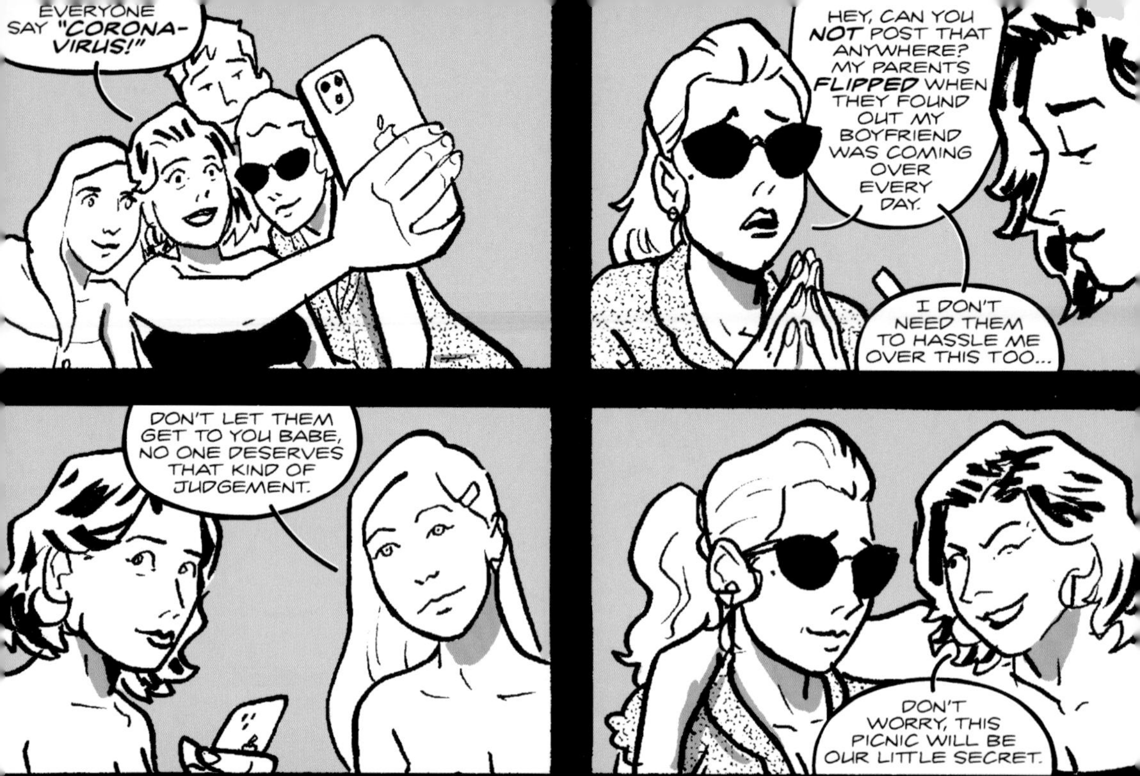
EVERYONE SAY "CORONA-VIRUS!"
HEY, CAN YOU NOT POST THAT ANYWHERE? MY PARENTS FLIPPED WHEN THEY FOUND OUT MY BOYFRIEND WAS COMING OVER EVERY DAY.
I DON'T NEED THEM TO HASSLE ME OVER THIS TOO...
DON'T LET THEM GET TO YOU BABE, NO ONE DESERVES THAT KIND OF JUDGEMENT.
DON'T WORRY, THIS PICNIC WILL BE OUR LITTLE SECRET.

DESPITE EVIDENCE, NYPD POLICE COMMISSIONER DENIES RACIAL BIAS IN CORONAVIRUS SOCIAL DISTANCING POLICIES.

THE NEW YORK TIMES

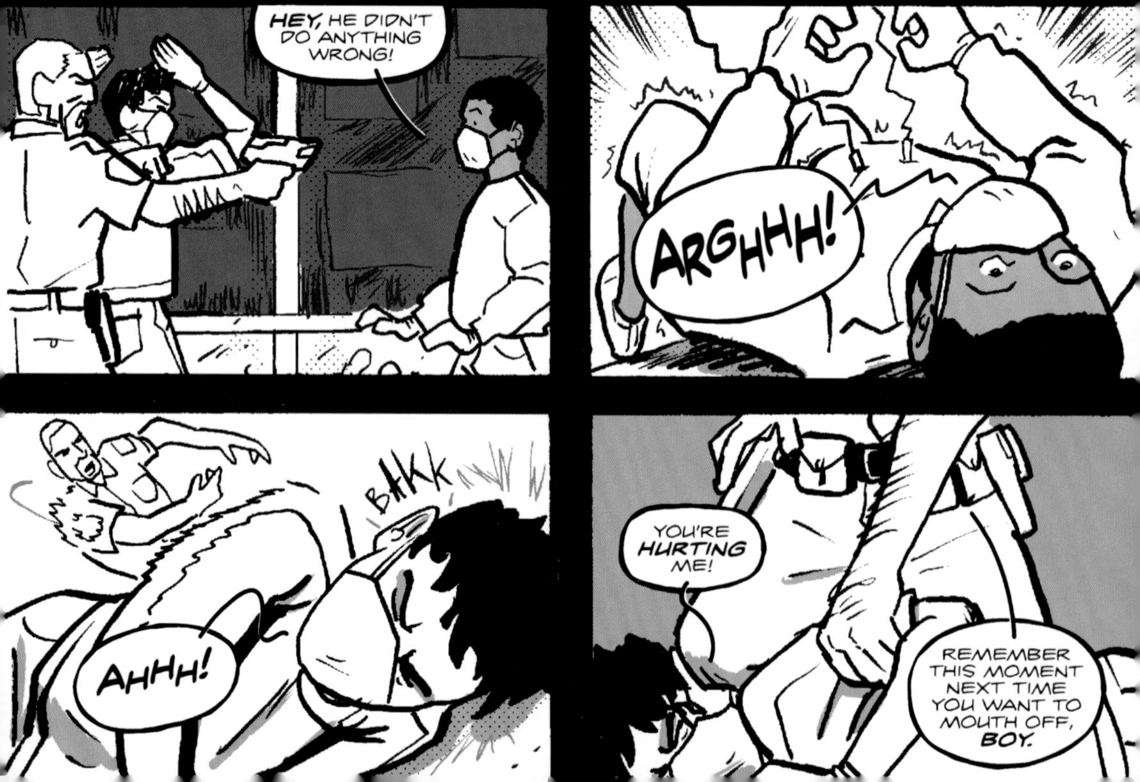
HEY, HE DIDN'T DO ANYTHING WRONG!
ARGHHH!
BAKK
AHHH!
YOU'RE HURTING ME!
REMEMBER THIS MOMENT NEXT TIME YOU WANT TO MOUTH OFF, BOY.

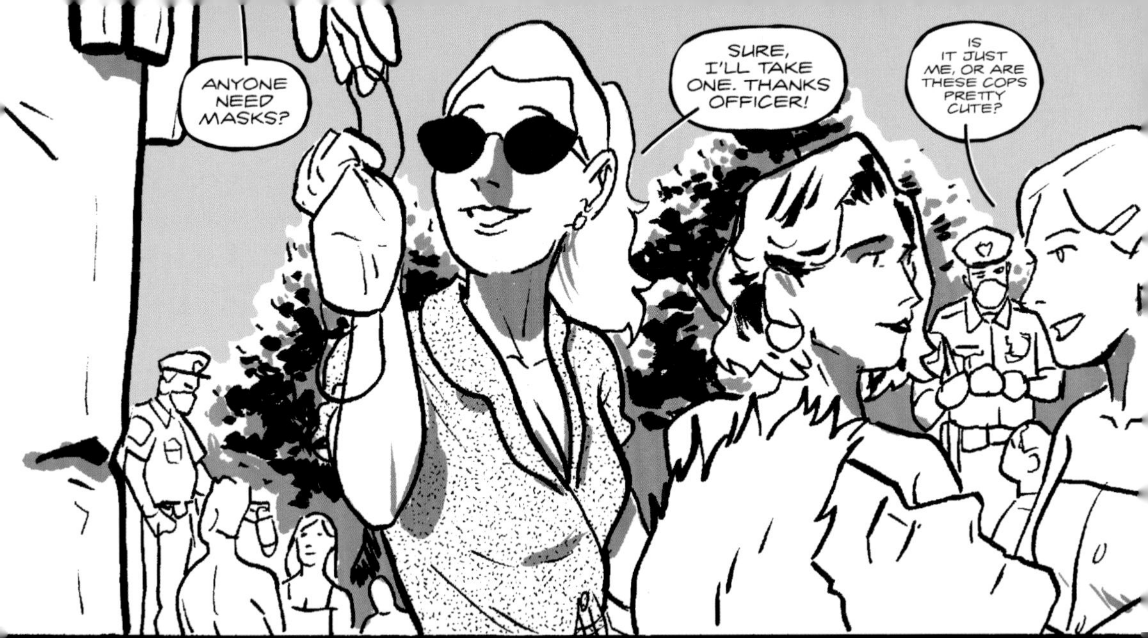
ANYONE NEED MASKS?
SURE, I'LL TAKE ONE. THANKS OFFICER!
IS IT JUST ME, OR ARE THESE COPS PRETTY CUTE?

INSPIRED BY TRUE EVENTS
NEW YORK CITY, *AMERIKKKA*

WRITTEN BY **JULIO ANTA**

ILLUSTRATED BY **JACOBY SALCEDO**

LETTERED BY **HASSAN OTSMANE-ELHAOU**

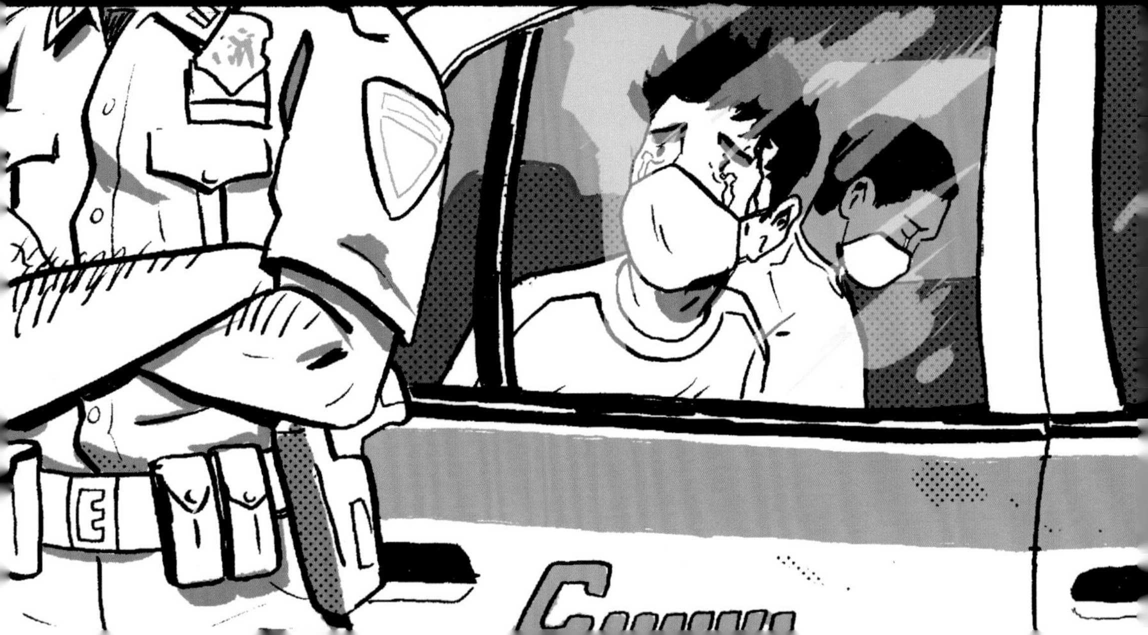

Early in the pandemic, I was terrified that both my parents would die of COVID.

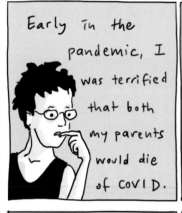

One horrible day in March, I learned within minutes that they'd both been exposed.

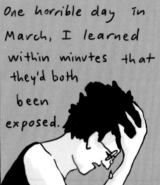

Mercifully, neither was infected and both are still alive. My mom is even thriving.

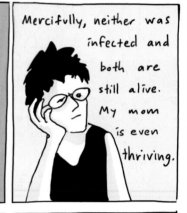

But I received news yesterday of a beloved uncle's death after a long struggle with Alzheimer's disease.

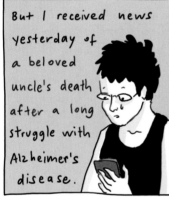

He made his career as a lawyer in the US Justice Department, but his passion was theater. He was a brilliant comic actor with an acerbic wit. I always felt we shared a special bond. The last time we saw one another, he could no longer speak. So —

we made faces instead.

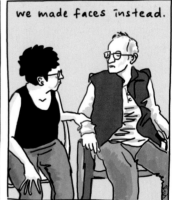

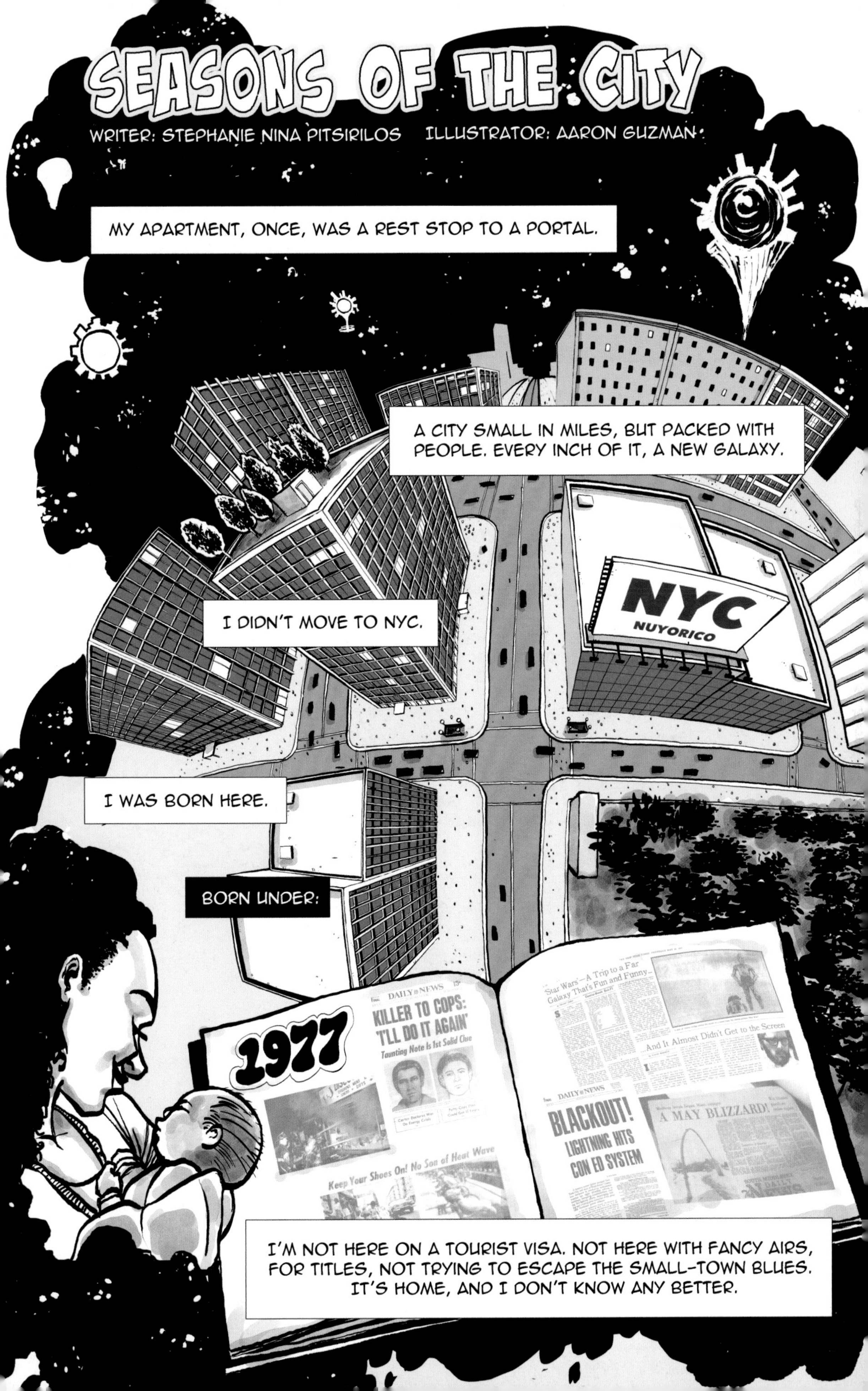
SEASONS OF THE CITY
WRITER: STEPHANIE NINA PITSIRILOS ILLUSTRATOR: AARON GUZMAN
MY APARTMENT, ONCE, WAS A REST STOP TO A PORTAL.
A CITY SMALL IN MILES, BUT PACKED WITH PEOPLE. EVERY INCH OF IT, A NEW GALAXY.
NYC
NUYORICO
I DIDN'T MOVE TO NYC.
I WAS BORN HERE.
BORN UNDER:
1977
DAILY NEWS
KILLER TO COPS: 'I'LL DO IT AGAIN'
Taunting Note Is 1st Solid Clue
Keep Your Shoes On! No Son of Heat Wave
'Star Wars'—A Trip to a Far Galaxy That's Fun and Funny...
...And It Almost Didn't Get to the Screen
DAILY NEWS
BLACKOUT! LIGHTNING HITS CON ED SYSTEM
A MAY BLIZZARD!
I'M NOT HERE ON A TOURIST VISA. NOT HERE WITH FANCY AIRS, FOR TITLES, NOT TRYING TO ESCAPE THE SMALL-TOWN BLUES. IT'S HOME, AND I DON'T KNOW ANY BETTER.

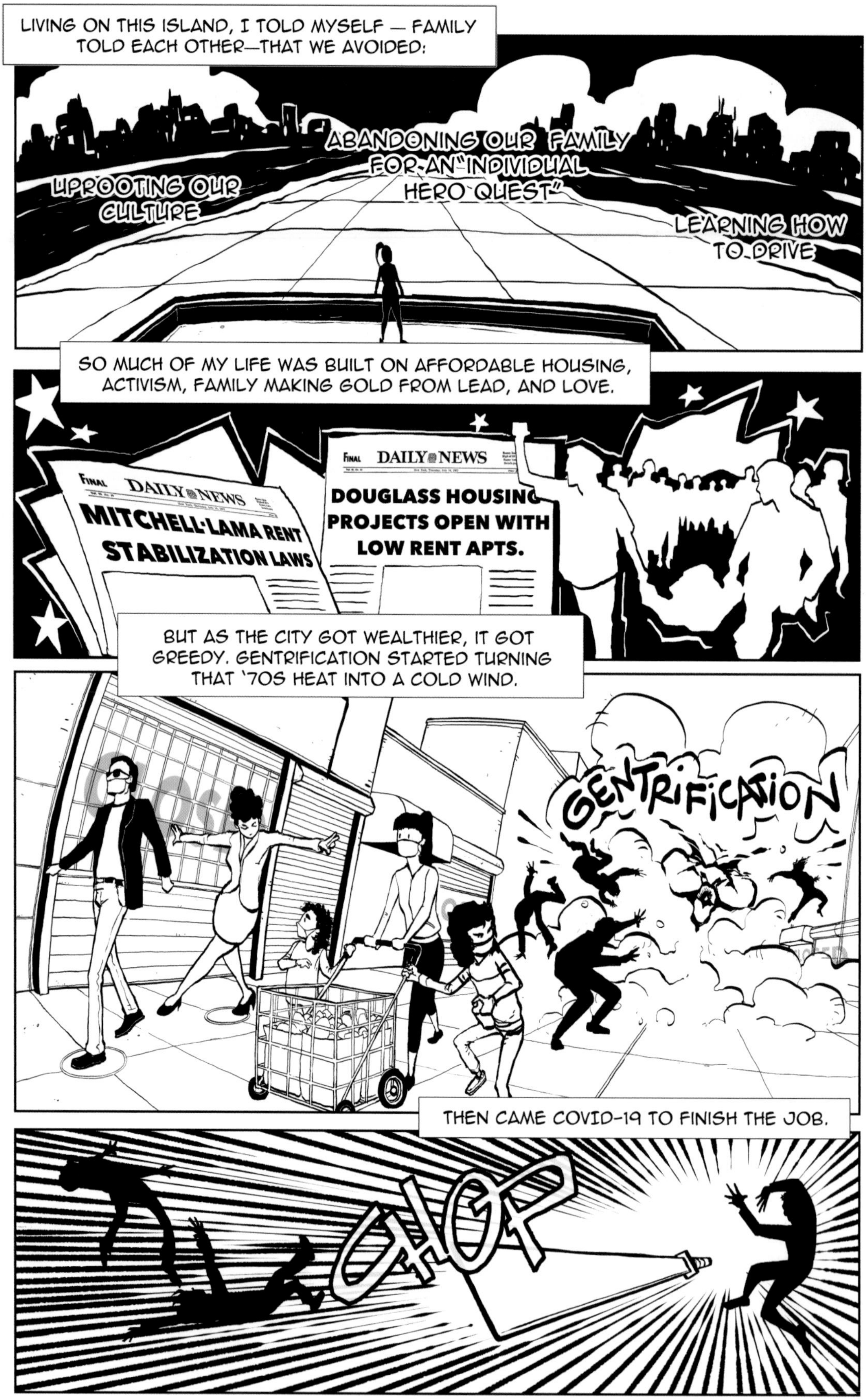
LIVING ON THIS ISLAND, I TOLD MYSELF — FAMILY TOLD EACH OTHER—THAT WE AVOIDED:
UPROOTING OUR CULTURE
ABANDONING OUR FAMILY FOR AN "INDIVIDUAL HERO QUEST"
LEARNING HOW TO DRIVE
SO MUCH OF MY LIFE WAS BUILT ON AFFORDABLE HOUSING, ACTIVISM, FAMILY MAKING GOLD FROM LEAD, AND LOVE.
FINAL DAILY NEWS
MITCHELL-LAMA RENT STABILIZATION LAWS
FINAL DAILY NEWS
DOUGLASS HOUSING PROJECTS OPEN WITH LOW RENT APTS.
BUT AS THE CITY GOT WEALTHIER, IT GOT GREEDY. GENTRIFICATION STARTED TURNING THAT '70S HEAT INTO A COLD WIND.
GENTRIFICATION
THEN CAME COVID-19 TO FINISH THE JOB.
CHOP

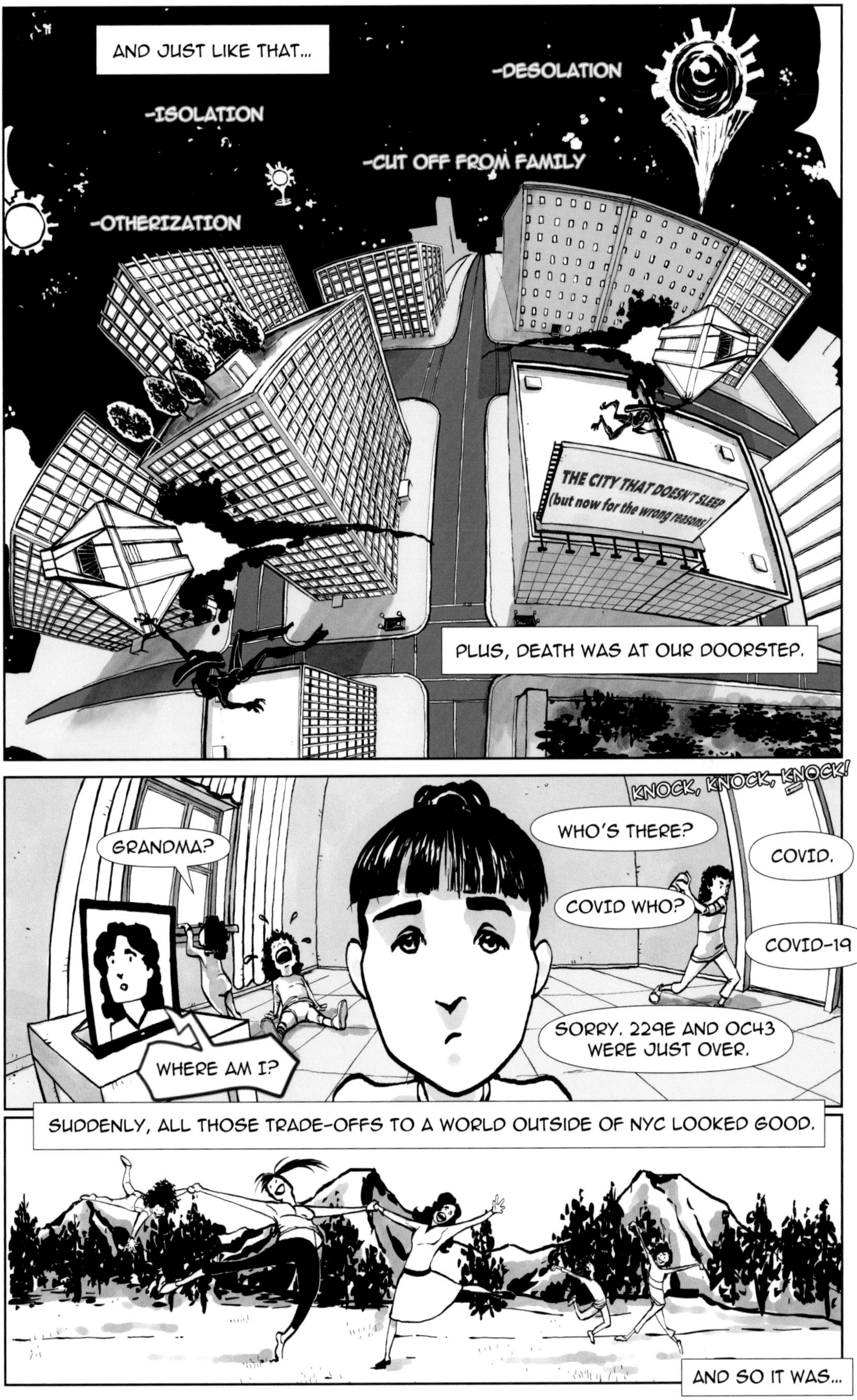
AND JUST LIKE THAT...
-ISOLATION
-DESOLATION
-CUT OFF FROM FAMILY
-OTHERIZATION
THE CITY THAT DOESN'T SLEEP
(but now for the wrong reasons)
PLUS, DEATH WAS AT OUR DOORSTEP.
KNOCK, KNOCK, KNOCK!
WHO'S THERE?
COVID.
COVID WHO?
COVID-19
SORRY. 229E AND OC43 WERE JUST OVER.
GRANDMA?
WHERE AM I?
SUDDENLY, ALL THOSE TRADE-OFFS TO A WORLD OUTSIDE OF NYC LOOKED GOOD.
AND SO IT WAS...

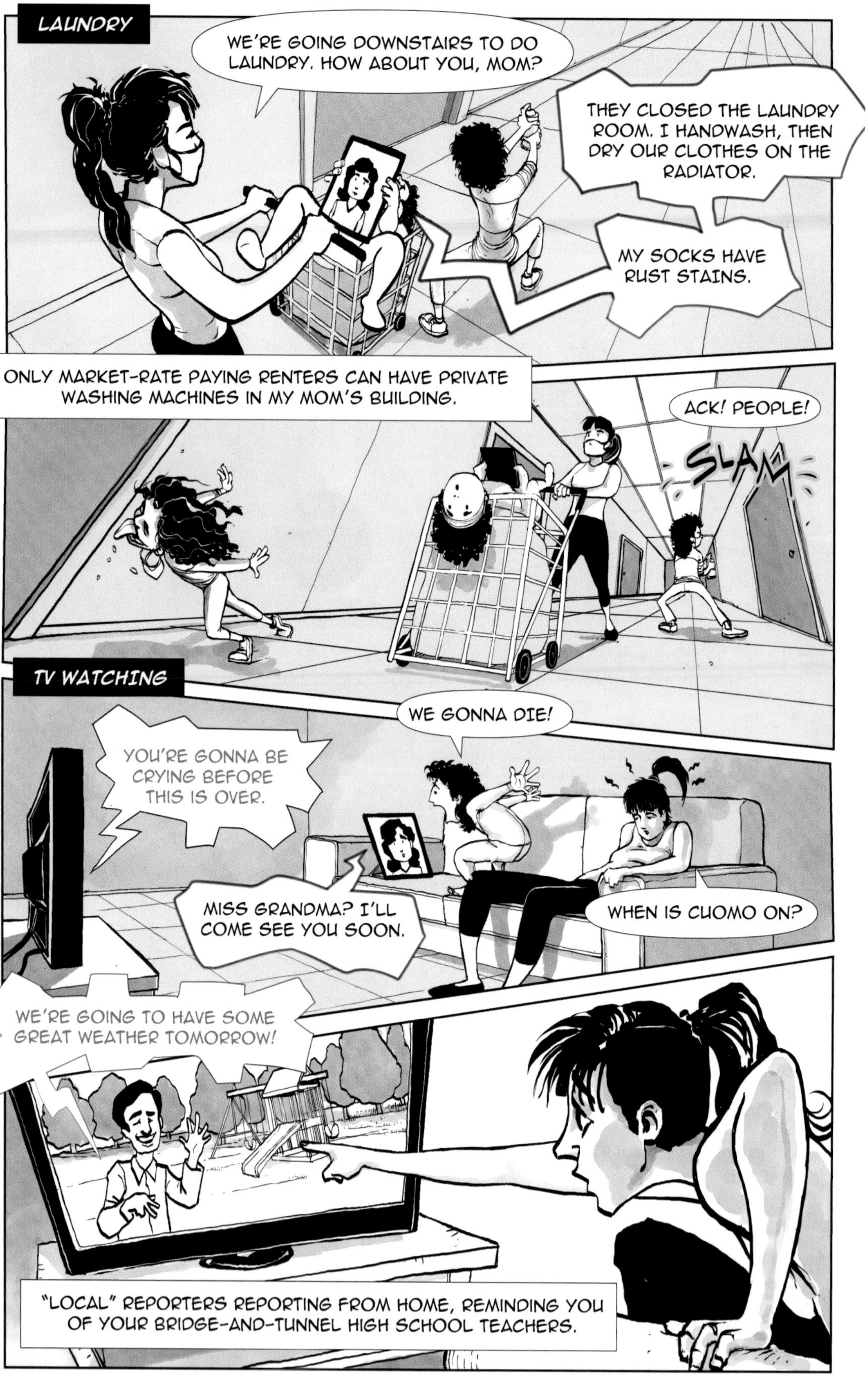
LAUNDRY
WE'RE GOING DOWNSTAIRS TO DO LAUNDRY. HOW ABOUT YOU, MOM?
THEY CLOSED THE LAUNDRY ROOM. I HANDWASH, THEN DRY OUR CLOTHES ON THE RADIATOR.
MY SOCKS HAVE RUST STAINS.
ONLY MARKET-RATE PAYING RENTERS CAN HAVE PRIVATE WASHING MACHINES IN MY MOM'S BUILDING.
ACK! PEOPLE!
SLAM
TV WATCHING
WE GONNA DIE!
YOU'RE GONNA BE CRYING BEFORE THIS IS OVER.
MISS GRANDMA? I'LL COME SEE YOU SOON.
WHEN IS CUOMO ON?
WE'RE GOING TO HAVE SOME GREAT WEATHER TOMORROW!
"LOCAL" REPORTERS REPORTING FROM HOME, REMINDING YOU OF YOUR BRIDGE-AND-TUNNEL HIGH SCHOOL TEACHERS.

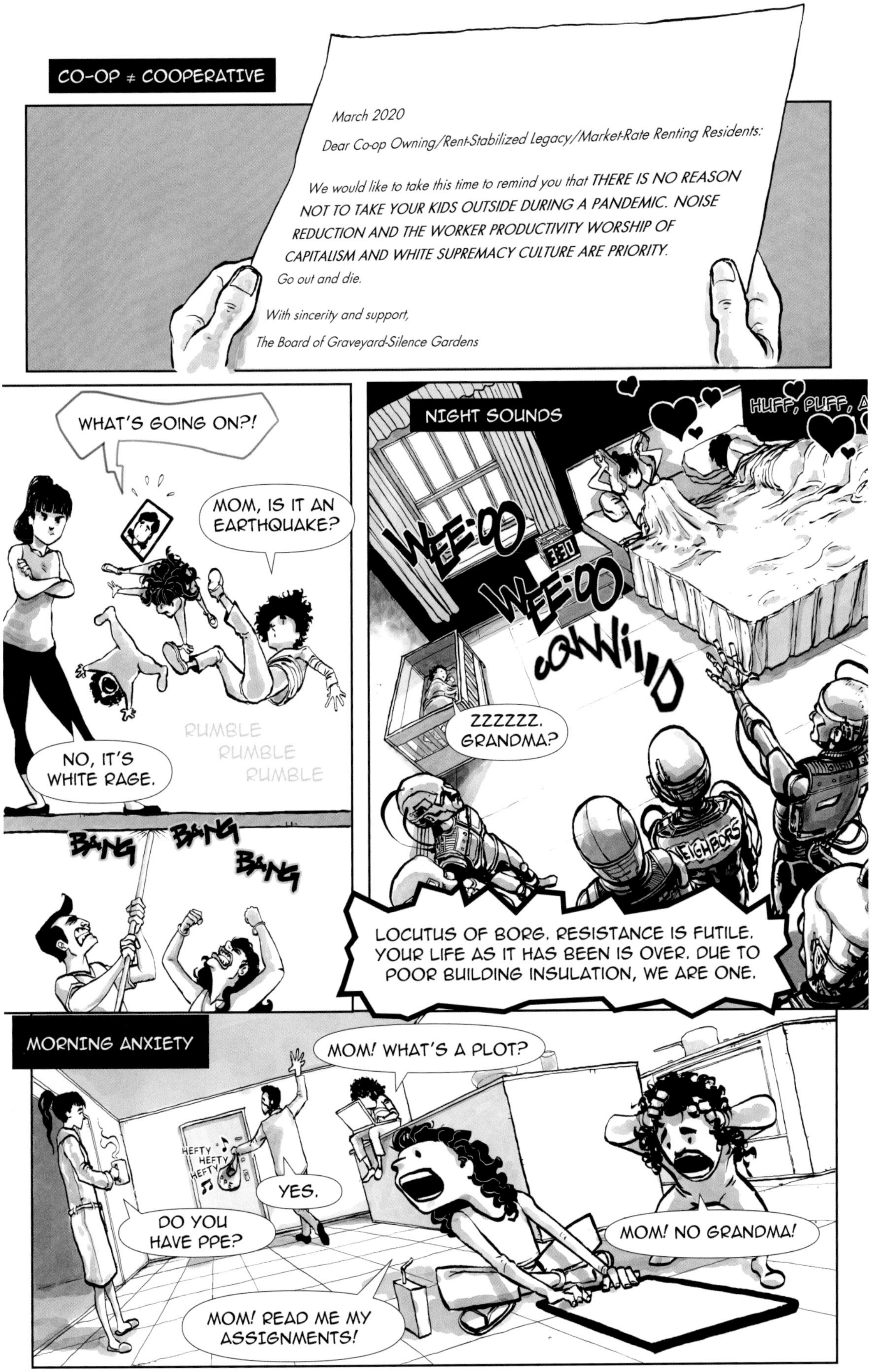

CO-OP ≠ COOPERATIVE
March 2020
Dear Co-op Owning/Rent-Stabilized Legacy/Market-Rate Renting Residents:
We would like to take this time to remind you that THERE IS NO REASON NOT TO TAKE YOUR KIDS OUTSIDE DURING A PANDEMIC. NOISE REDUCTION AND THE WORKER PRODUCTIVITY WORSHIP OF CAPITALISM AND WHITE SUPREMACY CULTURE ARE PRIORITY.
Go out and die.
With sincerity and support,
The Board of Graveyard-Silence Gardens
WHAT'S GOING ON?!
MOM, IS IT AN EARTHQUAKE?
NO, IT'S WHITE RAGE.
RUMBLE
RUMBLE
RUMBLE
BANG
BANG
BANG
NIGHT SOUNDS
HUFF, PUFF,
WEE-OO
3:30
WEE-OO
ZZZZZZ. GRANDMA?
NEIGHBORS
LOCUTUS OF BORG. RESISTANCE IS FUTILE. YOUR LIFE AS IT HAS BEEN IS OVER. DUE TO POOR BUILDING INSULATION, WE ARE ONE.
MORNING ANXIETY
MOM! WHAT'S A PLOT?
HEFTY
HEFTY
HEFTY
YES.
DO YOU HAVE PPE?
MOM! NO GRANDMA!
MOM! READ ME MY ASSIGNMENTS!

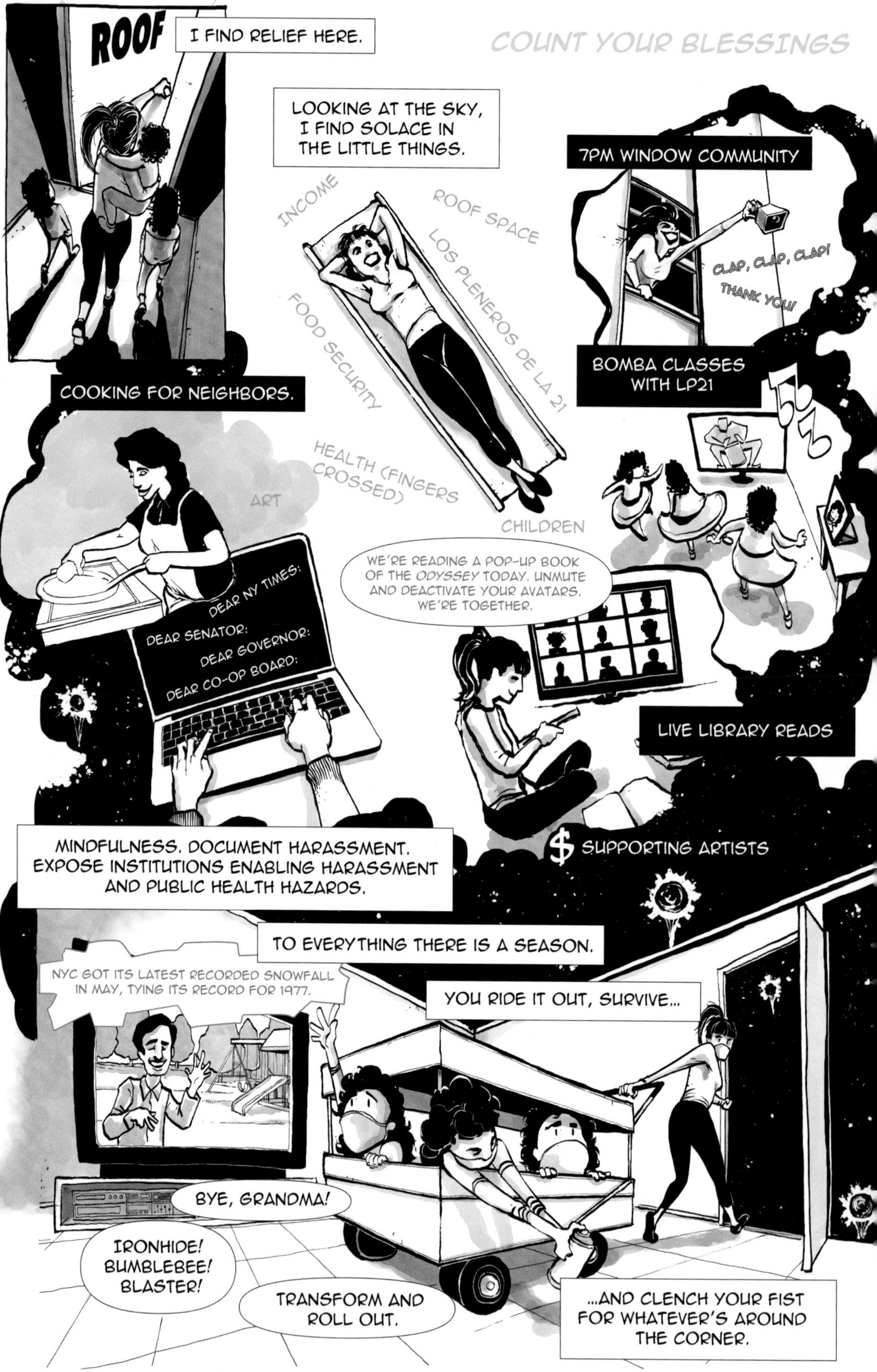
COUNT YOUR BLESSINGS
ROOF
I FIND RELIEF HERE.
LOOKING AT THE SKY, I FIND SOLACE IN THE LITTLE THINGS.
INCOME
ROOF SPACE
LOS PLENEROS DE LA 21
FOOD SECURITY
HEALTH (FINGERS CROSSED)
ART
CHILDREN
7PM WINDOW COMMUNITY
CLAP, CLAP, CLAP!
THANK YOU!
BOMBA CLASSES WITH LP21
COOKING FOR NEIGHBORS.
DEAR NY TIMES:
DEAR SENATOR:
DEAR GOVERNOR:
DEAR CO-OP BOARD:
WE'RE READING A POP-UP BOOK OF THE *ODYSSEY* TODAY. UNMUTE AND DEACTIVATE YOUR AVATARS. WE'RE TOGETHER.
LIVE LIBRARY READS
MINDFULNESS. DOCUMENT HARASSMENT. EXPOSE INSTITUTIONS ENABLING HARASSMENT AND PUBLIC HEALTH HAZARDS.
$ SUPPORTING ARTISTS
TO EVERYTHING THERE IS A SEASON.
NYC GOT ITS LATEST RECORDED SNOWFALL IN MAY, TYING ITS RECORD FOR 1977.
YOU RIDE IT OUT, SURVIVE...
BYE, GRANDMA!
IRONHIDE! BUMBLEBEE! BLASTER!
TRANSFORM AND ROLL OUT.
...AND CLENCH YOUR FIST FOR WHATEVER'S AROUND THE CORNER.

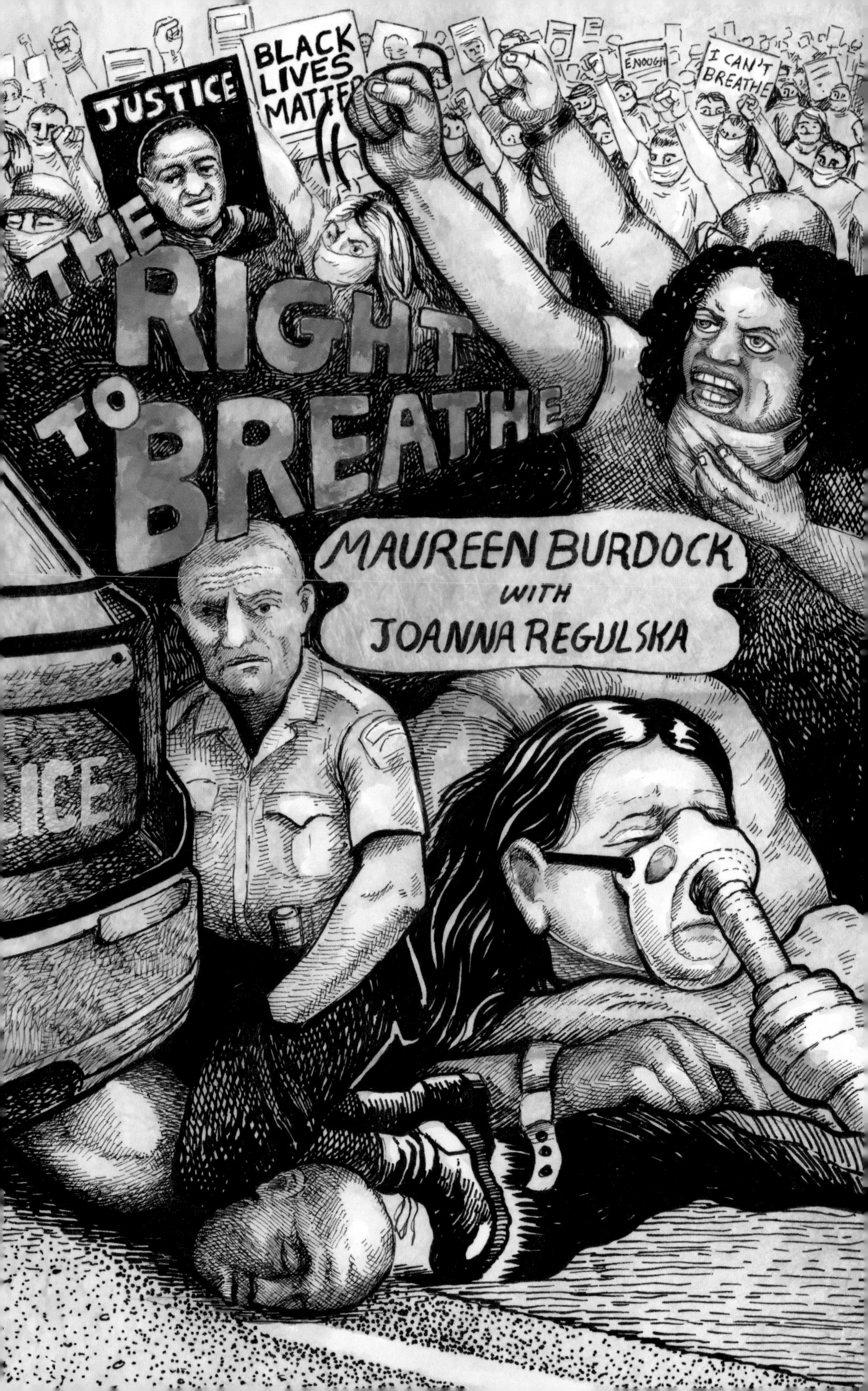
JUSTICE
BLACK LIVES MATTER
ENOUGH
I CAN'T BREATHE
THE RIGHT TO BREATHE
MAUREEN BURDOCK
WITH
JOANNA REGULSKA

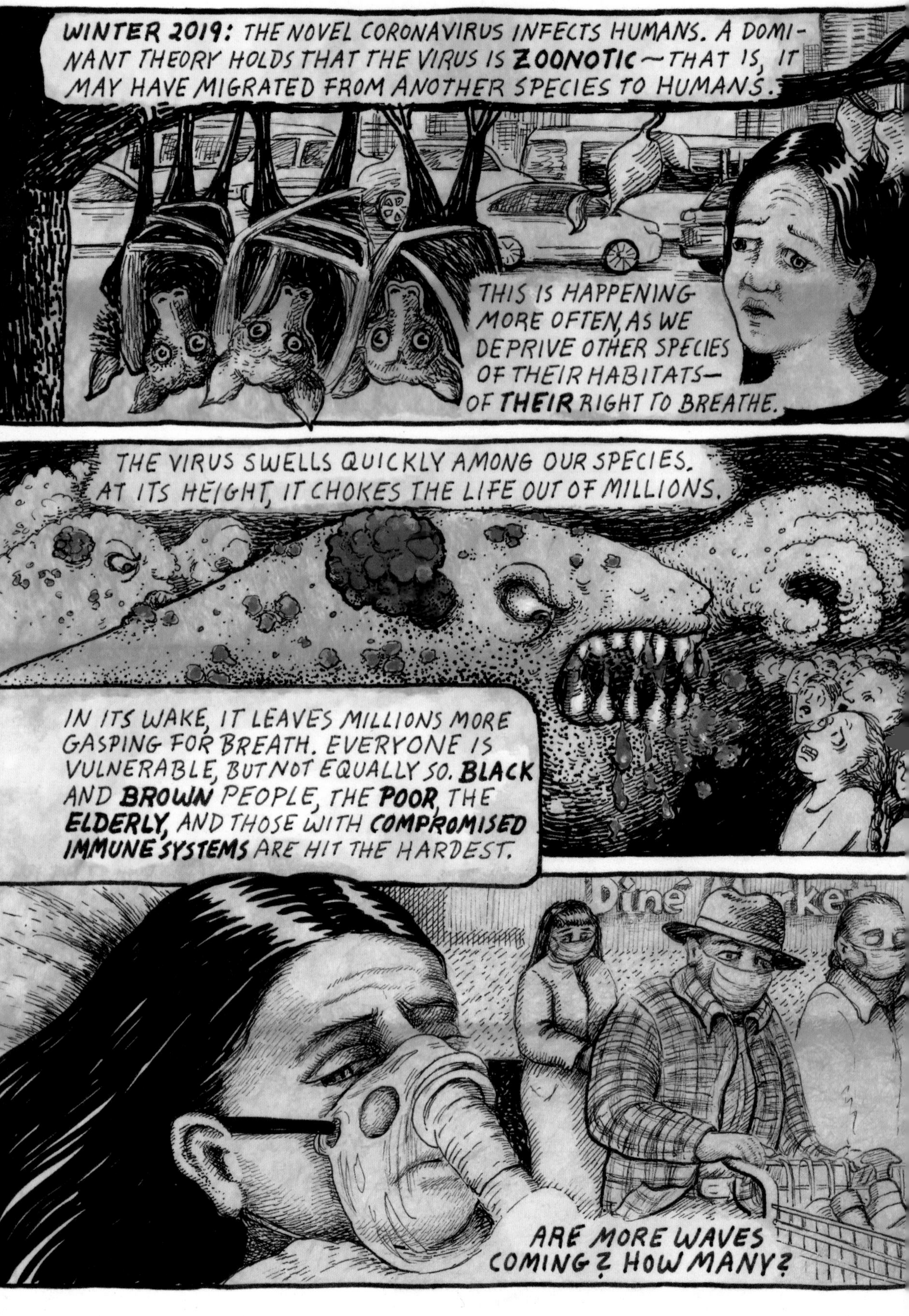
WINTER 2019: THE NOVEL CORONAVIRUS INFECTS HUMANS. A DOMINANT THEORY HOLDS THAT THE VIRUS IS ZOONOTIC—THAT IS, IT MAY HAVE MIGRATED FROM ANOTHER SPECIES TO HUMANS.
THIS IS HAPPENING MORE OFTEN, AS WE DEPRIVE OTHER SPECIES OF THEIR HABITATS—OF THEIR RIGHT TO BREATHE.
THE VIRUS SWELLS QUICKLY AMONG OUR SPECIES. AT ITS HEIGHT, IT CHOKES THE LIFE OUT OF MILLIONS.
IN ITS WAKE, IT LEAVES MILLIONS MORE GASPING FOR BREATH. EVERYONE IS VULNERABLE, BUT NOT EQUALLY SO. BLACK AND BROWN PEOPLE, THE POOR, THE ELDERLY, AND THOSE WITH COMPROMISED IMMUNE SYSTEMS ARE HIT THE HARDEST.
Diné
ARE MORE WAVES COMING? HOW MANY?

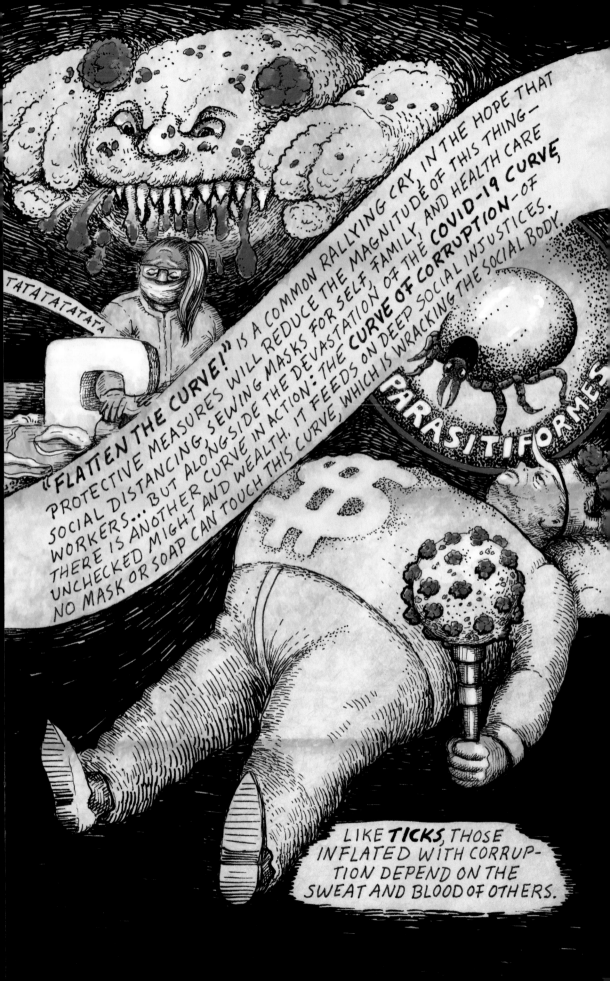

TATATATATATA

"FLATTEN THE CURVE!" IS A COMMON RALLYING CRY, IN THE HOPE THAT PROTECTIVE MEASURES WILL REDUCE THE MAGNITUDE OF THIS THING— SOCIAL DISTANCING, SEWING MASKS FOR SELF, FAMILY, AND HEALTH CARE WORKERS... BUT ALONGSIDE THE DEVASTATION OF THE COVID-19 CURVE, THERE IS ANOTHER CURVE IN ACTION: THE CURVE OF CORRUPTION—OF UNCHECKED MIGHT AND WEALTH, IT FEEDS ON DEEP SOCIAL INJUSTICES. NO MASK OR SOAP CAN TOUCH THIS CURVE, WHICH IS WRACKING THE SOCIAL BODY.

PARASITIFORMES

LIKE TICKS, THOSE INFLATED WITH CORRUPTION DEPEND ON THE SWEAT AND BLOOD OF OTHERS.

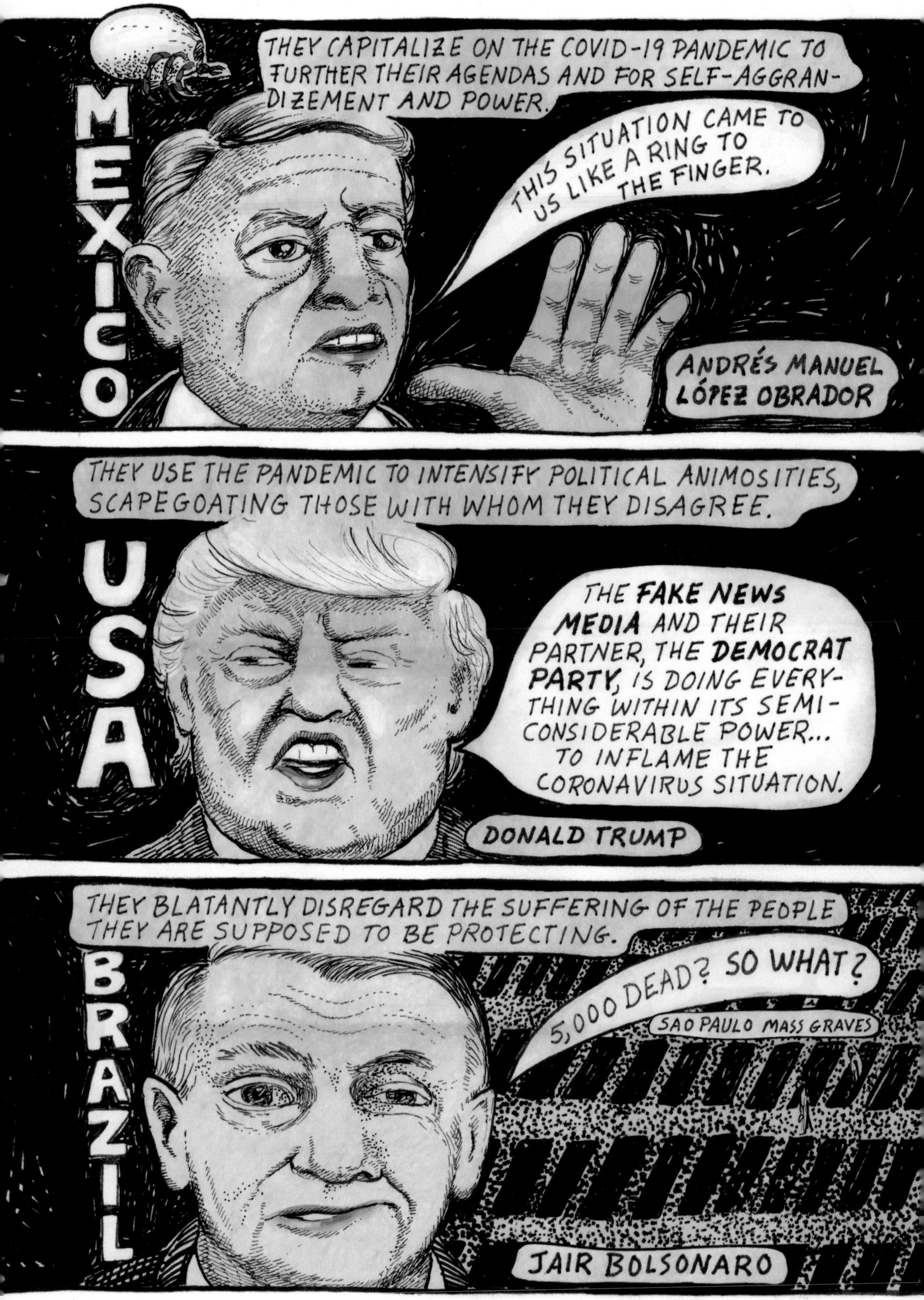
MEXICO
THEY CAPITALIZE ON THE COVID-19 PANDEMIC TO FURTHER THEIR AGENDAS AND FOR SELF-AGGRANDIZEMENT AND POWER.
THIS SITUATION CAME TO US LIKE A RING TO THE FINGER.
ANDRÉS MANUEL LÓPEZ OBRADOR
USA
THEY USE THE PANDEMIC TO INTENSIFY POLITICAL ANIMOSITIES, SCAPEGOATING THOSE WITH WHOM THEY DISAGREE.
THE **FAKE NEWS MEDIA** AND THEIR PARTNER, THE **DEMOCRAT PARTY**, IS DOING EVERYTHING WITHIN ITS SEMI-CONSIDERABLE POWER... TO INFLAME THE CORONAVIRUS SITUATION.
DONALD TRUMP
BRAZIL
THEY BLATANTLY DISREGARD THE SUFFERING OF THE PEOPLE THEY ARE SUPPOSED TO BE PROTECTING.
5,000 DEAD? SO WHAT?
SAO PAULO MASS GRAVES
JAIR BOLSONARO

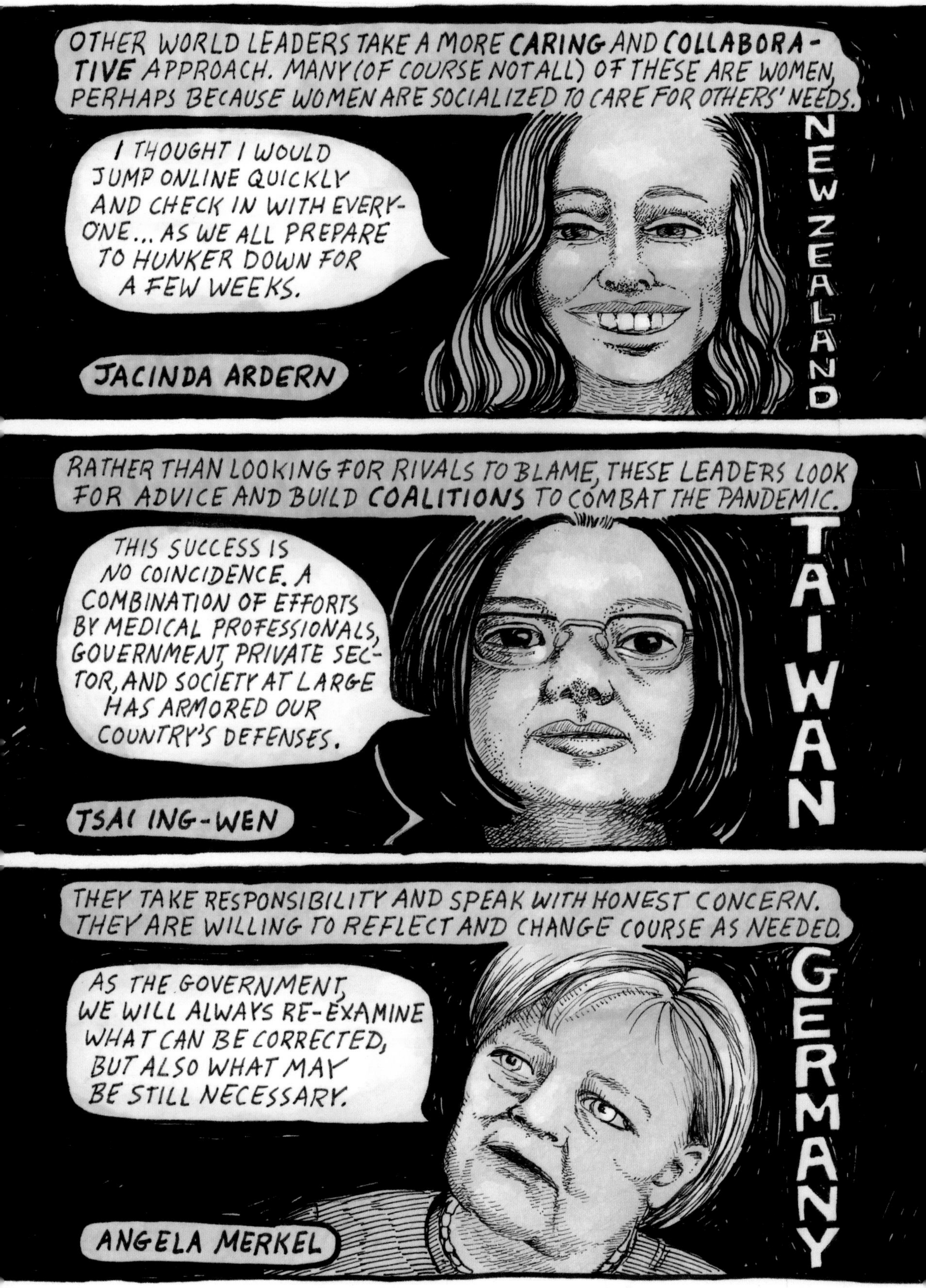
OTHER WORLD LEADERS TAKE A MORE CARING AND COLLABORATIVE APPROACH. MANY (OF COURSE NOT ALL) OF THESE ARE WOMEN, PERHAPS BECAUSE WOMEN ARE SOCIALIZED TO CARE FOR OTHERS' NEEDS.
I THOUGHT I WOULD JUMP ONLINE QUICKLY AND CHECK IN WITH EVERYONE... AS WE ALL PREPARE TO HUNKER DOWN FOR A FEW WEEKS.
JACINDA ARDERN
NEW ZEALAND
RATHER THAN LOOKING FOR RIVALS TO BLAME, THESE LEADERS LOOK FOR ADVICE AND BUILD COALITIONS TO COMBAT THE PANDEMIC.
THIS SUCCESS IS NO COINCIDENCE. A COMBINATION OF EFFORTS BY MEDICAL PROFESSIONALS, GOVERNMENT, PRIVATE SECTOR, AND SOCIETY AT LARGE HAS ARMORED OUR COUNTRY'S DEFENSES.
TSAI ING-WEN
TAIWAN
THEY TAKE RESPONSIBILITY AND SPEAK WITH HONEST CONCERN. THEY ARE WILLING TO REFLECT AND CHANGE COURSE AS NEEDED.
AS THE GOVERNMENT, WE WILL ALWAYS RE-EXAMINE WHAT CAN BE CORRECTED, BUT ALSO WHAT MAY BE STILL NECESSARY.
ANGELA MERKEL
GERMANY

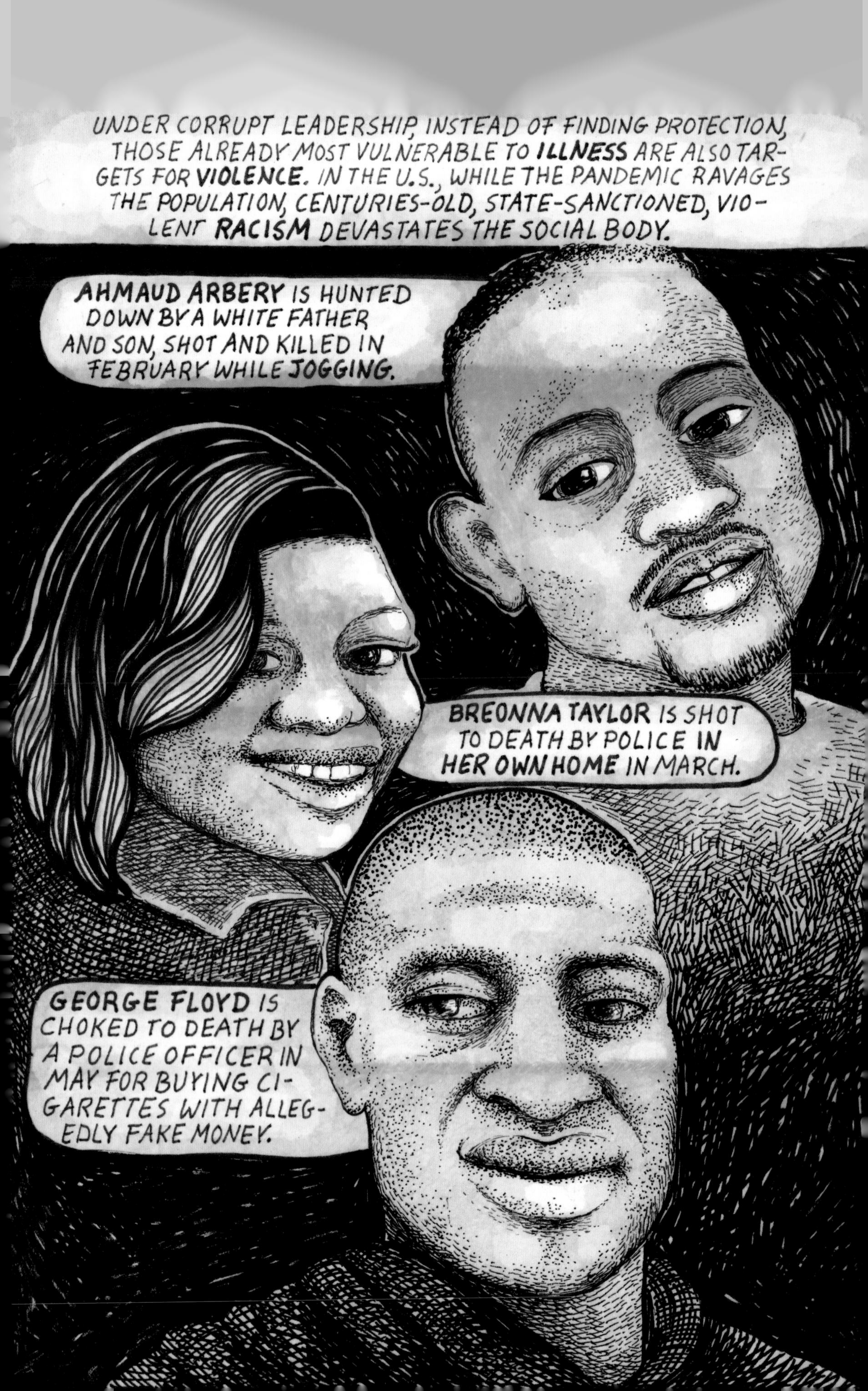
UNDER CORRUPT LEADERSHIP, INSTEAD OF FINDING PROTECTION, THOSE ALREADY MOST VULNERABLE TO **ILLNESS** ARE ALSO TARGETS FOR **VIOLENCE**. IN THE U.S., WHILE THE PANDEMIC RAVAGES THE POPULATION, CENTURIES-OLD, STATE-SANCTIONED, VIOLENT **RACISM** DEVASTATES THE SOCIAL BODY.
AHMAUD ARBERY IS HUNTED DOWN BY A WHITE FATHER AND SON, SHOT AND KILLED IN FEBRUARY WHILE **JOGGING**.
BREONNA TAYLOR IS SHOT TO DEATH BY POLICE **IN HER OWN HOME** IN MARCH.
GEORGE FLOYD IS CHOKED TO DEATH BY A POLICE OFFICER IN MAY FOR BUYING CIGARETTES WITH ALLEGEDLY FAKE MONEY.

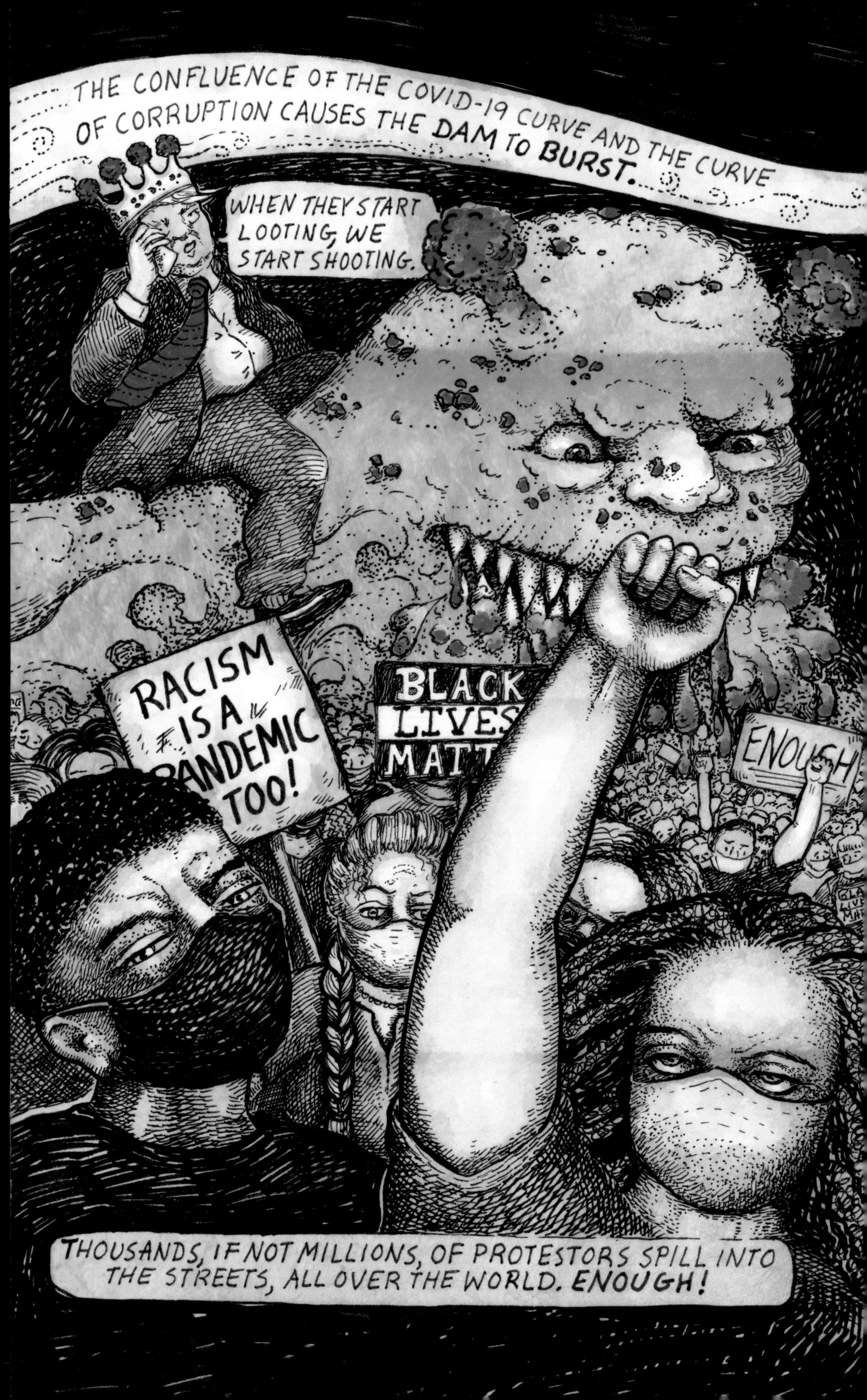
THE CONFLUENCE OF THE COVID-19 CURVE AND THE CURVE OF CORRUPTION CAUSES THE DAM TO BURST.
WHEN THEY START LOOTING, WE START SHOOTING.
RACISM IS A ANDEMIC TOO!
BLACK LIVES MATT
ENOUGH
THOUSANDS, IF NOT MILLIONS, OF PROTESTORS SPILL INTO THE STREETS, ALL OVER THE WORLD. ENOUGH!

ALONG WITH PROTESTING, EACH SMALL ACT OF TAKING NOTICE AND OF CARING INTENSIFIES THIS GLOBAL GROUNDSWELL.

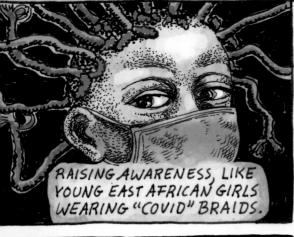

RAISING AWARENESS, LIKE YOUNG EAST AFRICAN GIRLS WEARING "COVID" BRAIDS.

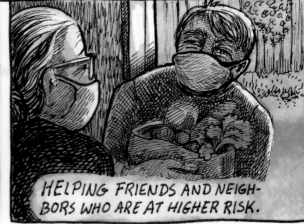

HELPING FRIENDS AND NEIGHBORS WHO ARE AT HIGHER RISK.

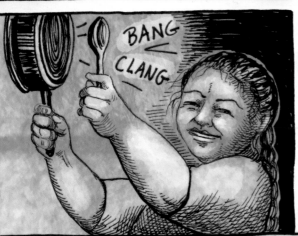

BANG
CLANG

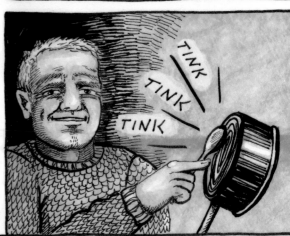

TINK
TINK
TINK

CHEERING ONE ANOTHER ON, MAKING NOISE IN SUPPORT OF OUR HEALTHCARE WORKERS.

TOGETHER, WE CAN *FLATTEN THE CURVE OF CORRUPTION AND THE CURVE OF COVID-19,* SO THAT EVERYONE CAN **BREATHE!**

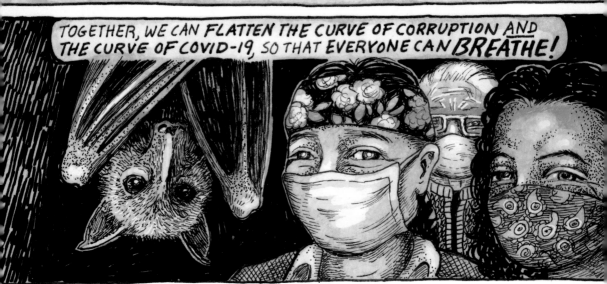

Pandemic precarities:
An account from the intersection of two worlds

KAY SOHINI

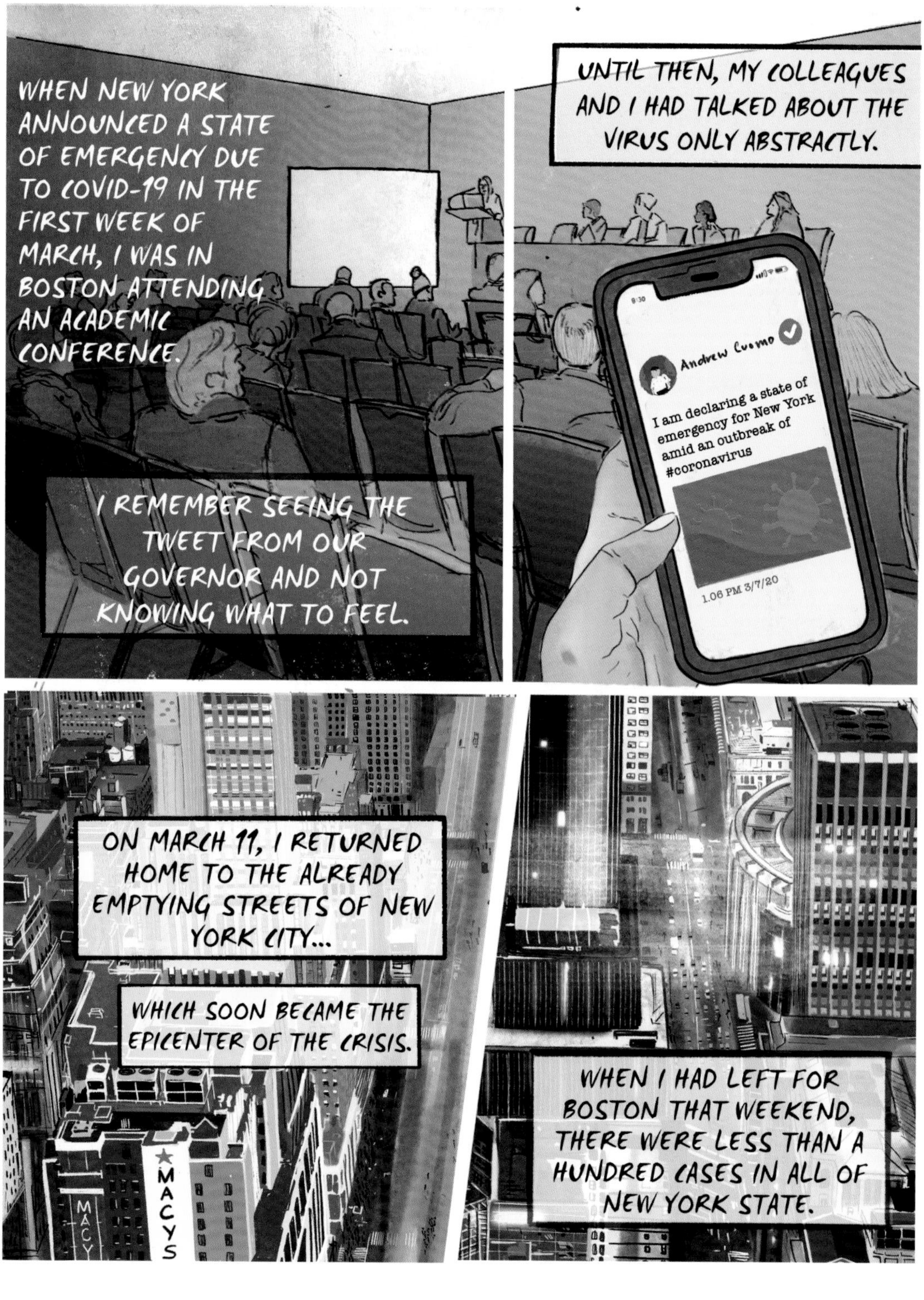
WHEN NEW YORK ANNOUNCED A STATE OF EMERGENCY DUE TO COVID-19 IN THE FIRST WEEK OF MARCH, I WAS IN BOSTON ATTENDING AN ACADEMIC CONFERENCE.
I REMEMBER SEEING THE TWEET FROM OUR GOVERNOR AND NOT KNOWING WHAT TO FEEL.
UNTIL THEN, MY COLLEAGUES AND I HAD TALKED ABOUT THE VIRUS ONLY ABSTRACTLY.
Andrew Cuomo
I am declaring a state of emergency for New York amid an outbreak of #coronavirus
1.06 PM 3/7/20
ON MARCH 11, I RETURNED HOME TO THE ALREADY EMPTYING STREETS OF NEW YORK CITY...
WHICH SOON BECAME THE EPICENTER OF THE CRISIS.
MACYS
MACYS
WHEN I HAD LEFT FOR BOSTON THAT WEEKEND, THERE WERE LESS THAN A HUNDRED CASES IN ALL OF NEW YORK STATE.

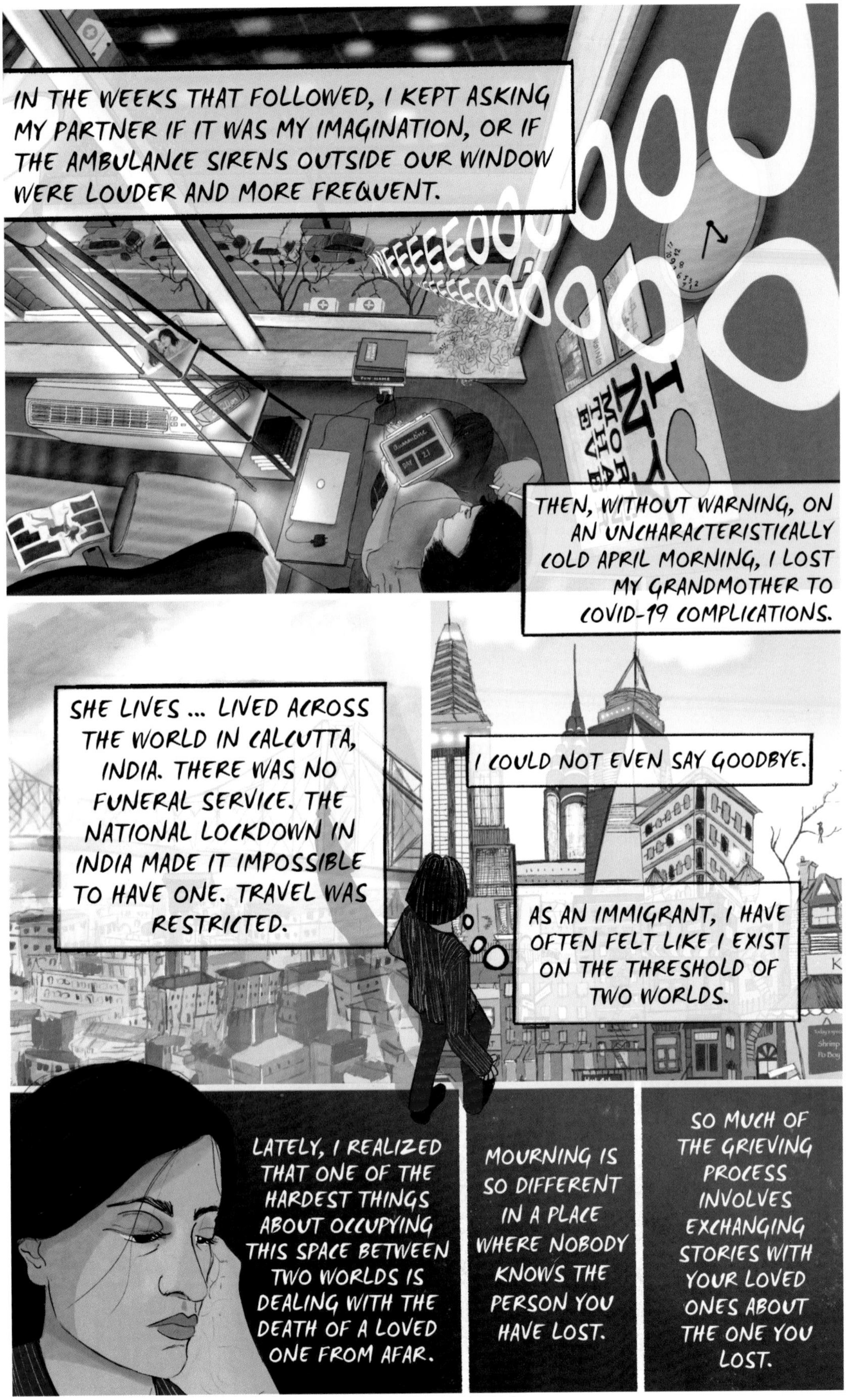
IN THE WEEKS THAT FOLLOWED, I KEPT ASKING MY PARTNER IF IT WAS MY IMAGINATION, OR IF THE AMBULANCE SIRENS OUTSIDE OUR WINDOW WERE LOUDER AND MORE FREQUENT.
WEEEEEOOOOOOO
THEN, WITHOUT WARNING, ON AN UNCHARACTERISTICALLY COLD APRIL MORNING, I LOST MY GRANDMOTHER TO COVID-19 COMPLICATIONS.
SHE LIVES ... LIVED ACROSS THE WORLD IN CALCUTTA, INDIA. THERE WAS NO FUNERAL SERVICE. THE NATIONAL LOCKDOWN IN INDIA MADE IT IMPOSSIBLE TO HAVE ONE. TRAVEL WAS RESTRICTED.
I COULD NOT EVEN SAY GOODBYE.
AS AN IMMIGRANT, I HAVE OFTEN FELT LIKE I EXIST ON THE THRESHOLD OF TWO WORLDS.
LATELY, I REALIZED THAT ONE OF THE HARDEST THINGS ABOUT OCCUPYING THIS SPACE BETWEEN TWO WORLDS IS DEALING WITH THE DEATH OF A LOVED ONE FROM AFAR.
MOURNING IS SO DIFFERENT IN A PLACE WHERE NOBODY KNOWS THE PERSON YOU HAVE LOST.
SO MUCH OF THE GRIEVING PROCESS INVOLVES EXCHANGING STORIES WITH YOUR LOVED ONES ABOUT THE ONE YOU LOST.

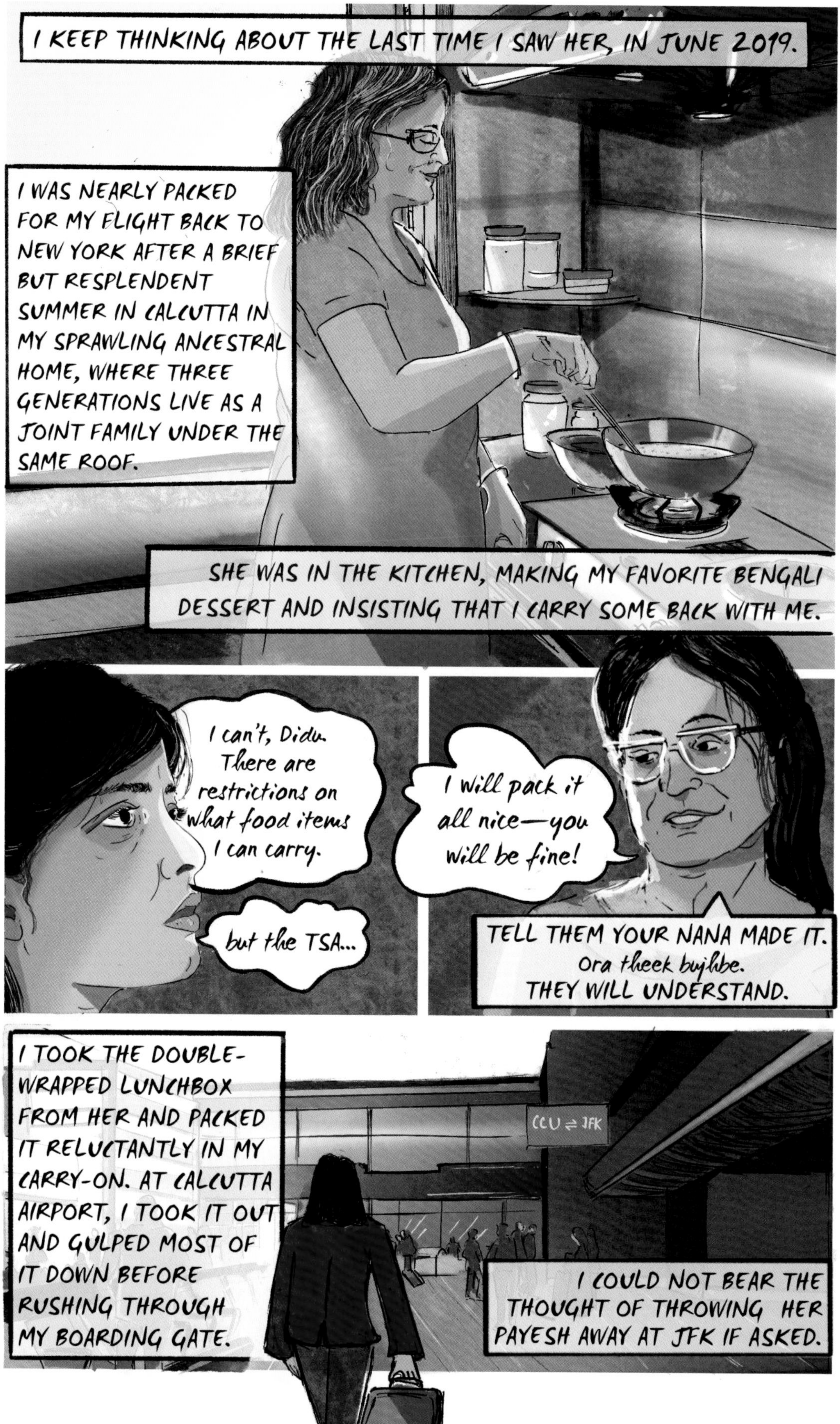
I KEEP THINKING ABOUT THE LAST TIME I SAW HER, IN JUNE 2019.
I WAS NEARLY PACKED FOR MY FLIGHT BACK TO NEW YORK AFTER A BRIEF BUT RESPLENDENT SUMMER IN CALCUTTA IN MY SPRAWLING ANCESTRAL HOME, WHERE THREE GENERATIONS LIVE AS A JOINT FAMILY UNDER THE SAME ROOF.
SHE WAS IN THE KITCHEN, MAKING MY FAVORITE BENGALI DESSERT AND INSISTING THAT I CARRY SOME BACK WITH ME.
I can't, Didu. There are restrictions on what food items I can carry.
but the TSA...
I will pack it all nice—you will be fine!
TELL THEM YOUR NANA MADE IT. Ora theek bujhbe. THEY WILL UNDERSTAND.
I TOOK THE DOUBLE-WRAPPED LUNCHBOX FROM HER AND PACKED IT RELUCTANTLY IN MY CARRY-ON. AT CALCUTTA AIRPORT, I TOOK IT OUT AND GULPED MOST OF IT DOWN BEFORE RUSHING THROUGH MY BOARDING GATE.
CCU ⇄ JFK
I COULD NOT BEAR THE THOUGHT OF THROWING HER PAYESH AWAY AT JFK IF ASKED.

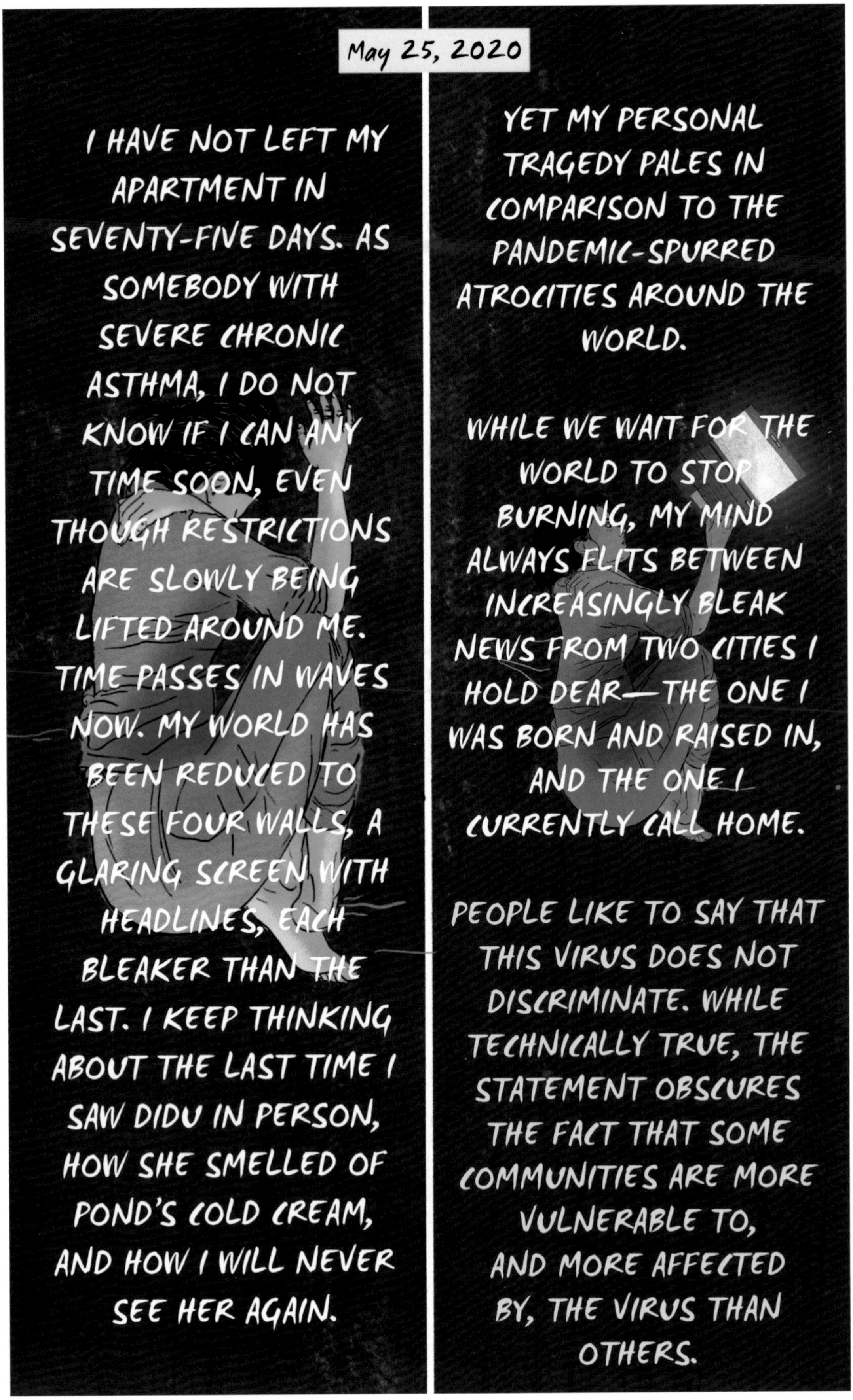
May 25, 2020
I HAVE NOT LEFT MY APARTMENT IN SEVENTY-FIVE DAYS. AS SOMEBODY WITH SEVERE CHRONIC ASTHMA, I DO NOT KNOW IF I CAN ANY TIME SOON, EVEN THOUGH RESTRICTIONS ARE SLOWLY BEING LIFTED AROUND ME. TIME PASSES IN WAVES NOW. MY WORLD HAS BEEN REDUCED TO THESE FOUR WALLS, A GLARING SCREEN WITH HEADLINES, EACH BLEAKER THAN THE LAST. I KEEP THINKING ABOUT THE LAST TIME I SAW DIDU IN PERSON, HOW SHE SMELLED OF POND'S COLD CREAM, AND HOW I WILL NEVER SEE HER AGAIN.
YET MY PERSONAL TRAGEDY PALES IN COMPARISON TO THE PANDEMIC-SPURRED ATROCITIES AROUND THE WORLD.
WHILE WE WAIT FOR THE WORLD TO STOP BURNING, MY MIND ALWAYS FLITS BETWEEN INCREASINGLY BLEAK NEWS FROM TWO CITIES I HOLD DEAR—THE ONE I WAS BORN AND RAISED IN, AND THE ONE I CURRENTLY CALL HOME.
PEOPLE LIKE TO SAY THAT THIS VIRUS DOES NOT DISCRIMINATE. WHILE TECHNICALLY TRUE, THE STATEMENT OBSCURES THE FACT THAT SOME COMMUNITIES ARE MORE VULNERABLE TO, AND MORE AFFECTED BY, THE VIRUS THAN OTHERS.

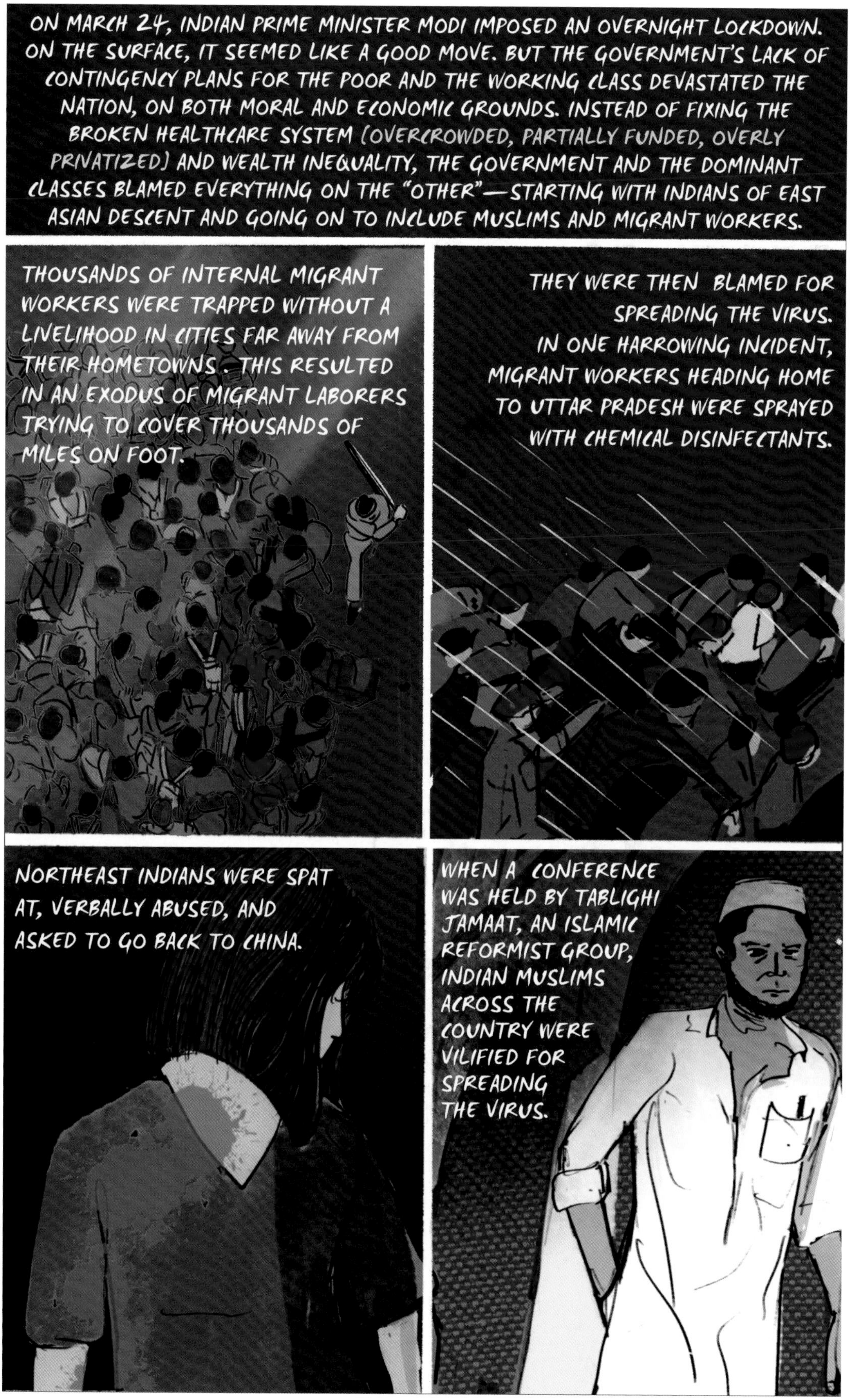
ON MARCH 24, INDIAN PRIME MINISTER MODI IMPOSED AN OVERNIGHT LOCKDOWN. ON THE SURFACE, IT SEEMED LIKE A GOOD MOVE. BUT THE GOVERNMENT'S LACK OF CONTINGENCY PLANS FOR THE POOR AND THE WORKING CLASS DEVASTATED THE NATION, ON BOTH MORAL AND ECONOMIC GROUNDS. INSTEAD OF FIXING THE BROKEN HEALTHCARE SYSTEM (OVERCROWDED, PARTIALLY FUNDED, OVERLY PRIVATIZED) AND WEALTH INEQUALITY, THE GOVERNMENT AND THE DOMINANT CLASSES BLAMED EVERYTHING ON THE "OTHER"—STARTING WITH INDIANS OF EAST ASIAN DESCENT AND GOING ON TO INCLUDE MUSLIMS AND MIGRANT WORKERS.
THOUSANDS OF INTERNAL MIGRANT WORKERS WERE TRAPPED WITHOUT A LIVELIHOOD IN CITIES FAR AWAY FROM THEIR HOMETOWNS. THIS RESULTED IN AN EXODUS OF MIGRANT LABORERS TRYING TO COVER THOUSANDS OF MILES ON FOOT.
THEY WERE THEN BLAMED FOR SPREADING THE VIRUS. IN ONE HARROWING INCIDENT, MIGRANT WORKERS HEADING HOME TO UTTAR PRADESH WERE SPRAYED WITH CHEMICAL DISINFECTANTS.
NORTHEAST INDIANS WERE SPAT AT, VERBALLY ABUSED, AND ASKED TO GO BACK TO CHINA.
WHEN A CONFERENCE WAS HELD BY TABLIGHI JAMAAT, AN ISLAMIC REFORMIST GROUP, INDIAN MUSLIMS ACROSS THE COUNTRY WERE VILIFIED FOR SPREADING THE VIRUS.

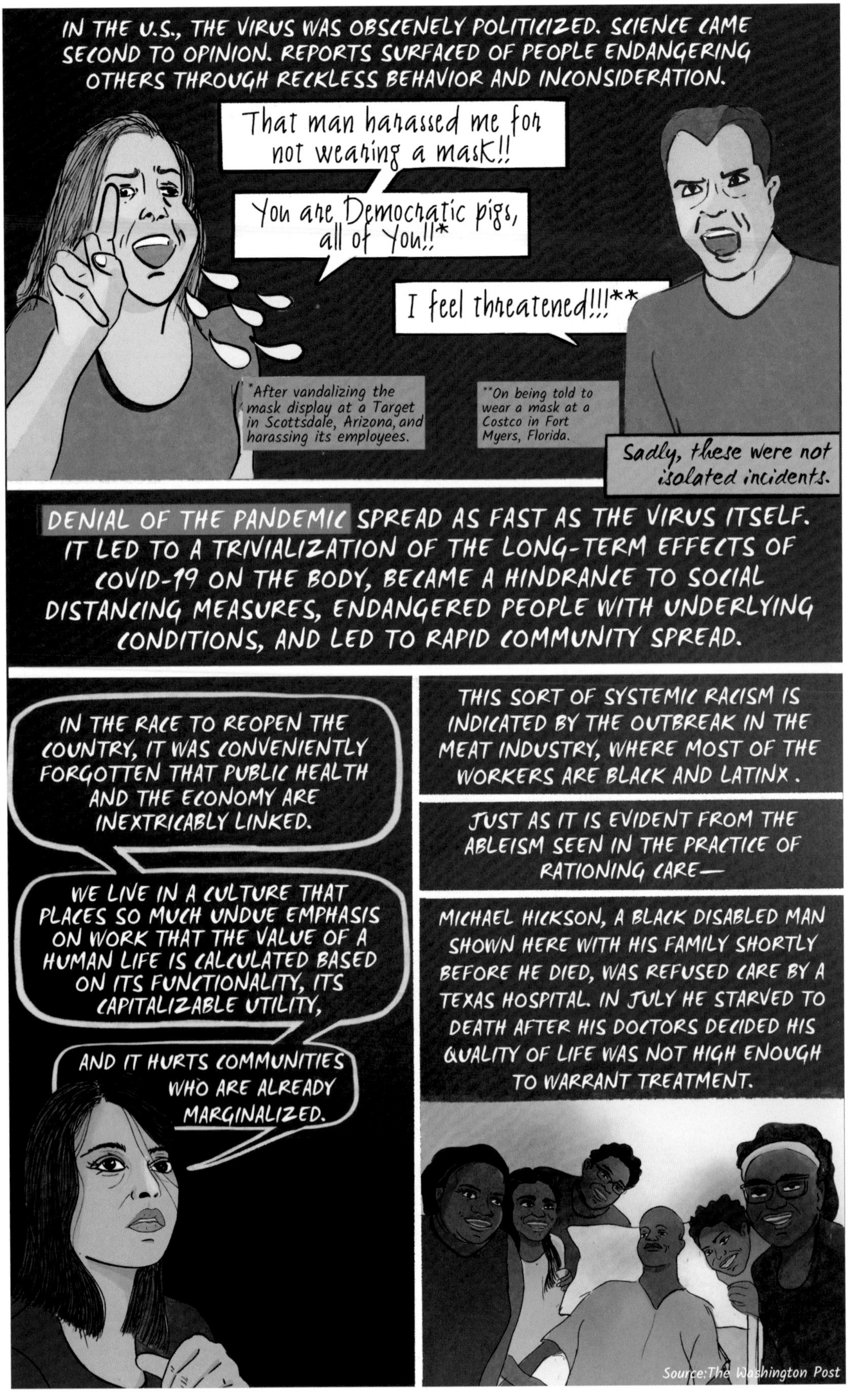
IN THE U.S., THE VIRUS WAS OBSCENELY POLITICIZED. SCIENCE CAME SECOND TO OPINION. REPORTS SURFACED OF PEOPLE ENDANGERING OTHERS THROUGH RECKLESS BEHAVIOR AND INCONSIDERATION.
That man harassed me for not wearing a mask!!
You are Democratic pigs, all of You!!*
I feel threatened!!!**
*After vandalizing the mask display at a Target in Scottsdale, Arizona, and harassing its employees.
**On being told to wear a mask at a Costco in Fort Myers, Florida.
Sadly, these were not isolated incidents.
DENIAL OF THE PANDEMIC SPREAD AS FAST AS THE VIRUS ITSELF. IT LED TO A TRIVIALIZATION OF THE LONG-TERM EFFECTS OF COVID-19 ON THE BODY, BECAME A HINDRANCE TO SOCIAL DISTANCING MEASURES, ENDANGERED PEOPLE WITH UNDERLYING CONDITIONS, AND LED TO RAPID COMMUNITY SPREAD.
IN THE RACE TO REOPEN THE COUNTRY, IT WAS CONVENIENTLY FORGOTTEN THAT PUBLIC HEALTH AND THE ECONOMY ARE INEXTRICABLY LINKED.
WE LIVE IN A CULTURE THAT PLACES SO MUCH UNDUE EMPHASIS ON WORK THAT THE VALUE OF A HUMAN LIFE IS CALCULATED BASED ON ITS FUNCTIONALITY, ITS CAPITALIZABLE UTILITY,
AND IT HURTS COMMUNITIES WHO ARE ALREADY MARGINALIZED.
THIS SORT OF SYSTEMIC RACISM IS INDICATED BY THE OUTBREAK IN THE MEAT INDUSTRY, WHERE MOST OF THE WORKERS ARE BLACK AND LATINX.
JUST AS IT IS EVIDENT FROM THE ABLEISM SEEN IN THE PRACTICE OF RATIONING CARE—
MICHAEL HICKSON, A BLACK DISABLED MAN SHOWN HERE WITH HIS FAMILY SHORTLY BEFORE HE DIED, WAS REFUSED CARE BY A TEXAS HOSPITAL. IN JULY HE STARVED TO DEATH AFTER HIS DOCTORS DECIDED HIS QUALITY OF LIFE WAS NOT HIGH ENOUGH TO WARRANT TREATMENT.
Source: The Washington Post

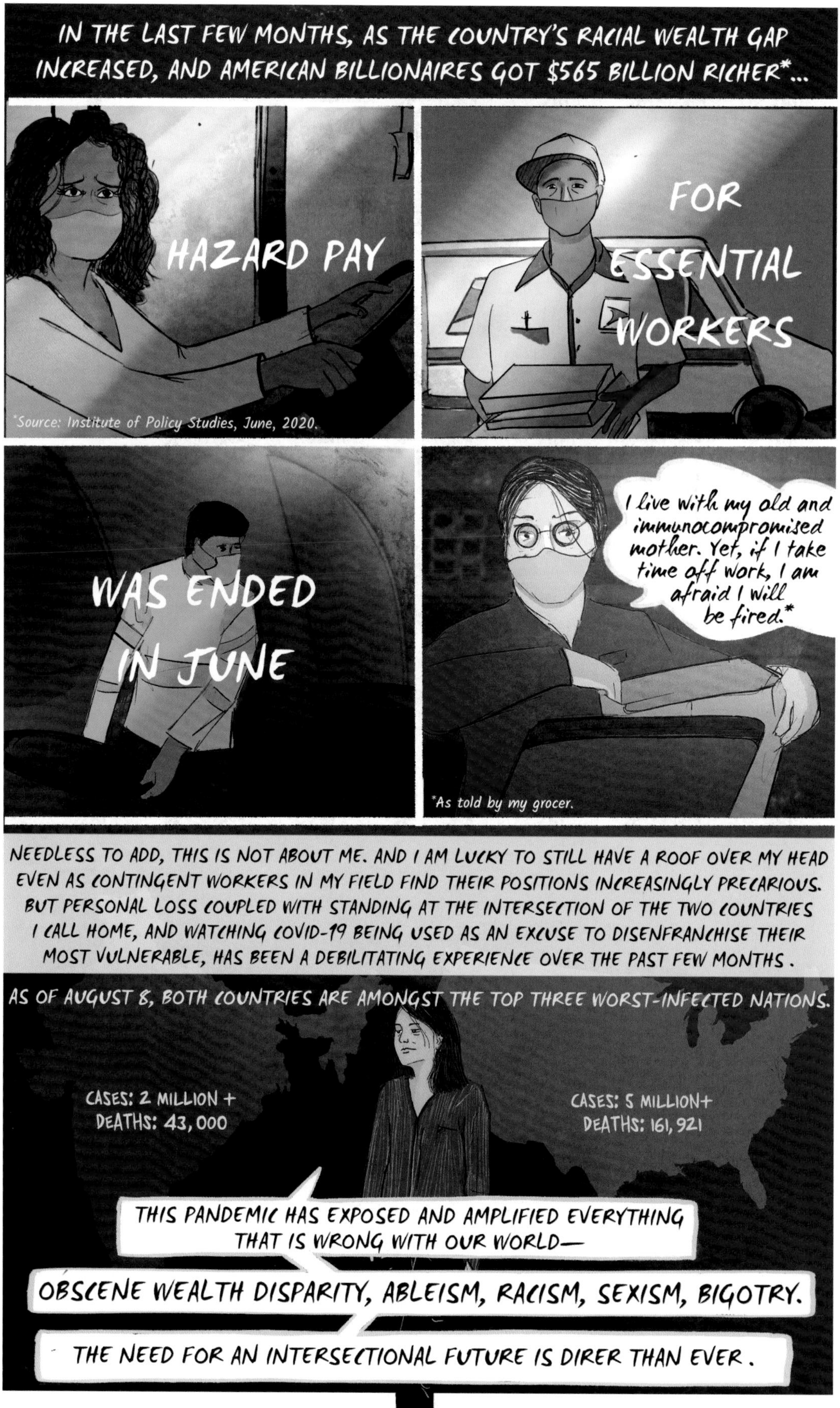
IN THE LAST FEW MONTHS, AS THE COUNTRY'S RACIAL WEALTH GAP INCREASED, AND AMERICAN BILLIONAIRES GOT $565 BILLION RICHER*...
HAZARD PAY
*Source: Institute of Policy Studies, June, 2020.
FOR ESSENTIAL WORKERS
WAS ENDED IN JUNE
I live with my old and immunocompromised mother. Yet, if I take time off work, I am afraid I will be fired.*
*As told by my grocer.
NEEDLESS TO ADD, THIS IS NOT ABOUT ME. AND I AM LUCKY TO STILL HAVE A ROOF OVER MY HEAD EVEN AS CONTINGENT WORKERS IN MY FIELD FIND THEIR POSITIONS INCREASINGLY PRECARIOUS. BUT PERSONAL LOSS COUPLED WITH STANDING AT THE INTERSECTION OF THE TWO COUNTRIES I CALL HOME, AND WATCHING COVID-19 BEING USED AS AN EXCUSE TO DISENFRANCHISE THEIR MOST VULNERABLE, HAS BEEN A DEBILITATING EXPERIENCE OVER THE PAST FEW MONTHS.
AS OF AUGUST 8, BOTH COUNTRIES ARE AMONGST THE TOP THREE WORST-INFECTED NATIONS.
CASES: 2 MILLION +
DEATHS: 43,000
CASES: 5 MILLION+
DEATHS: 161,921
THIS PANDEMIC HAS EXPOSED AND AMPLIFIED EVERYTHING THAT IS WRONG WITH OUR WORLD—
OBSCENE WEALTH DISPARITY, ABLEISM, RACISM, SEXISM, BIGOTRY.
THE NEED FOR AN INTERSECTIONAL FUTURE IS DIRER THAN EVER.

SAYING GOODBYE

INTERVIEW BY CHRISTOPHER HARLAND-DUNAWAY
ILLUSTRATED BY THI BUI
SCRIPT BY SARAH MIRK AND AMANDA PIKE

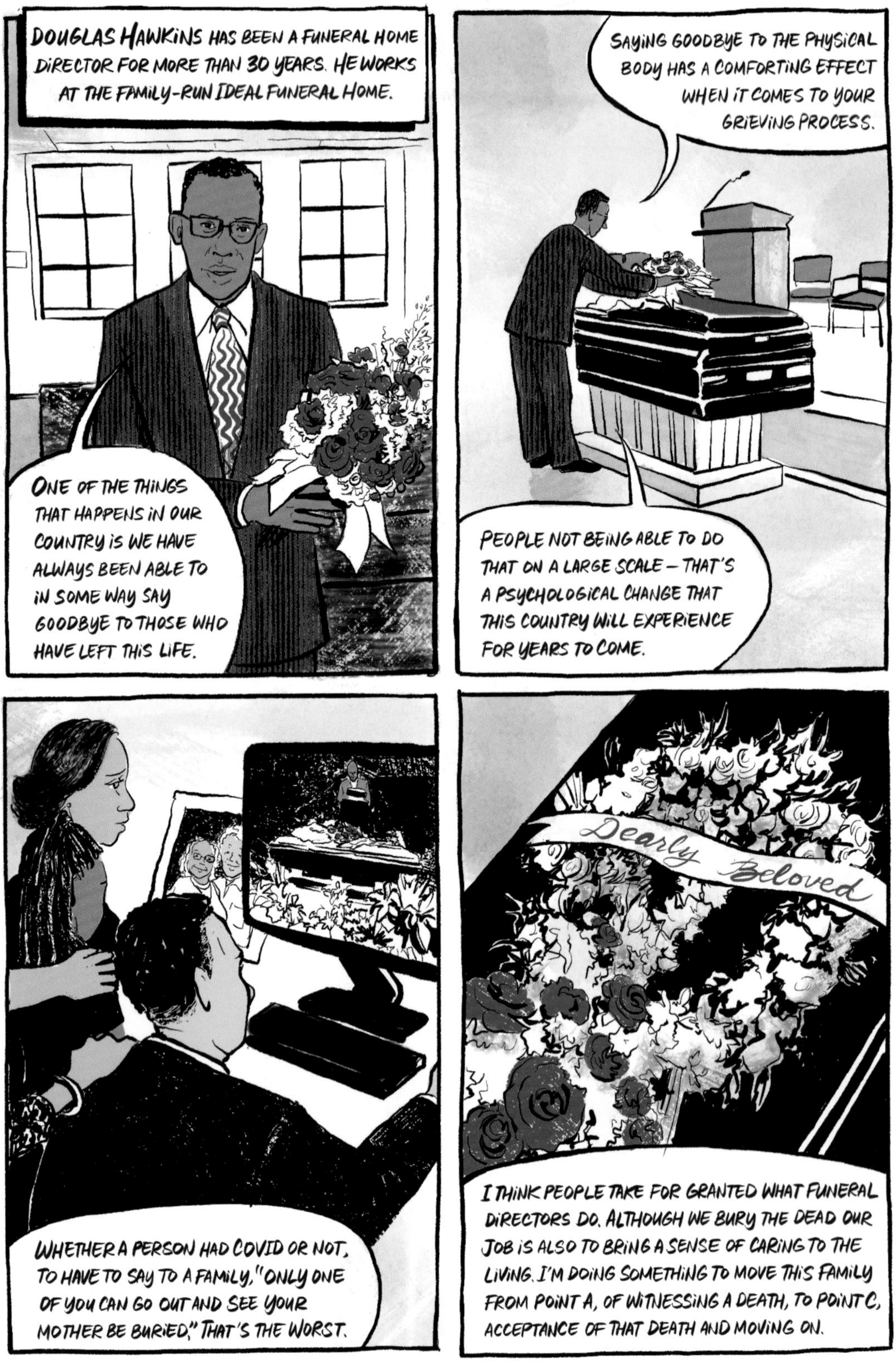
DOUGLAS HAWKINS HAS BEEN A FUNERAL HOME DIRECTOR FOR MORE THAN 30 YEARS. HE WORKS AT THE FAMILY-RUN IDEAL FUNERAL HOME.
ONE OF THE THINGS THAT HAPPENS IN OUR COUNTRY IS WE HAVE ALWAYS BEEN ABLE TO IN SOME WAY SAY GOODBYE TO THOSE WHO HAVE LEFT THIS LIFE.
SAYING GOODBYE TO THE PHYSICAL BODY HAS A COMFORTING EFFECT WHEN IT COMES TO YOUR GRIEVING PROCESS.
PEOPLE NOT BEING ABLE TO DO THAT ON A LARGE SCALE — THAT'S A PSYCHOLOGICAL CHANGE THAT THIS COUNTRY WILL EXPERIENCE FOR YEARS TO COME.
WHETHER A PERSON HAD COVID OR NOT, TO HAVE TO SAY TO A FAMILY, "ONLY ONE OF YOU CAN GO OUT AND SEE YOUR MOTHER BE BURIED," THAT'S THE WORST.
Dearly Beloved
I THINK PEOPLE TAKE FOR GRANTED WHAT FUNERAL DIRECTORS DO. ALTHOUGH WE BURY THE DEAD OUR JOB IS ALSO TO BRING A SENSE OF CARING TO THE LIVING. I'M DOING SOMETHING TO MOVE THIS FAMILY FROM POINT A, OF WITNESSING A DEATH, TO POINT C, ACCEPTANCE OF THAT DEATH AND MOVING ON.

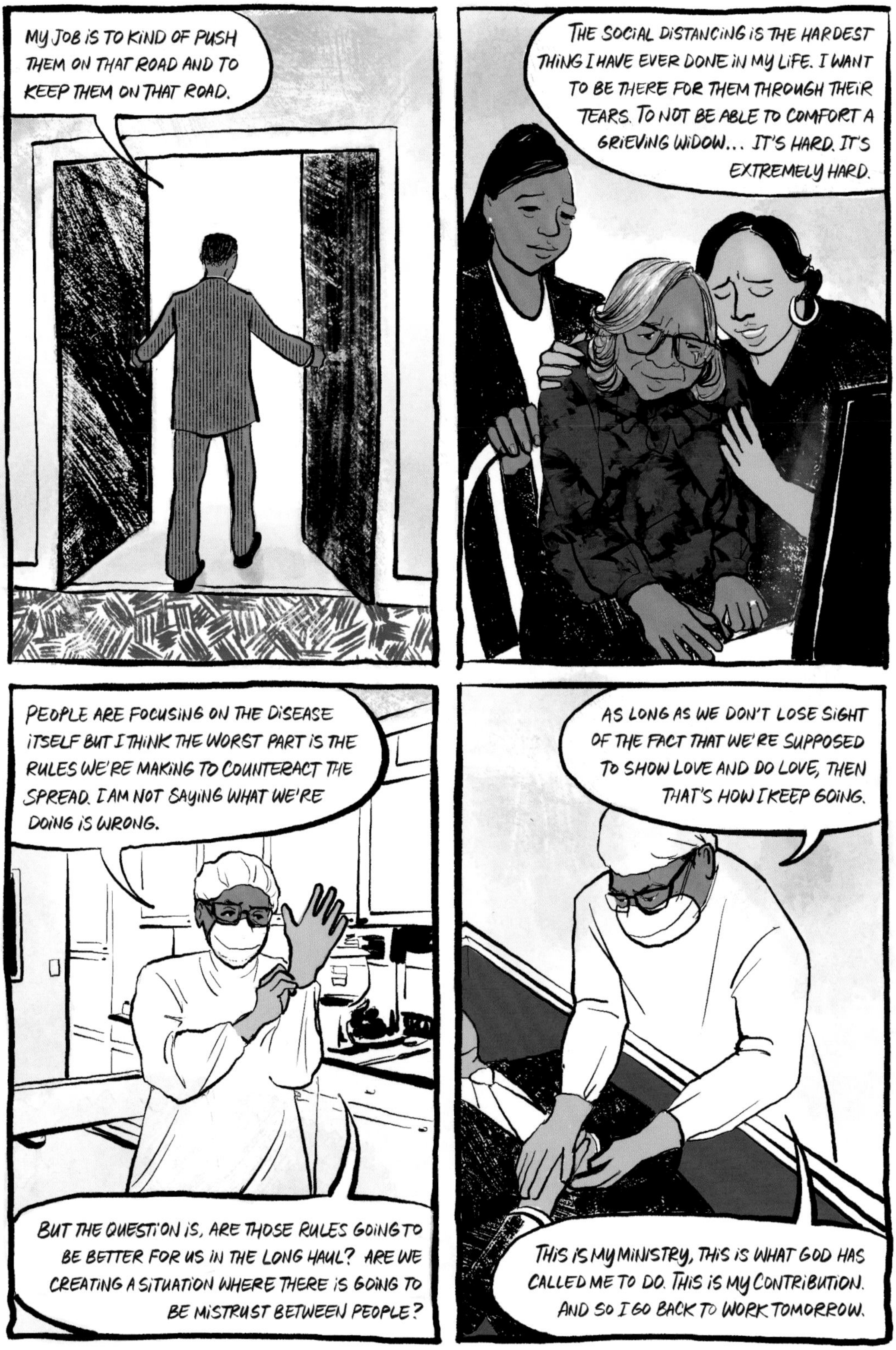
MY JOB IS TO KIND OF PUSH THEM ON THAT ROAD AND TO KEEP THEM ON THAT ROAD.
THE SOCIAL DISTANCING IS THE HARDEST THING I HAVE EVER DONE IN MY LIFE. I WANT TO BE THERE FOR THEM THROUGH THEIR TEARS. TO NOT BE ABLE TO COMFORT A GRIEVING WIDOW... IT'S HARD. IT'S EXTREMELY HARD.
PEOPLE ARE FOCUSING ON THE DISEASE ITSELF BUT I THINK THE WORST PART IS THE RULES WE'RE MAKING TO COUNTERACT THE SPREAD. I AM NOT SAYING WHAT WE'RE DOING IS WRONG.
BUT THE QUESTION IS, ARE THOSE RULES GOING TO BE BETTER FOR US IN THE LONG HAUL? ARE WE CREATING A SITUATION WHERE THERE IS GOING TO BE MISTRUST BETWEEN PEOPLE?
AS LONG AS WE DON'T LOSE SIGHT OF THE FACT THAT WE'RE SUPPOSED TO SHOW LOVE AND DO LOVE, THEN THAT'S HOW I KEEP GOING.
THIS IS MY MINISTRY, THIS IS WHAT GOD HAS CALLED ME TO DO. THIS IS MY CONTRIBUTION. AND SO I GO BACK TO WORK TOMORROW.

Originally published by Reveal from the Center for Investigative Reporting.

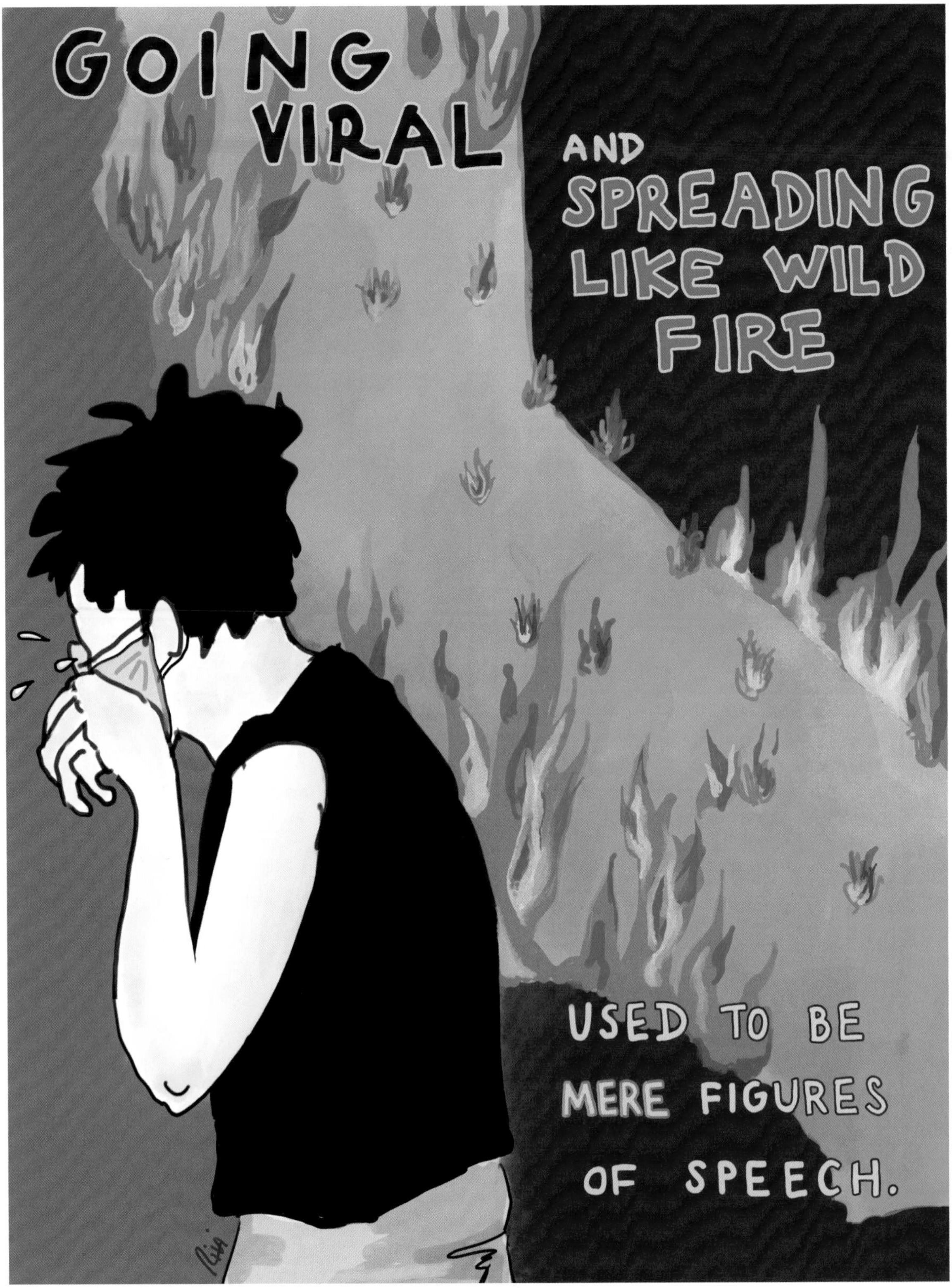
GOING VIRAL
AND SPREADING LIKE WILD FIRE
USED TO BE MERE FIGURES OF SPEECH.

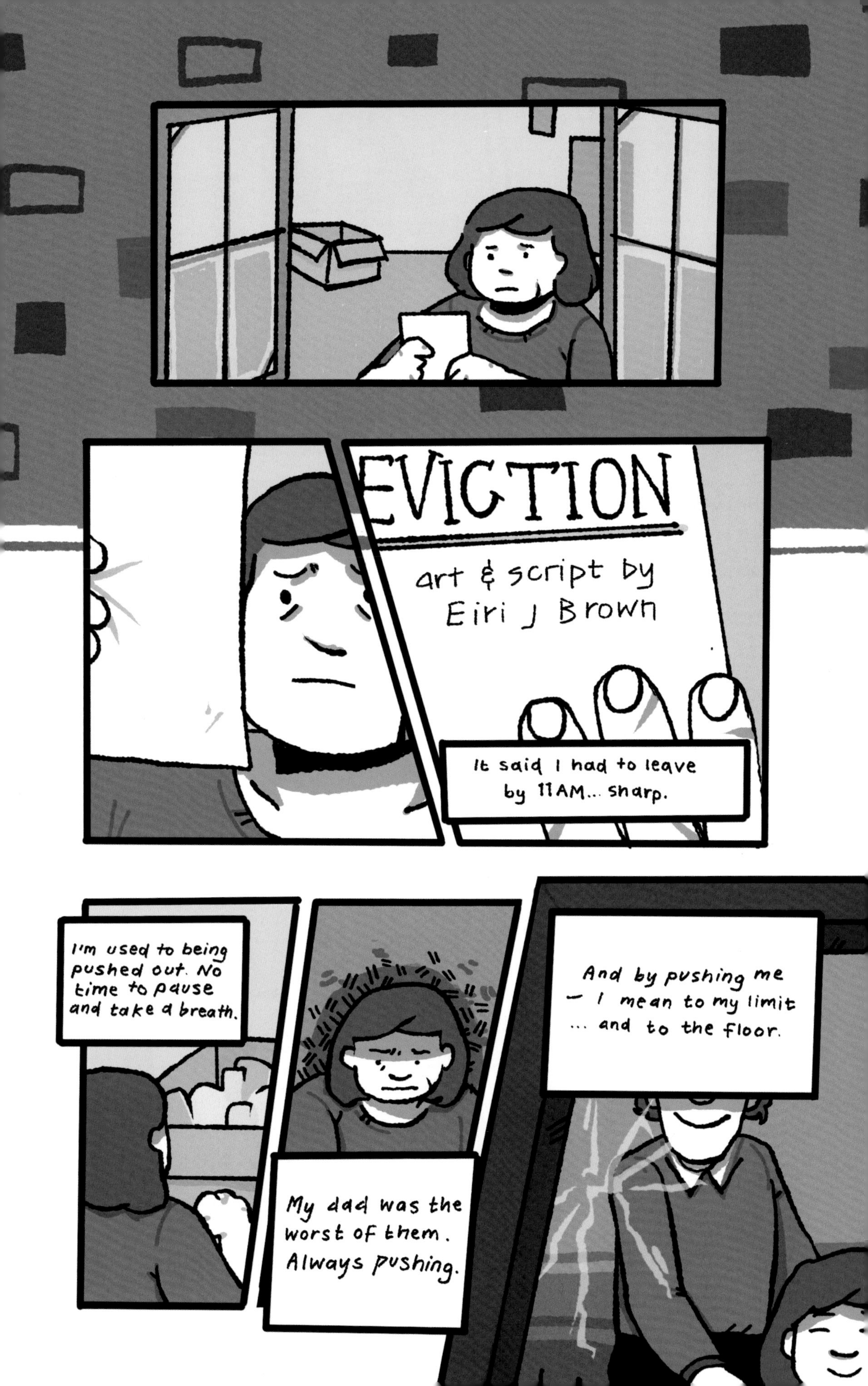
EVICTION
art & script by
Eiri J Brown
It said I had to leave by 11AM... sharp.
I'm used to being pushed out. No time to pause and take a breath.
My dad was the worst of them. Always pushing.
And by pushing me — I mean to my limit ... and to the floor.

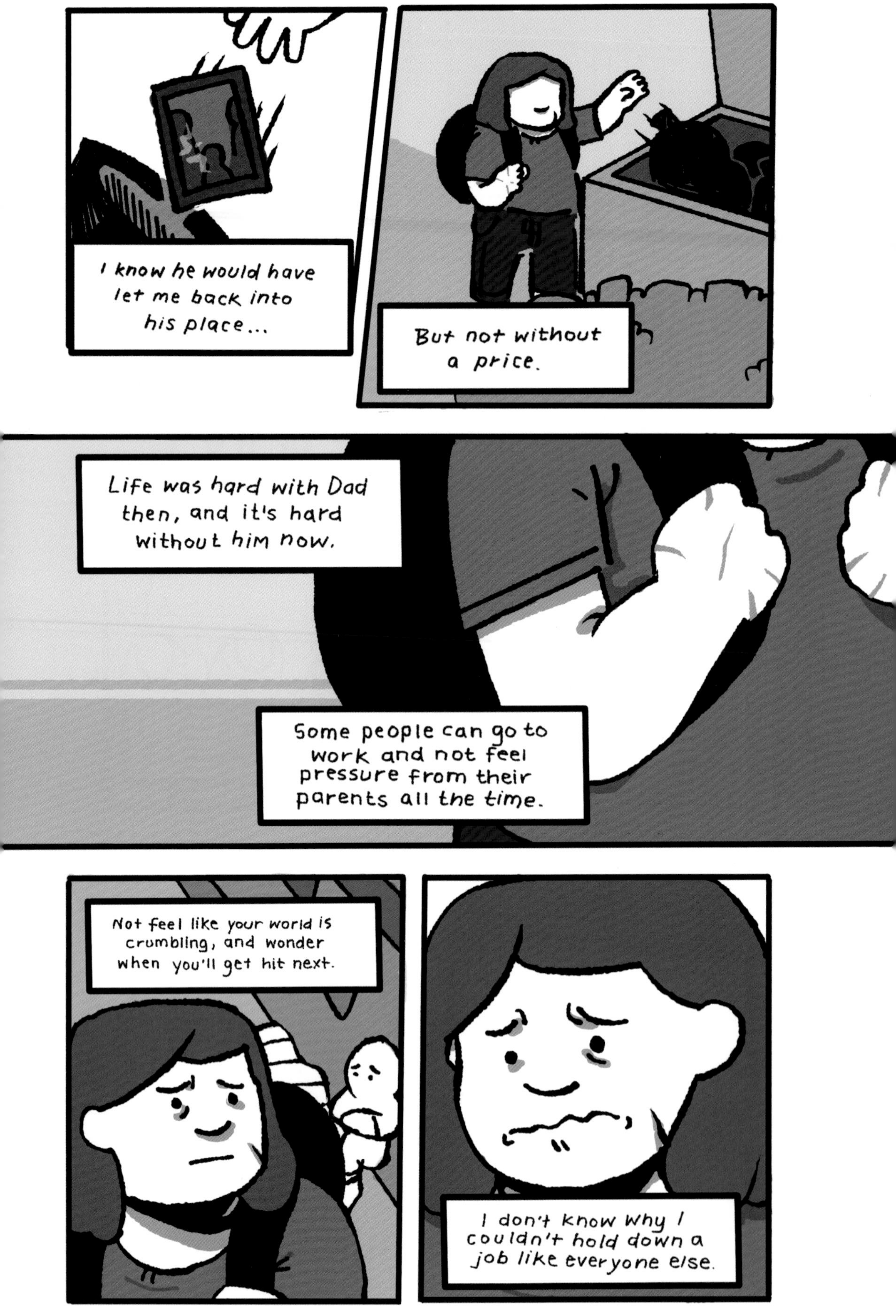
I know he would have let me back into his place...
But not without a price.
Life was hard with Dad then, and it's hard without him now.
Some people can go to work and not feel pressure from their parents all the time.
Not feel like your world is crumbling, and wonder when you'll get hit next.
I don't know why I couldn't hold down a job like everyone else.

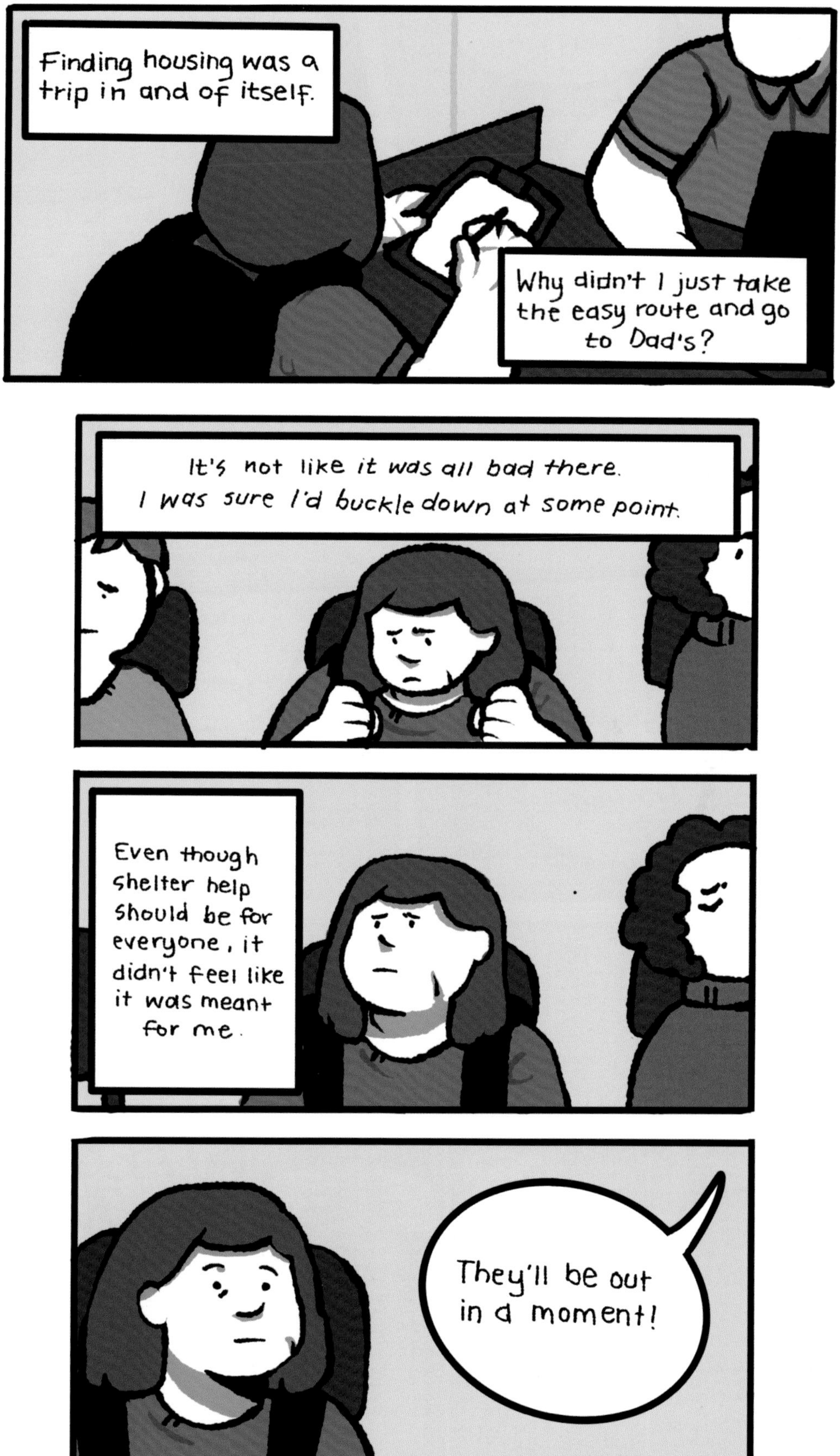
Finding housing was a trip in and of itself.
Why didn't I just take the easy route and go to Dad's?
It's not like it was all bad there. I was sure I'd buckle down at some point.
Even though shelter help should be for everyone, it didn't feel like it was meant for me.
They'll be out in a moment!

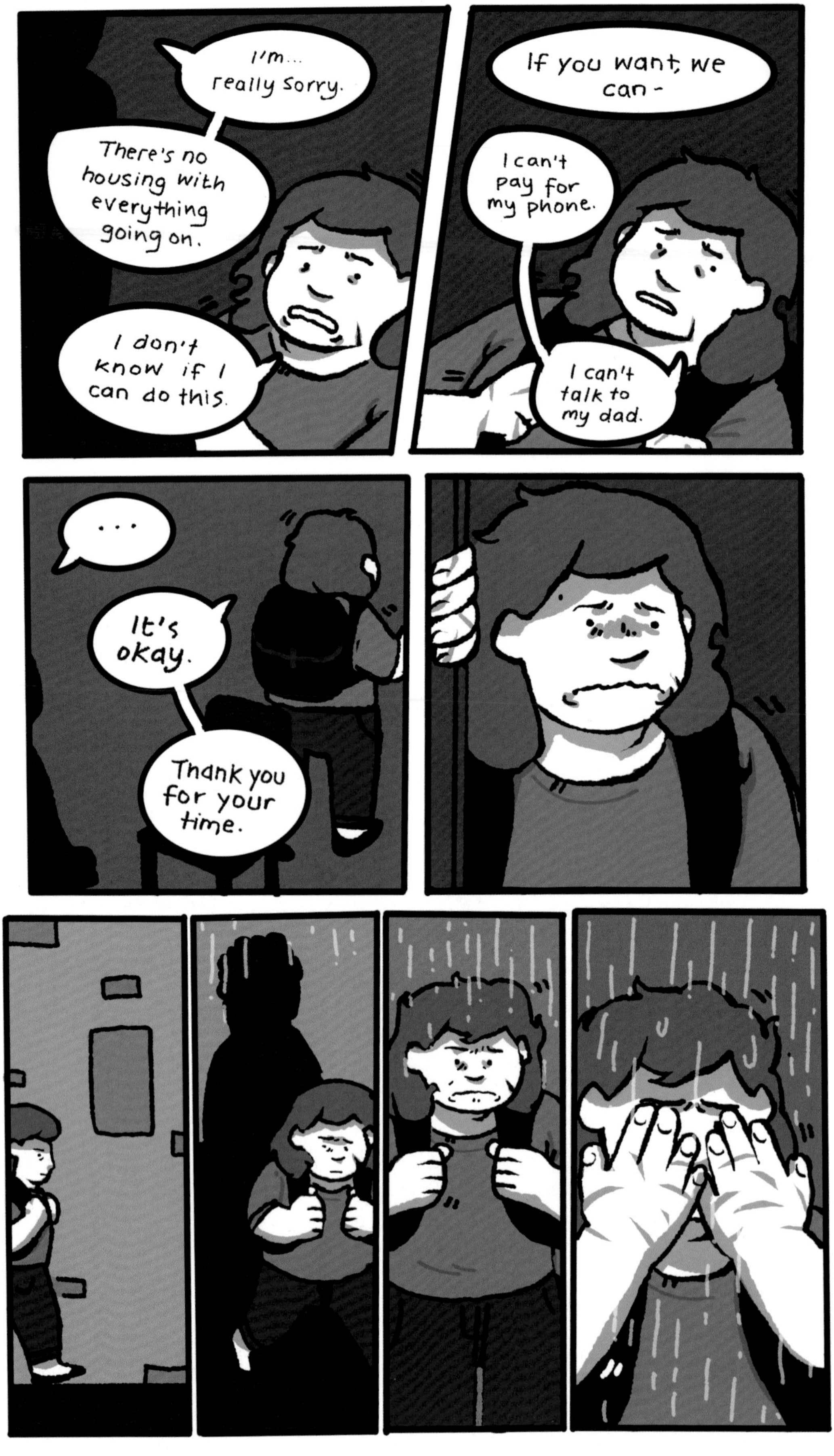
I'm... really sorry.
There's no housing with everything going on.
I don't know if I can do this.
If you want, we can-
I can't pay for my phone.
I can't talk to my dad.
...
It's okay.
Thank you for your time.

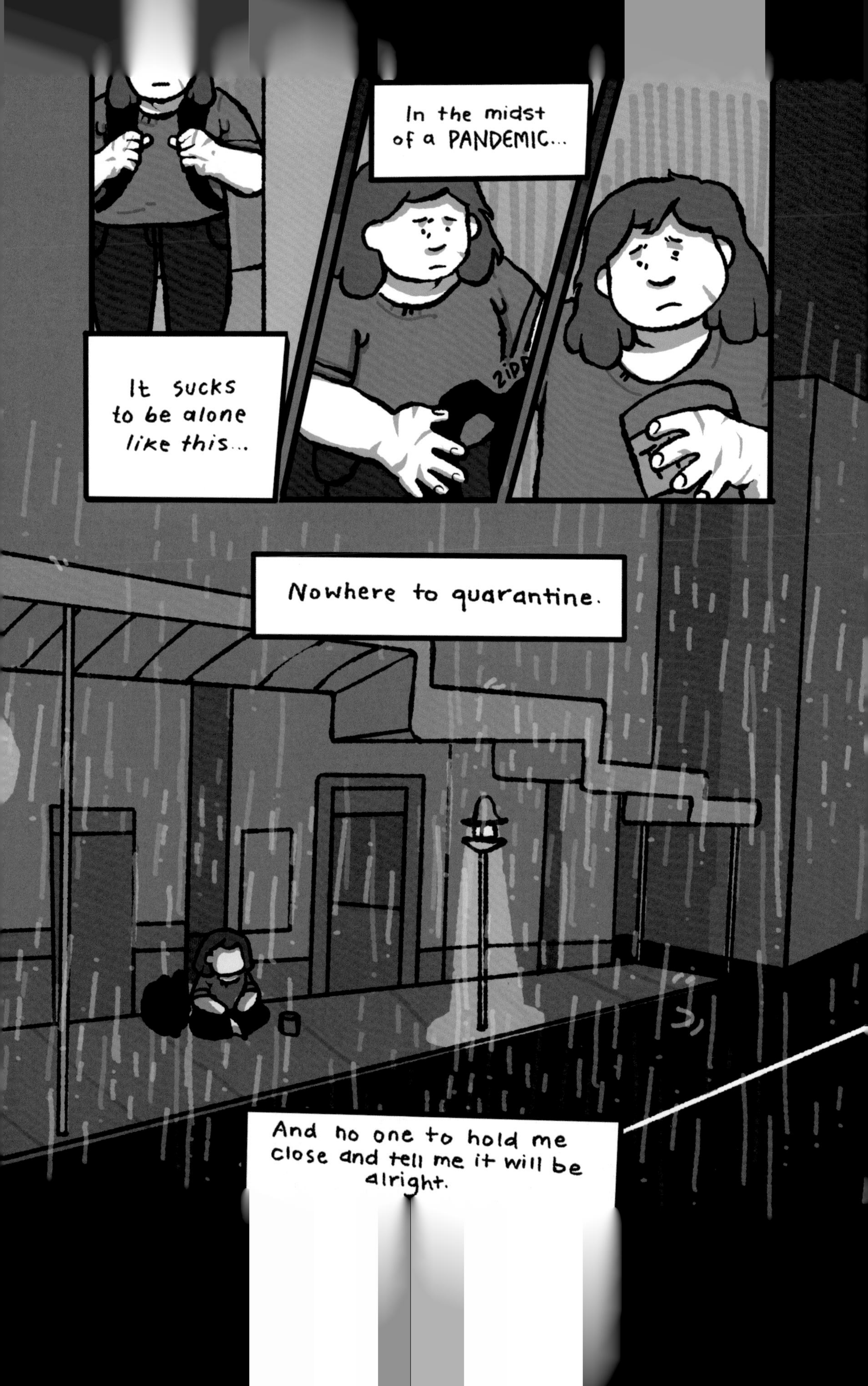
It sucks to be alone like this...
In the midst of a PANDEMIC...
ZIPP
Nowhere to quarantine.
And no one to hold me close and tell me it will be alright.

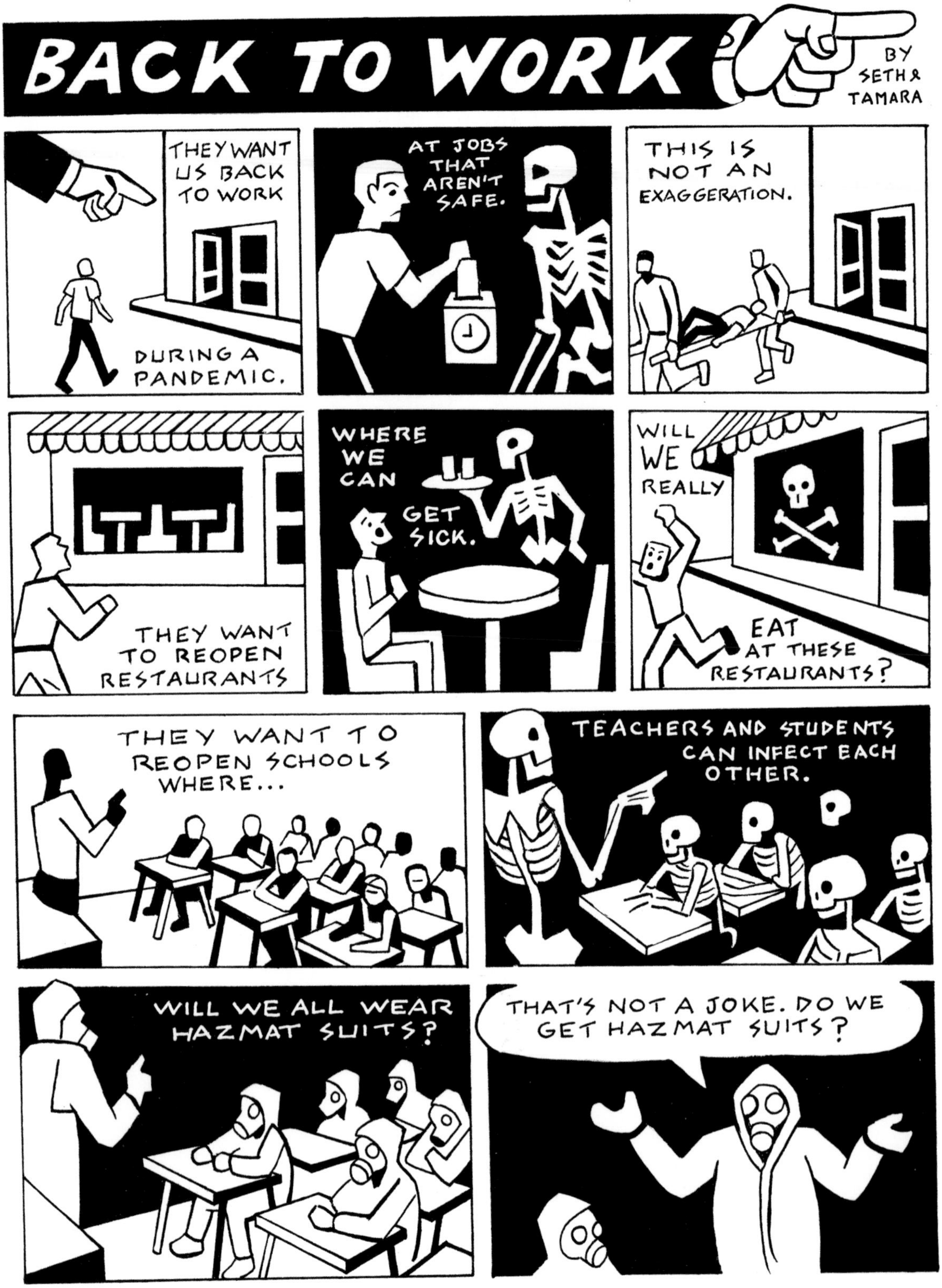
BACK TO WORK
BY SETH & TAMARA
THEY WANT US BACK TO WORK
DURING A PANDEMIC.
AT JOBS THAT AREN'T SAFE.
THIS IS NOT AN EXAGGERATION.
THEY WANT TO REOPEN RESTAURANTS
WHERE WE CAN
GET SICK.
WILL WE REALLY
EAT AT THESE RESTAURANTS?
THEY WANT TO REOPEN SCHOOLS WHERE...
TEACHERS AND STUDENTS CAN INFECT EACH OTHER.
WILL WE ALL WEAR HAZMAT SUITS?
THAT'S NOT A JOKE. DO WE GET HAZMAT SUITS?

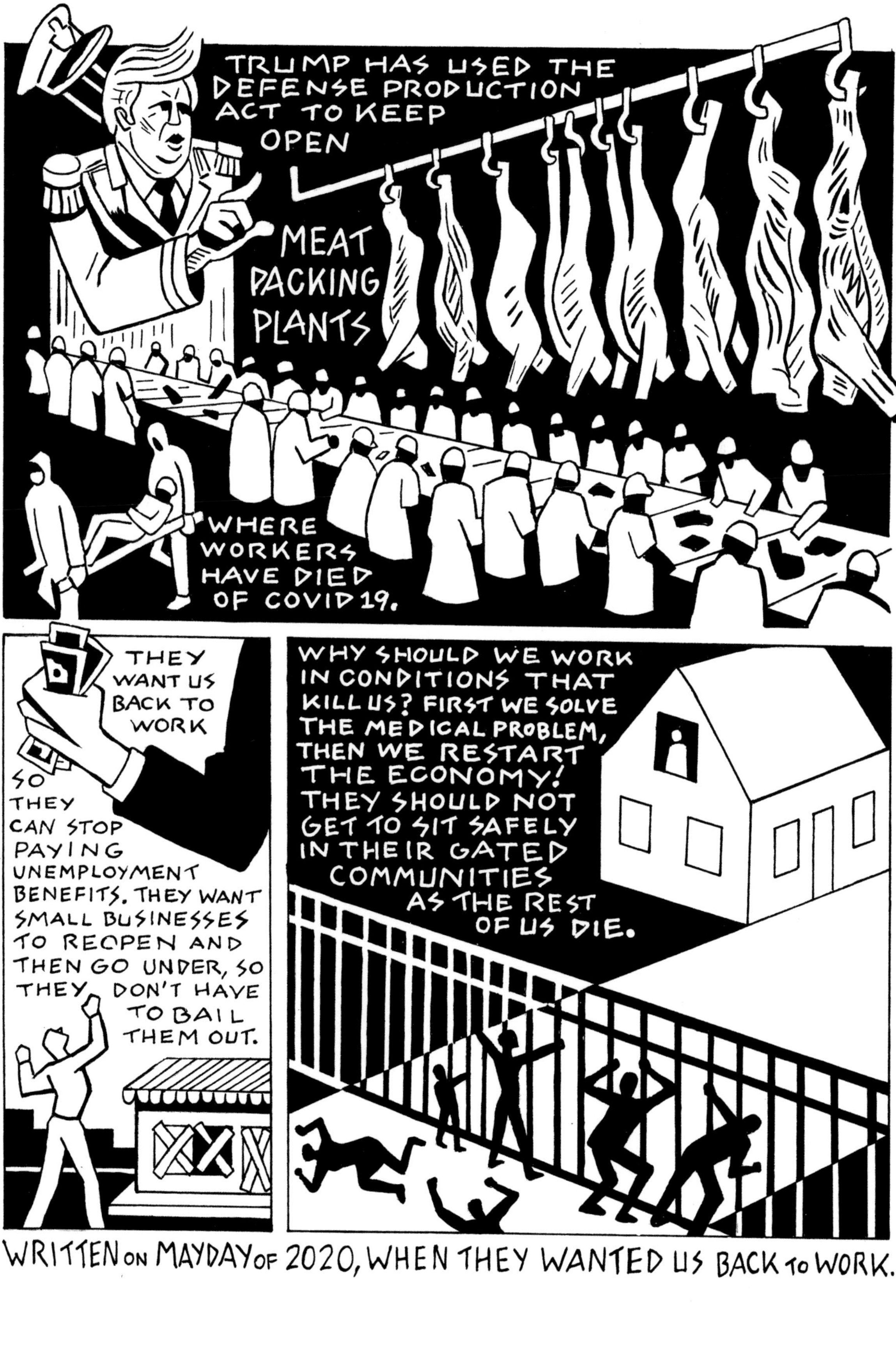
TRUMP HAS USED THE DEFENSE PRODUCTION ACT TO KEEP OPEN
MEAT PACKING PLANTS
WHERE WORKERS HAVE DIED OF COVID19.
THEY WANT US BACK TO WORK
SO THEY CAN STOP PAYING UNEMPLOYMENT BENEFITS. THEY WANT SMALL BUSINESSES TO REOPEN AND THEN GO UNDER, SO THEY DON'T HAVE TO BAIL THEM OUT.
WHY SHOULD WE WORK IN CONDITIONS THAT KILL US? FIRST WE SOLVE THE MEDICAL PROBLEM, THEN WE RESTART THE ECONOMY! THEY SHOULD NOT GET TO SIT SAFELY IN THEIR GATED COMMUNITIES AS THE REST OF US DIE.

WRITTEN ON MAYDAY OF 2020, WHEN THEY WANTED US BACK TO WORK.

MAXIMUM OCCUPANCY 1
16
OTIS
mundane
hazards

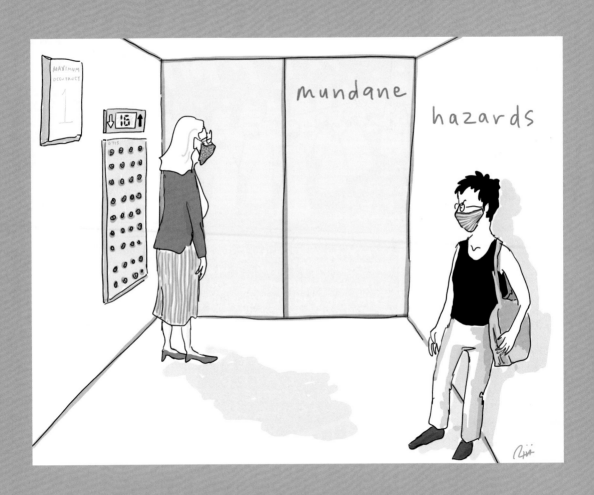

In general practice, Covid 19 is forcing family doctors to adopt the

NEW MODEL CONSULTATION

By Dr Ian Williams, a.k.a. The Bad Doctor Covid lockdown 2020

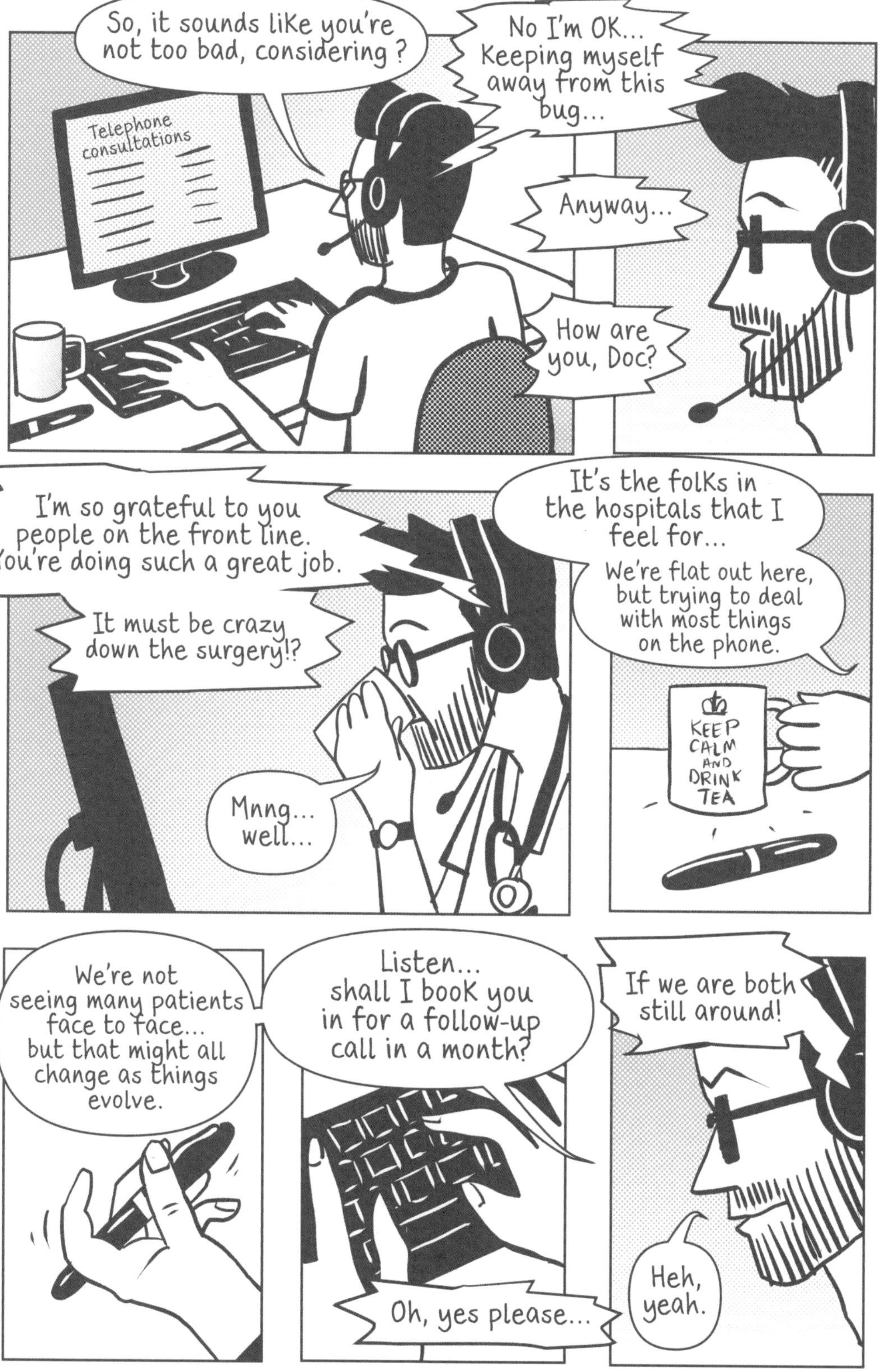

So, it sounds like you're not too bad, considering?
Telephone consultations
No I'm OK... Keeping myself away from this bug...
Anyway...
How are you, Doc?
I'm so grateful to you people on the front line. You're doing such a great job.
It must be crazy down the surgery!?
Mnng... well...
It's the folks in the hospitals that I feel for...
We're flat out here, but trying to deal with most things on the phone.
KEEP CALM AND DRINK TEA
We're not seeing many patients face to face... but that might all change as things evolve.
Listen... shall I book you in for a follow-up call in a month?
Oh, yes please...
If we are both still around!
Heh, yeah.

Most people are profoundly grateful just to speak to a doctor on the phone. The occasional patient, however, seems oblivious to the NEW REALITY of the pandemic...

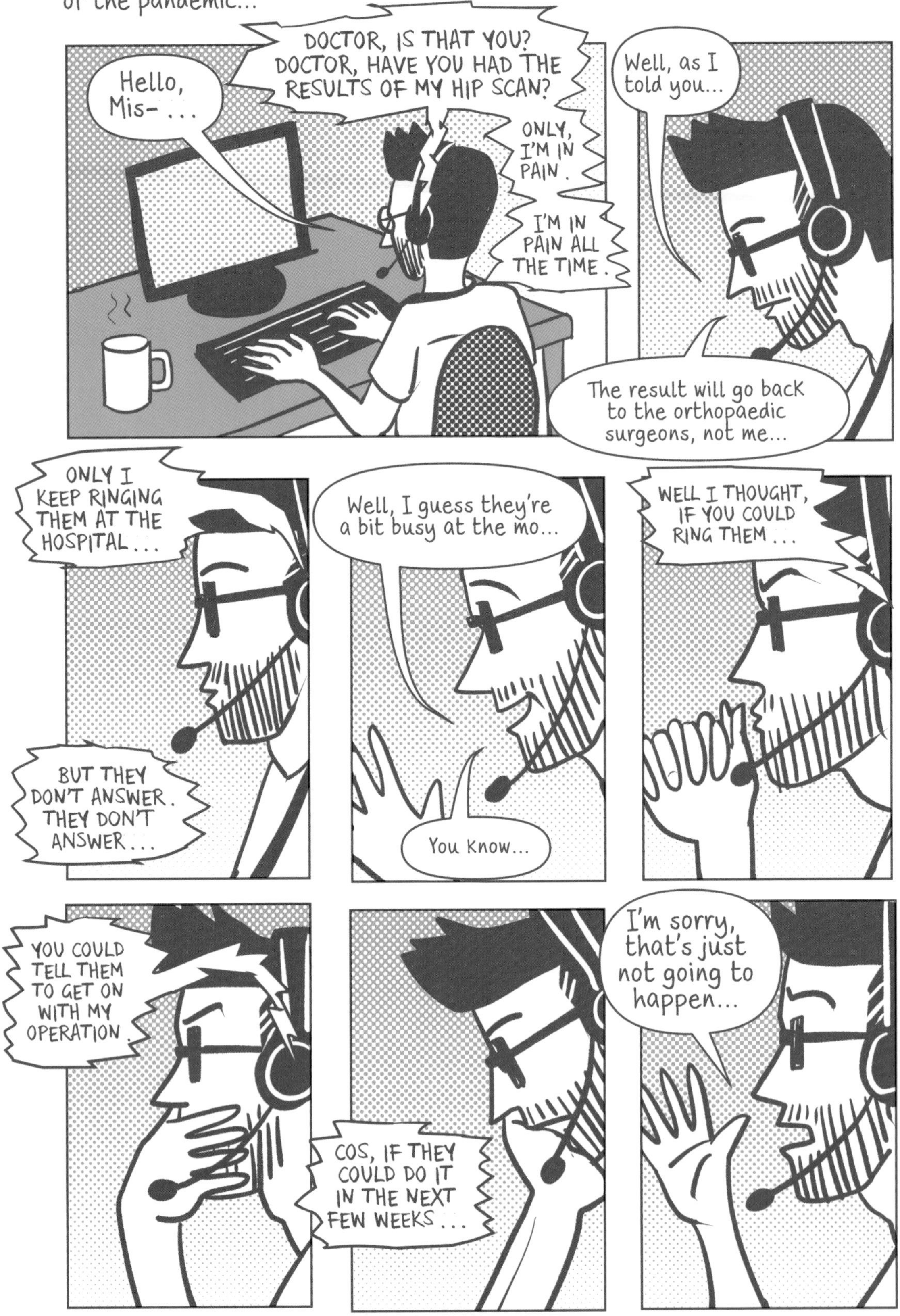
Hello, Mis- . . .
DOCTOR, IS THAT YOU? DOCTOR, HAVE YOU HAD THE RESULTS OF MY HIP SCAN?
ONLY, I'M IN PAIN.
I'M IN PAIN ALL THE TIME.
Well, as I told you...
The result will go back to the orthopaedic surgeons, not me...
ONLY I KEEP RINGING THEM AT THE HOSPITAL . . .
BUT THEY DON'T ANSWER. THEY DON'T ANSWER . . .
Well, I guess they're a bit busy at the mo...
You know...
WELL I THOUGHT, IF YOU COULD RING THEM . . .
YOU COULD TELL THEM TO GET ON WITH MY OPERATION.
COS, IF THEY COULD DO IT IN THE NEXT FEW WEEKS . . .
I'm sorry, that's just not going to happen...

With a couple of comorbidities, this lady should be shielding. But, trapped in her world of medical dependency, she cannot help but demand action.

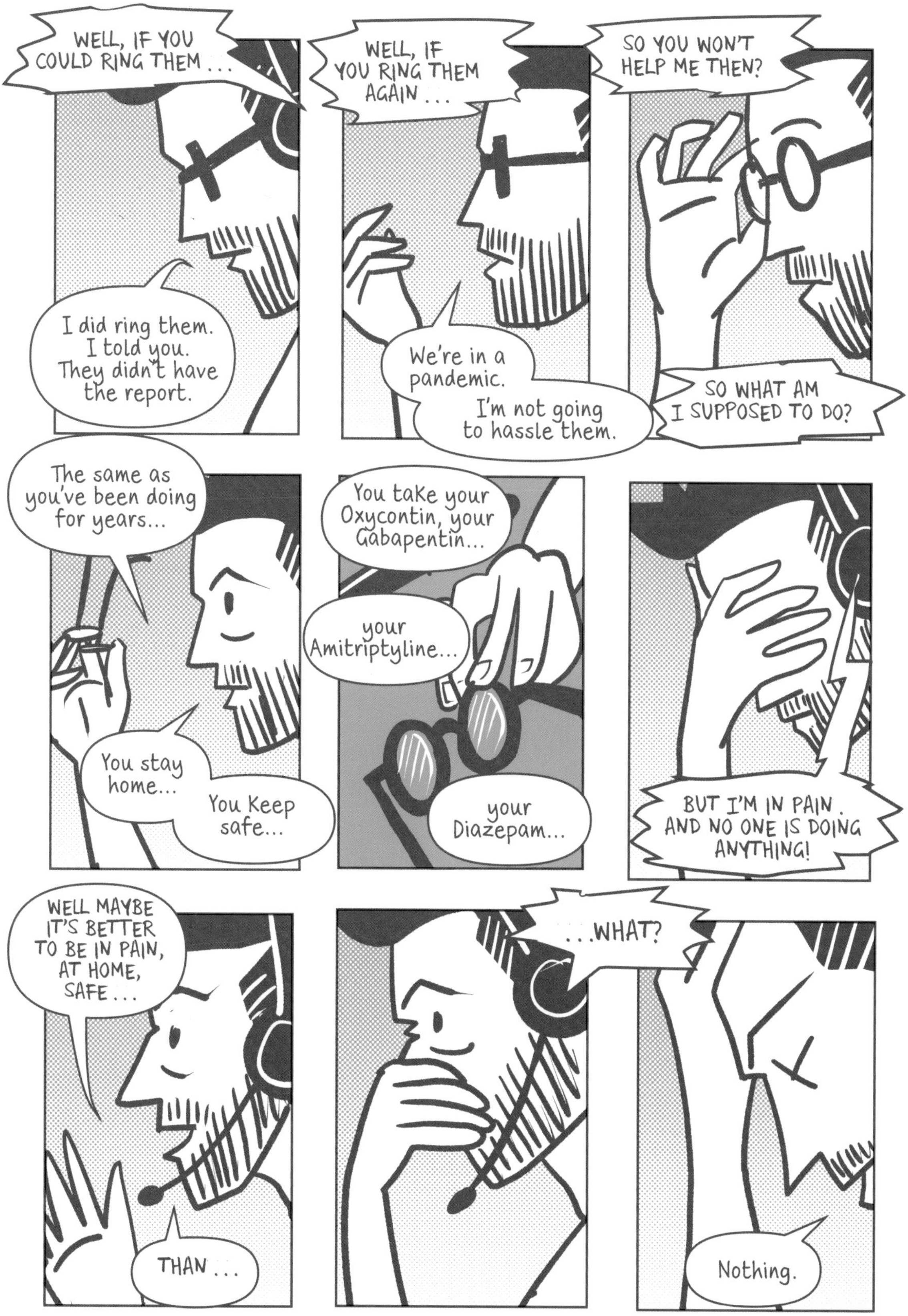
WELL, IF YOU COULD RING THEM . . .
I did ring them. I told you. They didn't have the report.
WELL, IF YOU RING THEM AGAIN . . .
We're in a pandemic.
I'm not going to hassle them.
SO YOU WON'T HELP ME THEN?
SO WHAT AM I SUPPOSED TO DO?
The same as you've been doing for years...
You stay home...
You Keep safe...
You take your Oxycontin, your Gabapentin...
your Amitriptyline...
your Diazepam...
BUT I'M IN PAIN. AND NO ONE IS DOING ANYTHING!
WELL MAYBE IT'S BETTER TO BE IN PAIN, AT HOME, SAFE . . .
THAN . . .
. . .WHAT?
Nothing.

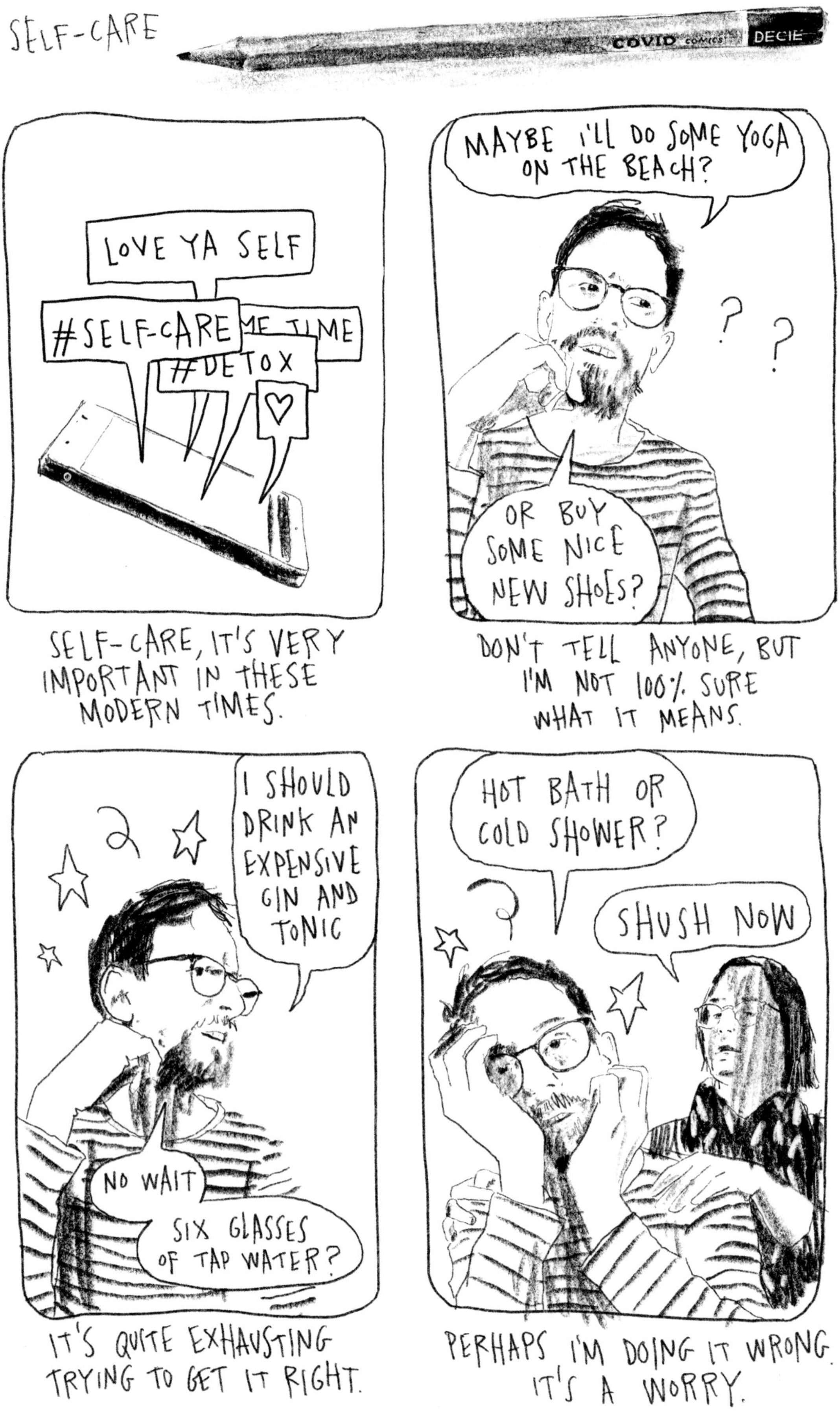
SELF-CARE
COVID
DECIE
LOVE YA SELF
#SELF-CARE
ME TIME
#DETOX
SELF-CARE, IT'S VERY IMPORTANT IN THESE MODERN TIMES.
MAYBE I'LL DO SOME YOGA ON THE BEACH?
OR BUY SOME NICE NEW SHOES?
DON'T TELL ANYONE, BUT I'M NOT 100% SURE WHAT IT MEANS.
I SHOULD DRINK AN EXPENSIVE GIN AND TONIC
NO WAIT
SIX GLASSES OF TAP WATER?
IT'S QUITE EXHAUSTING TRYING TO GET IT RIGHT.
HOT BATH OR COLD SHOWER?
SHUSH NOW
PERHAPS I'M DOING IT WRONG. IT'S A WORRY.

A NEW REALITY

by Annie Zhu & Richard You Wu

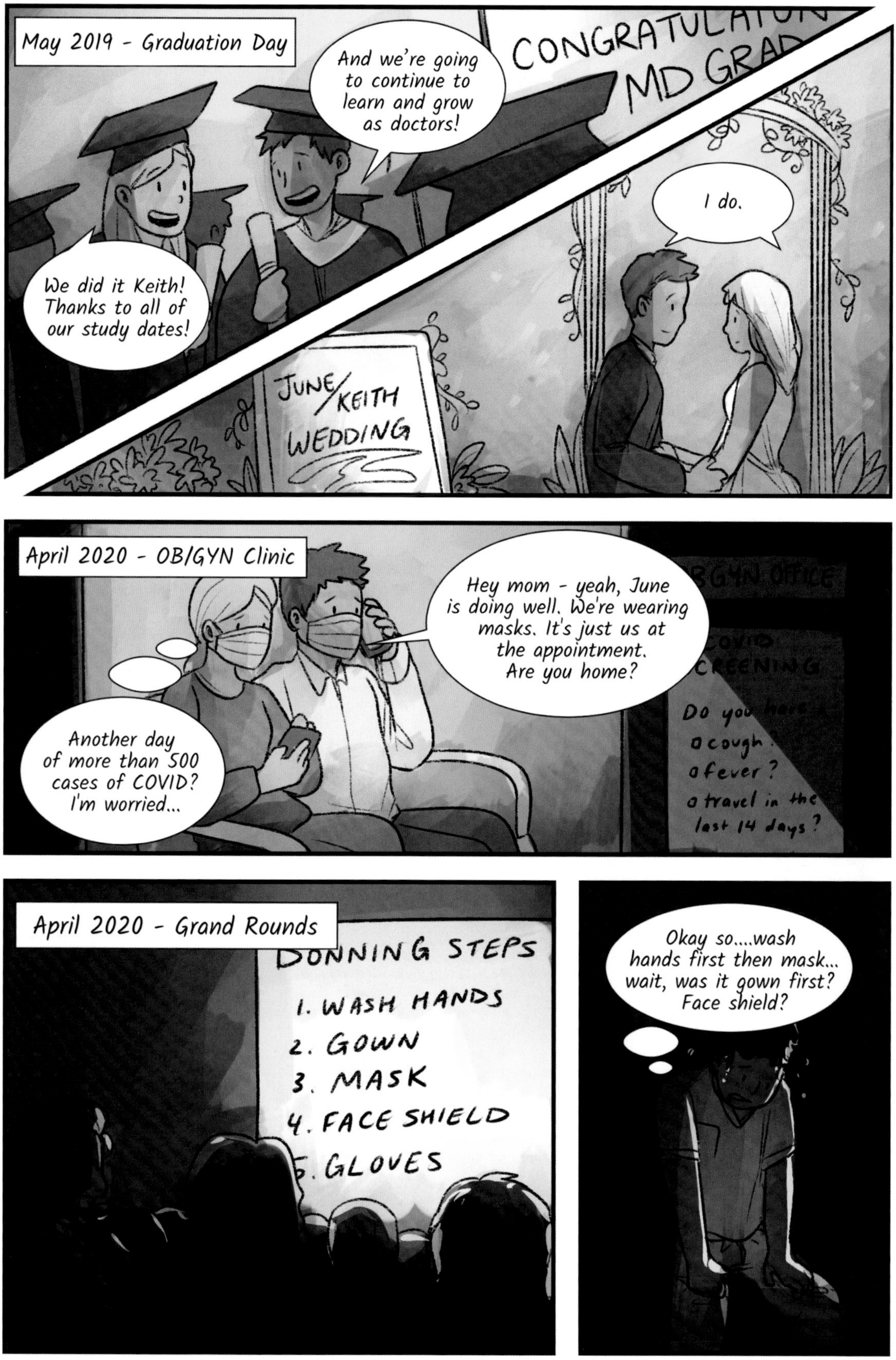

May 2019 - Graduation Day
And we're going to continue to learn and grow as doctors!
CONGRATULATION MD GRAD
We did it Keith! Thanks to all of our study dates!
I do.
JUNE/KEITH WEDDING
April 2020 - OB/GYN Clinic
Hey mom - yeah, June is doing well. We're wearing masks. It's just us at the appointment. Are you home?
Another day of more than 500 cases of COVID? I'm worried...
COVID SCREENING
o cough
o fever?
o travel in the last 14 days?
April 2020 - Grand Rounds
DONNING STEPS
1. WASH HANDS
2. GOWN
3. MASK
4. FACE SHIELD
5. GLOVES
Okay so....wash hands first then mask... wait, was it gown first? Face shield?

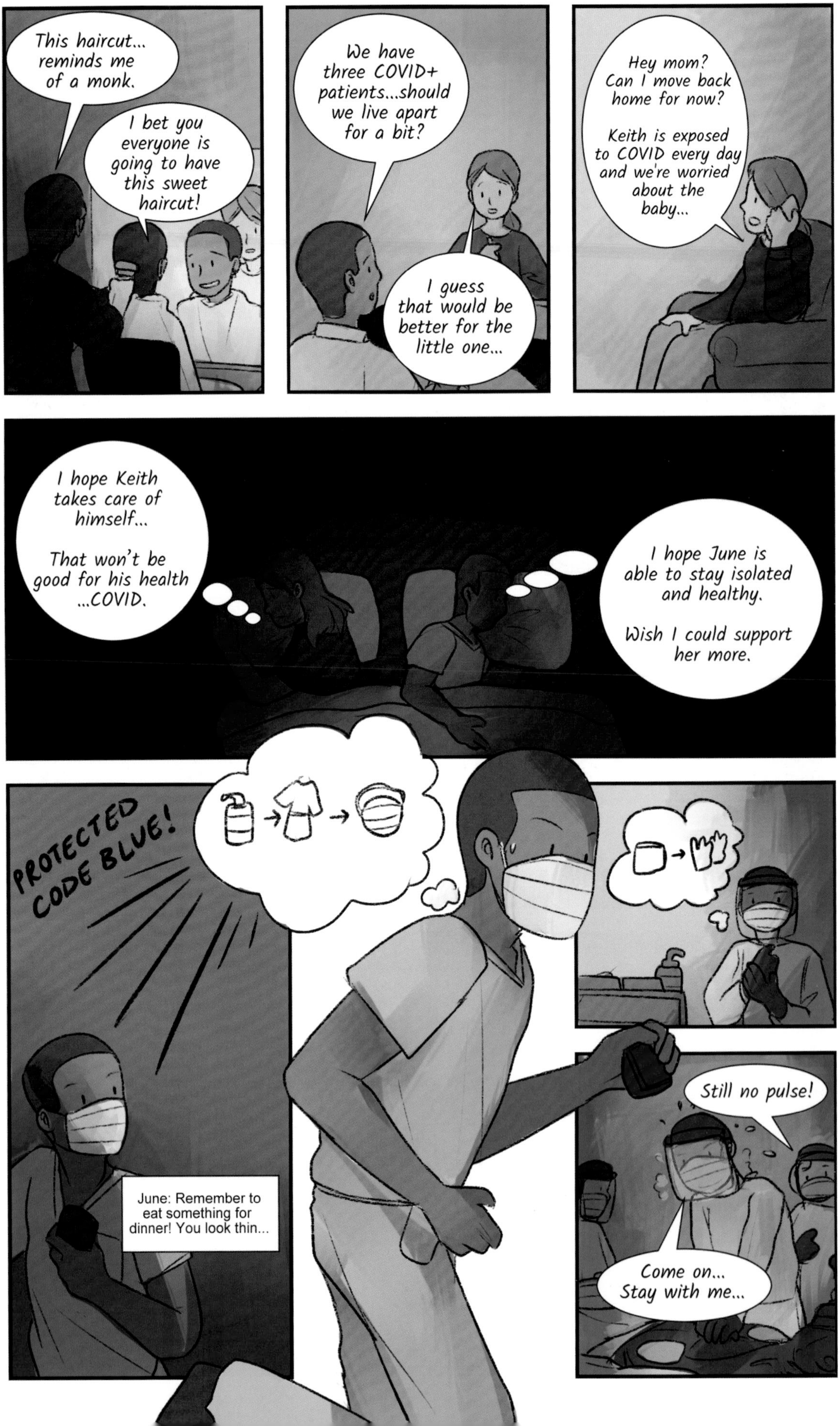
This haircut... reminds me of a monk.
I bet you everyone is going to have this sweet haircut!
We have three COVID+ patients...should we live apart for a bit?
I guess that would be better for the little one...
Hey mom? Can I move back home for now?
Keith is exposed to COVID every day and we're worried about the baby...
I hope Keith takes care of himself...
That won't be good for his health ...COVID.
I hope June is able to stay isolated and healthy.
Wish I could support her more.
PROTECTED CODE BLUE!
June: Remember to eat something for dinner! You look thin...
Still no pulse!
Come on... Stay with me...

I worry about Keith being on the front lines...
TELE HEALTH
CALL: KEITH
ACCEPT
DECLINE
PPE SHORTAGE
Just had a really difficult code. Young guy. We did everything but...
I'm sorry...that's always hard to go through. But you did your best... were you protected at least?
Yeah... But with the PPE... it's harder. And I feel disconnected from my patients. If they can't see my face, can they trust me?
PPE DONATION
What a great idea! Asking people to donate extra PPE if they have supplies...
Mom, I'm going to ask our local vendors for spare PPE.
That would help Keith and the others.
ACHOOOOOO!
#*@%!
Hey mom, I'm...really scared.
COVID ASSESSMENT CENTRE

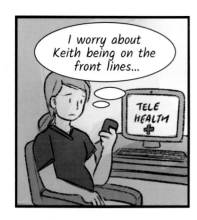

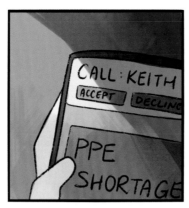

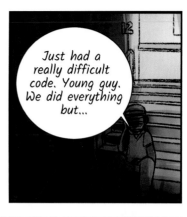

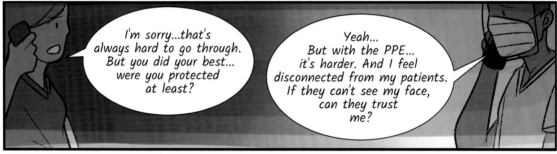

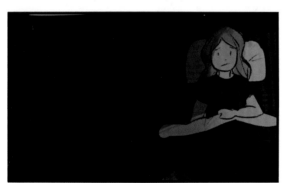

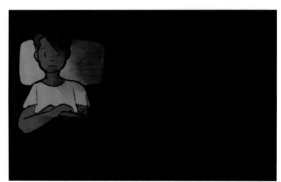

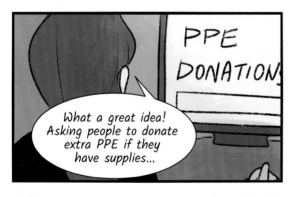

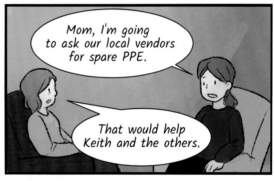

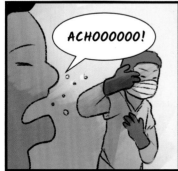

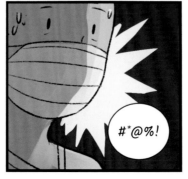

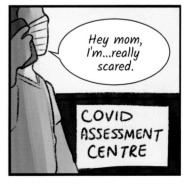

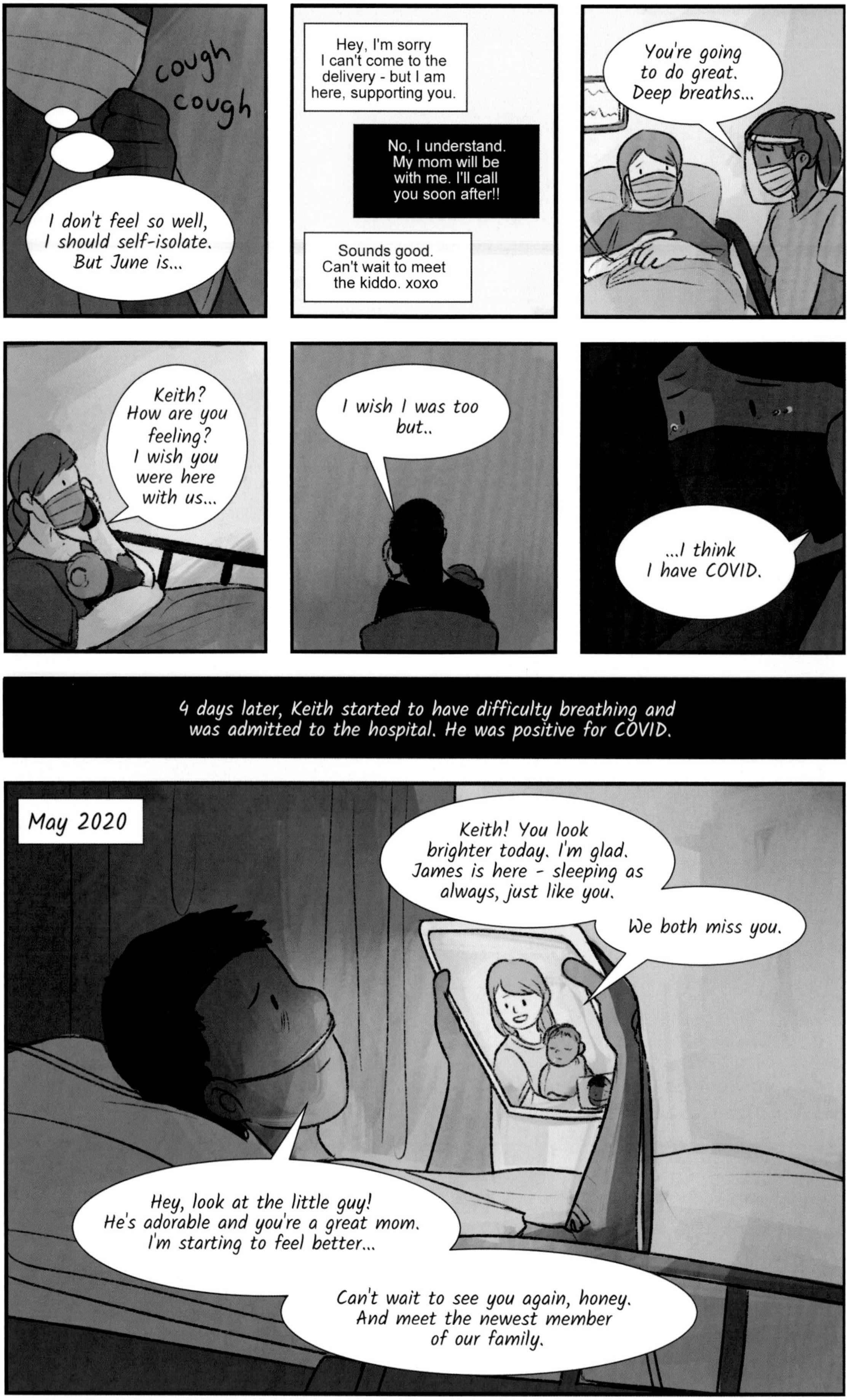
cough
cough
I don't feel so well, I should self-isolate. But June is...
Hey, I'm sorry I can't come to the delivery - but I am here, supporting you.
No, I understand. My mom will be with me. I'll call you soon after!!
Sounds good. Can't wait to meet the kiddo. xoxo
You're going to do great. Deep breaths...
Keith? How are you feeling? I wish you were here with us...
I wish I was too but..
...I think I have COVID.
4 days later, Keith started to have difficulty breathing and was admitted to the hospital. He was positive for COVID.
May 2020
Keith! You look brighter today. I'm glad. James is here - sleeping as always, just like you.
We both miss you.
Hey, look at the little guy! He's adorable and you're a great mom. I'm starting to feel better...
Can't wait to see you again, honey. And meet the newest member of our family.

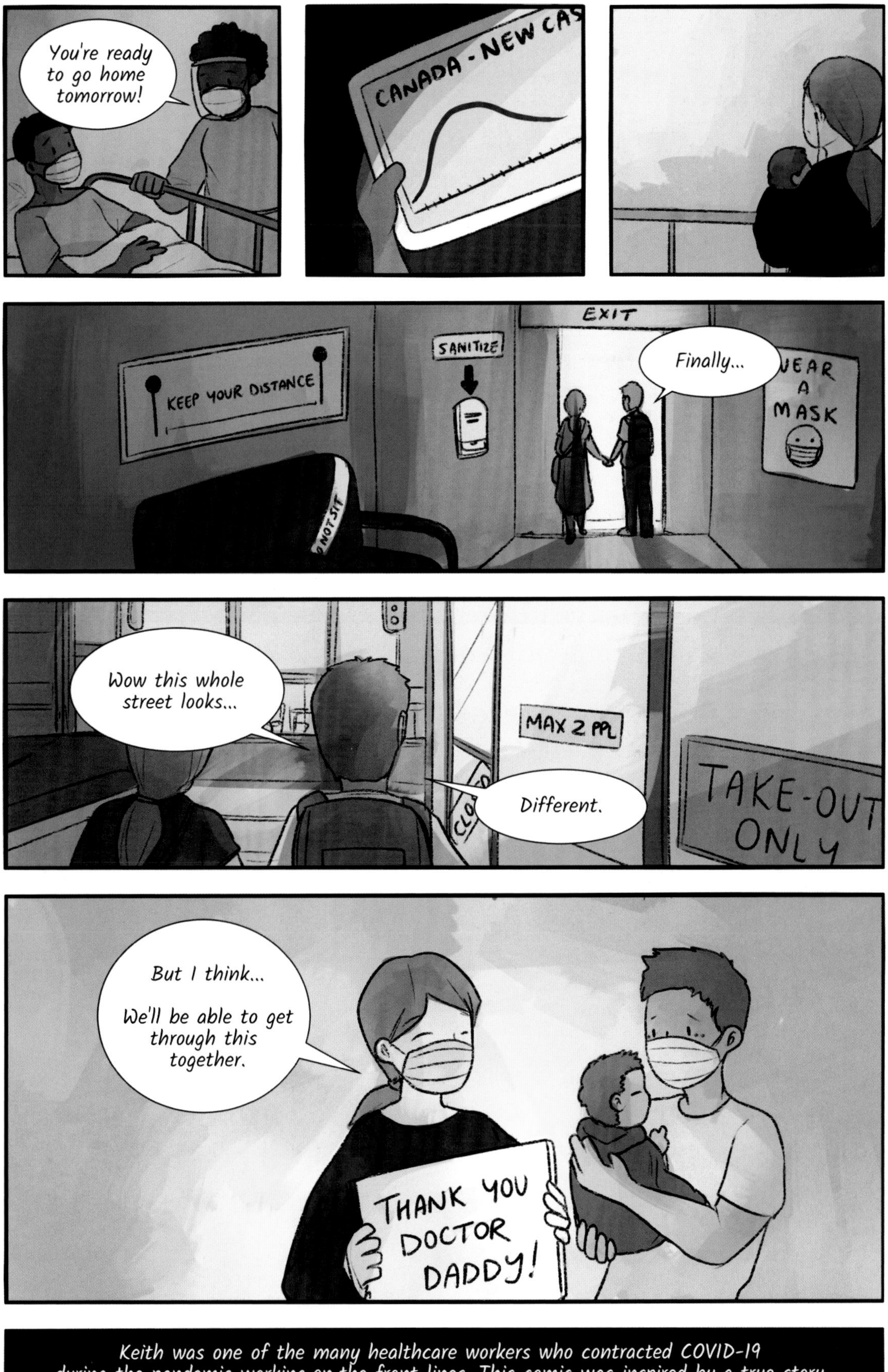
You're ready to go home tomorrow!
CANADA
KEEP YOUR DISTANCE
SANITIZE
EXIT
Finally...
MASK
NOT SIT
Wow this whole street looks...
MAX 2 PPL
Different.
TAKE-OUT ONLY
But I think...
We'll be able to get through this together.
THANK YOU DOCTOR DADDY!

Keith was one of the many healthcare workers who contracted COVID-19 during the pandemic working on the front lines. This comic was inspired by a true story although the names and anecdotes were altered and fictionalized. COVID-19 affects us all, regardless of who we are. It's important that we all do our part to keep our loved ones and members of our community safe.

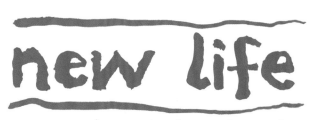

new life

by roland burkart
translation natascha hoffmeyer

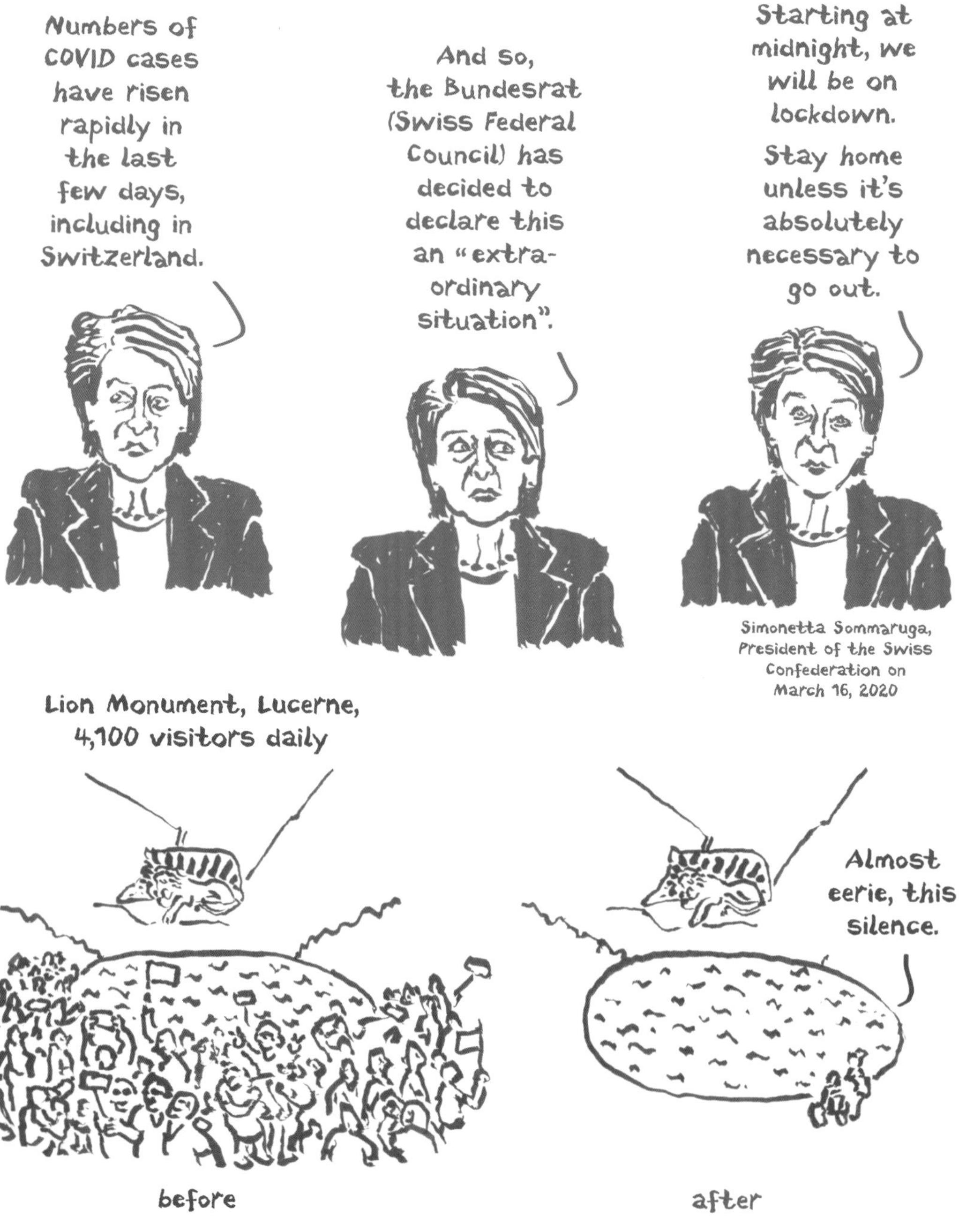
Numbers of COVID cases have risen rapidly in the last few days, including in Switzerland.
And so, the Bundesrat (Swiss Federal Council) has decided to declare this an "extra-ordinary situation".
Starting at midnight, we will be on lockdown.
Stay home unless it's absolutely necessary to go out.
Simonetta Sommaruga, President of the Swiss Confederation on March 16, 2020
Lion Monument, Lucerne, 4,100 visitors daily
Almost eerie, this silence.
before
after

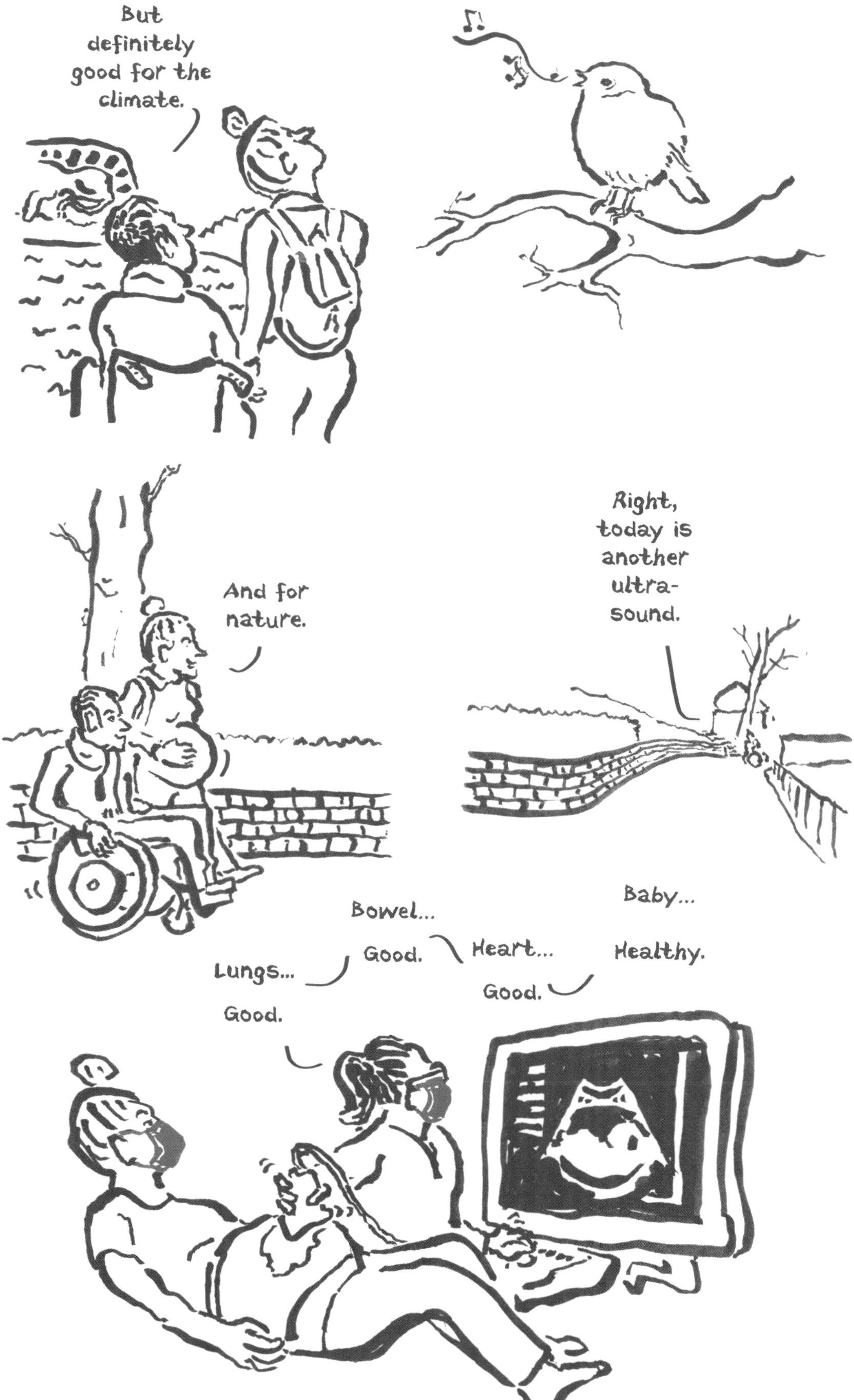
But definitely good for the climate.
And for nature.
Right, today is another ultra-sound.
Lungs...
Good.
Bowel...
Good.
Heart...
Good.
Baby...
Healthy.

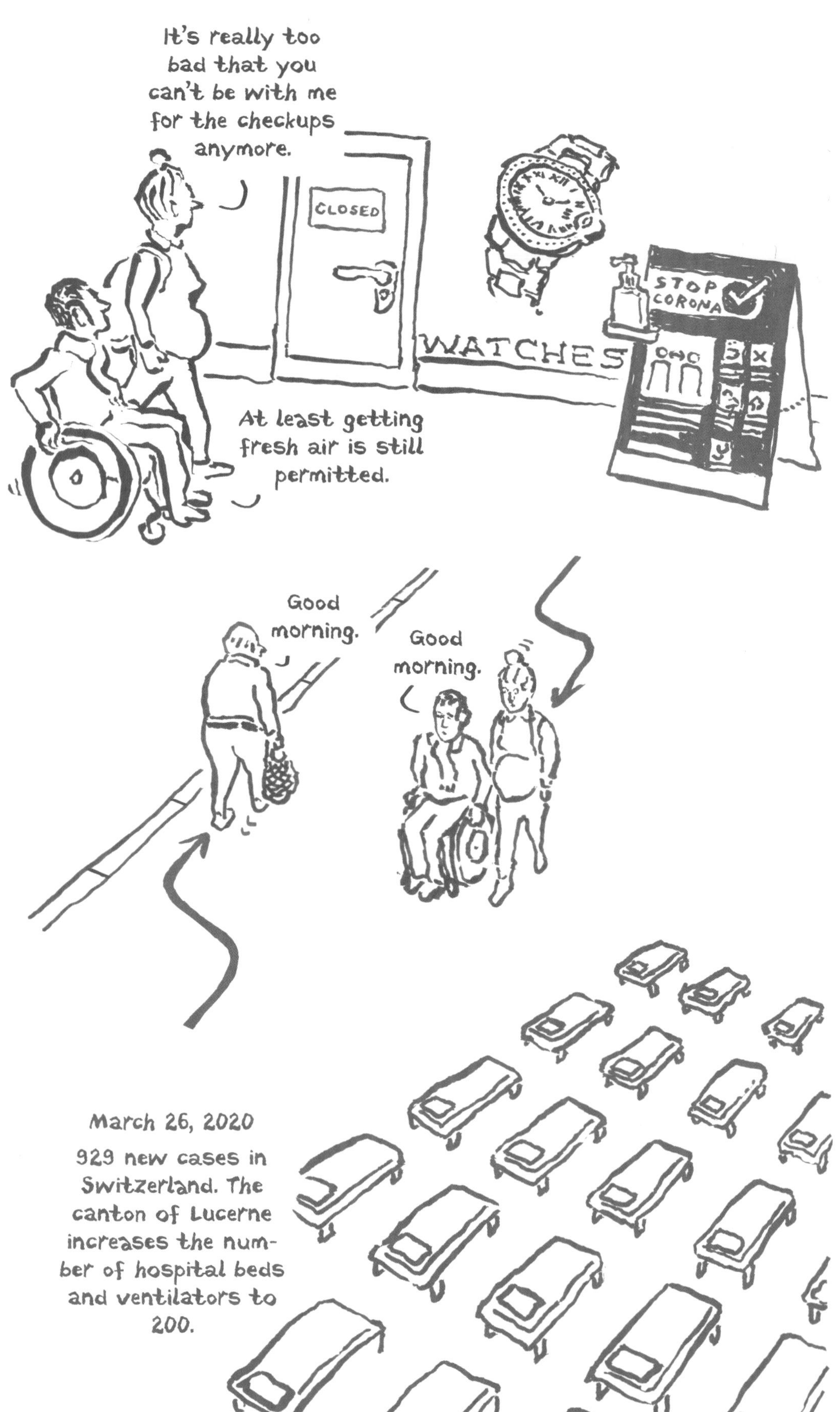
It's really too bad that you can't be with me for the checkups anymore.
CLOSED
WATCHES
STOP CORONA
At least getting fresh air is still permitted.
Good morning.
Good morning.
March 26, 2020
929 new cases in Switzerland. The canton of Lucerne increases the number of hospital beds and ventilators to 200.

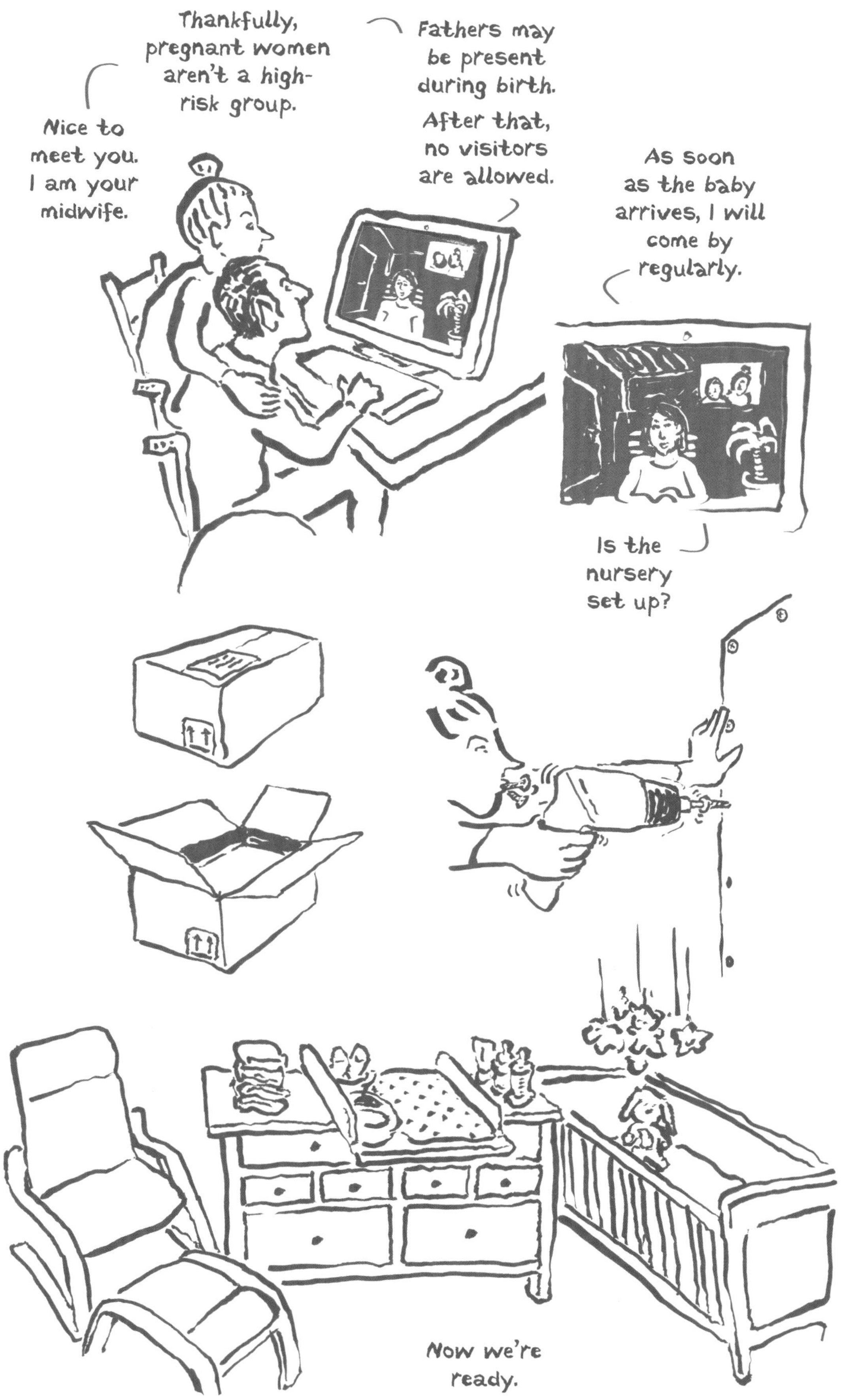
Nice to meet you. I am your midwife.
Thankfully, pregnant women aren't a high-risk group.
Fathers may be present during birth.
After that, no visitors are allowed.
As soon as the baby arrives, I will come by regularly.
Is the nursery set up?
Now we're ready.

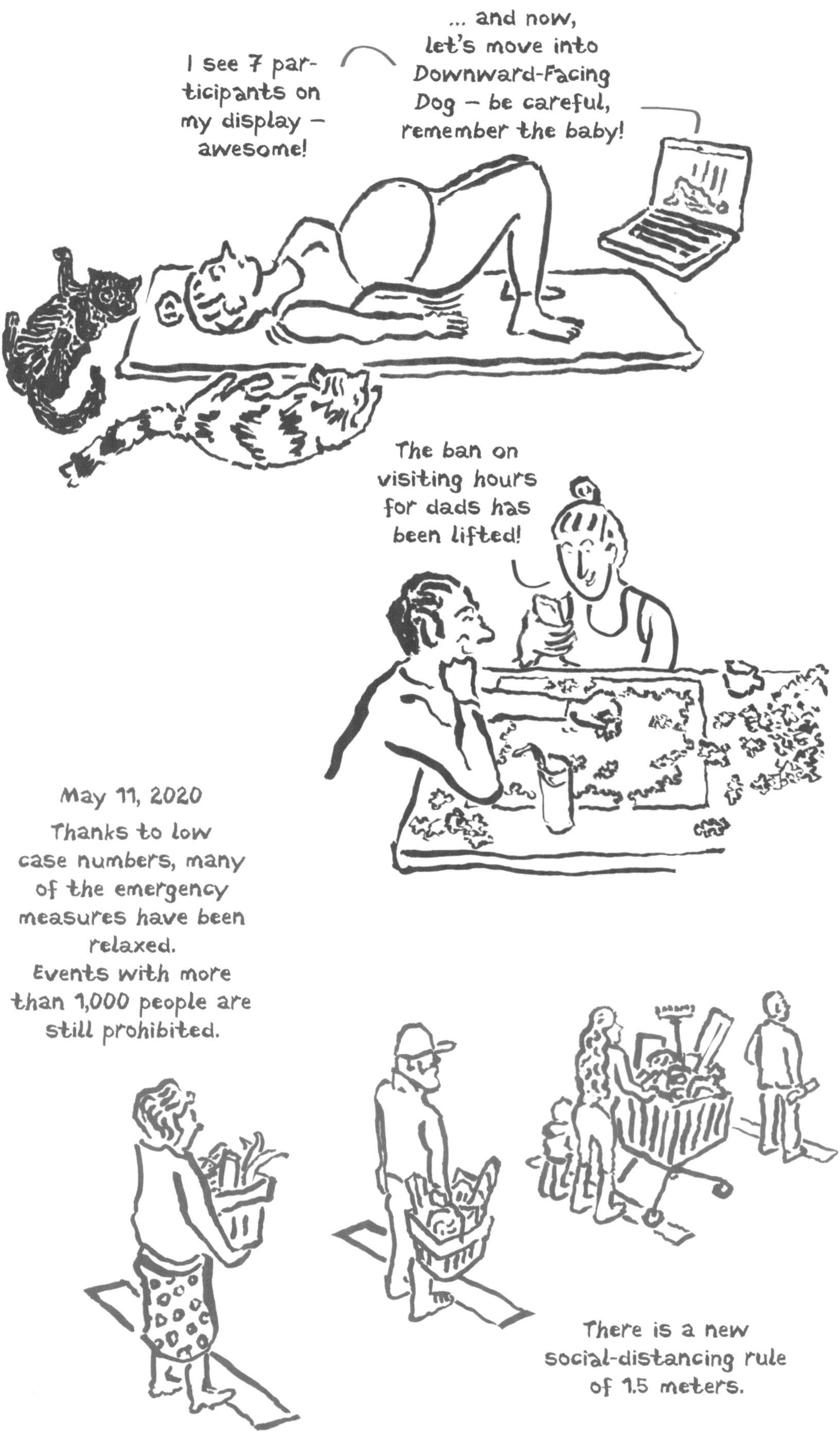

I see 7 participants on my display – awesome!
... and now, let's move into Downward-Facing Dog – be careful, remember the baby!
The ban on visiting hours for dads has been lifted!
May 11, 2020
Thanks to low case numbers, many of the emergency measures have been relaxed.
Events with more than 1,000 people are still prohibited.
There is a new social-distancing rule of 1.5 meters.

Now push!

It's a girl!

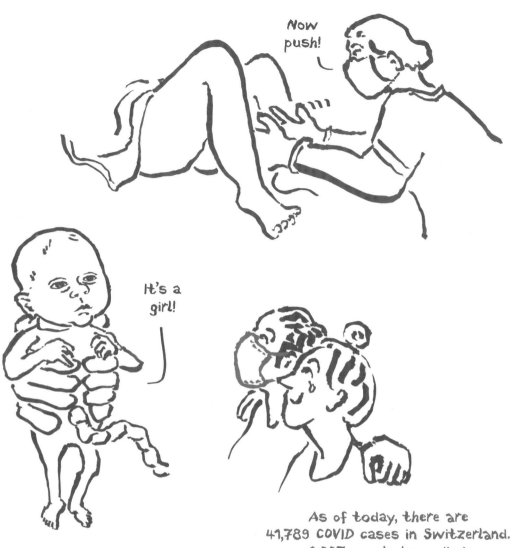

As of today, there are
41,789 COVID cases in Switzerland.
2,007 people have died.
Case numbers are slowly rising again.

Is she asleep yet?
Yes.
Uh, no – she just opened her eyes again.

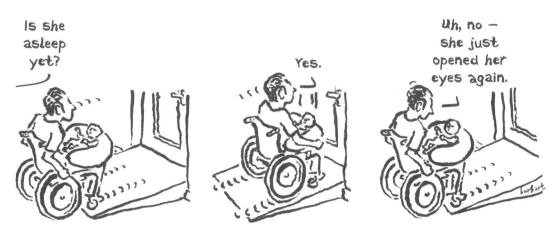

Despite the stress of COVID-19, there is new life in Switzerland: As of Sept. 1, 2020, more than 39,400 babies have been born during this pandemic.

What the hell?!?! What do you mean we're all expelled?!?! Every single person at the frat party was wearing a mask!
DEAN'S OFFICE

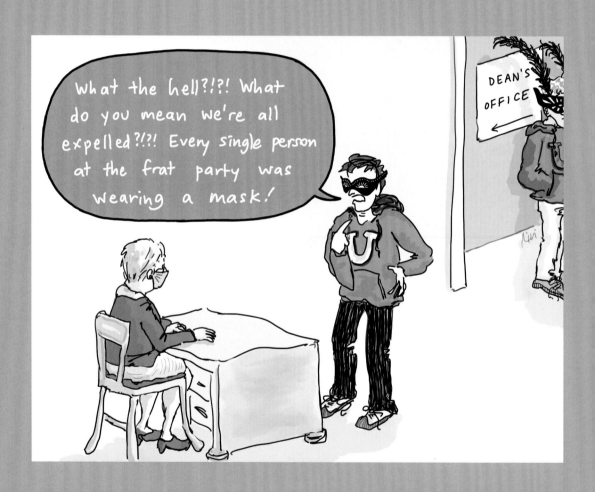

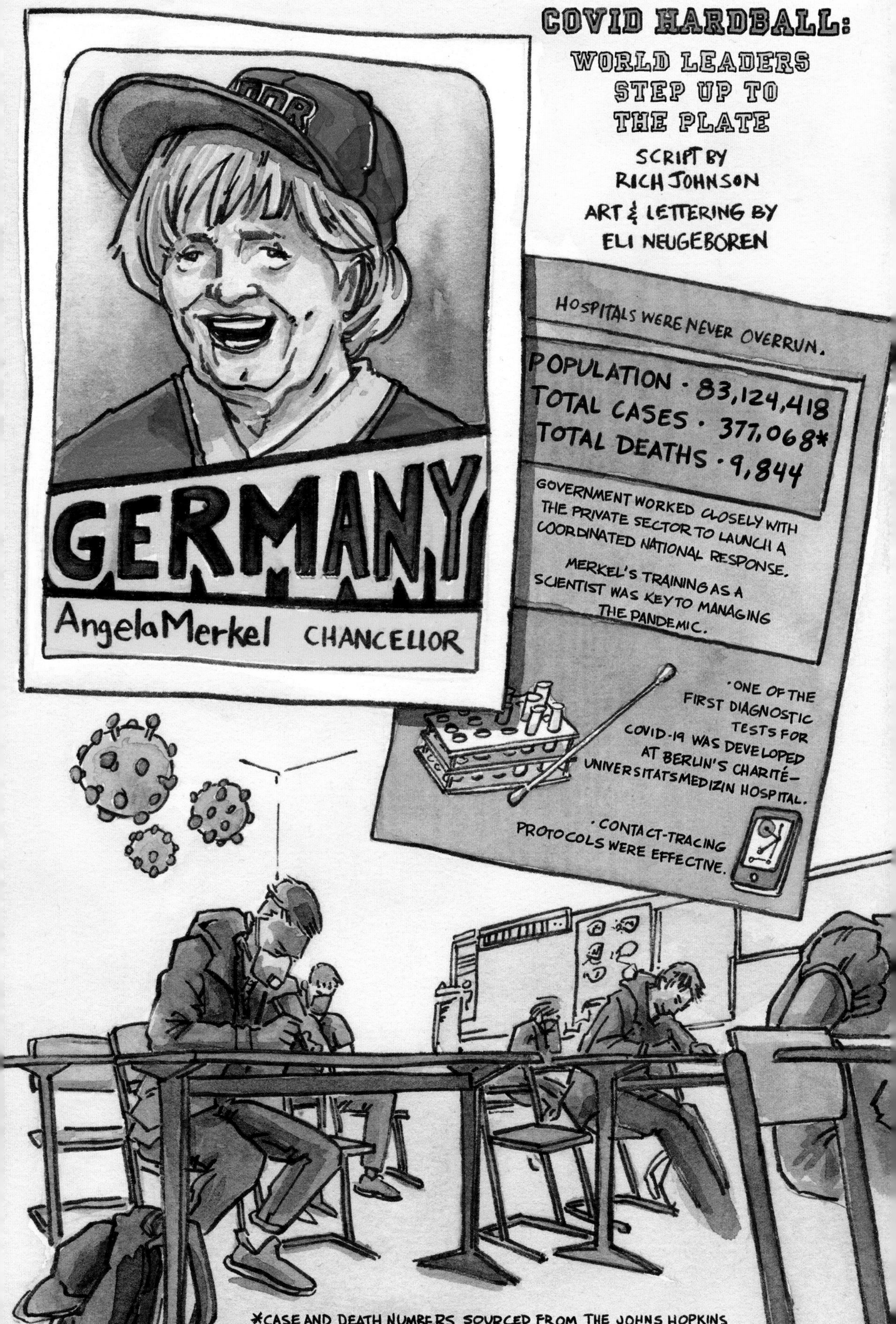
COVID HARDBALL:
WORLD LEADERS STEP UP TO THE PLATE
SCRIPT BY RICH JOHNSON
ART & LETTERING BY ELI NEUGEBOREN
DDR
GERMANY
Angela Merkel CHANCELLOR
HOSPITALS WERE NEVER OVERRUN.
POPULATION · 83,124,418
TOTAL CASES · 377,068*
TOTAL DEATHS · 9,844
GOVERNMENT WORKED CLOSELY WITH THE PRIVATE SECTOR TO LAUNCH A COORDINATED NATIONAL RESPONSE.
MERKEL'S TRAINING AS A SCIENTIST WAS KEY TO MANAGING THE PANDEMIC.
· ONE OF THE FIRST DIAGNOSTIC TESTS FOR COVID-19 WAS DEVELOPED AT BERLIN'S CHARITÉ–UNIVERSITATSMEDIZIN HOSPITAL.
· CONTACT-TRACING PROTOCOLS WERE EFFECTIVE.
*CASE AND DEATH NUMBERS SOURCED FROM THE JOHNS HOPKINS CORONAVIRUS RESOURCE CENTER ON OCTOBER 20, 2020, AT HTTPS://CORONAVIRUS.JHU.EDU/MAP.HTML

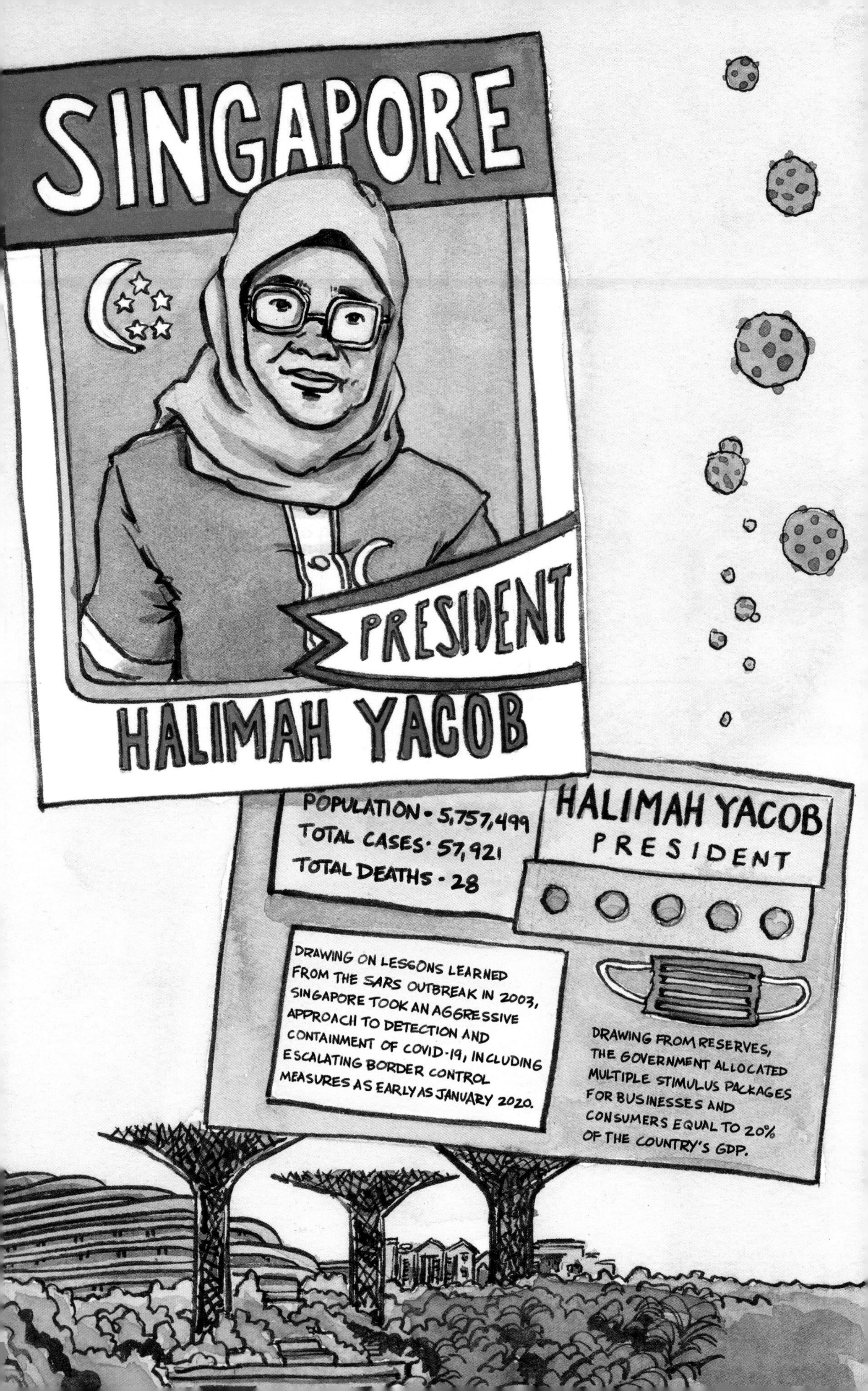
SINGAPORE
PRESIDENT
HALIMAH YACOB
POPULATION • 5,757,499
TOTAL CASES • 57,921
TOTAL DEATHS • 28
HALIMAH YACOB
PRESIDENT
DRAWING ON LESSONS LEARNED FROM THE SARS OUTBREAK IN 2003, SINGAPORE TOOK AN AGGRESSIVE APPROACH TO DETECTION AND CONTAINMENT OF COVID-19, INCLUDING ESCALATING BORDER CONTROL MEASURES AS EARLY AS JANUARY 2020.
DRAWING FROM RESERVES, THE GOVERNMENT ALLOCATED MULTIPLE STIMULUS PACKAGES FOR BUSINESSES AND CONSUMERS EQUAL TO 20% OF THE COUNTRY'S GDP.

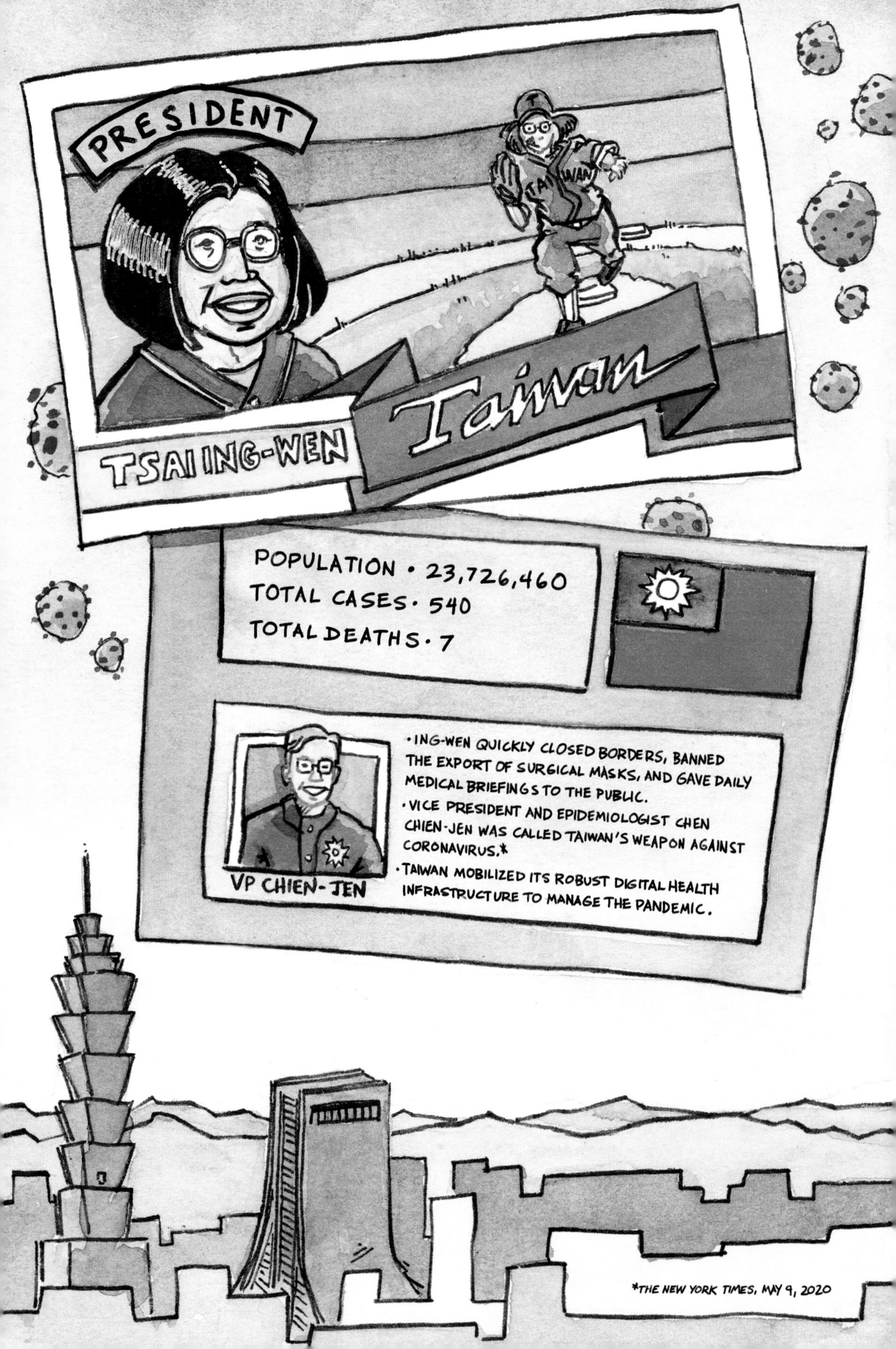
PRESIDENT
TAIWAN
TSAI ING-WEN
Taiwan
POPULATION · 23,726,460
TOTAL CASES · 540
TOTAL DEATHS · 7
VP CHIEN-JEN
· ING-WEN QUICKLY CLOSED BORDERS, BANNED THE EXPORT OF SURGICAL MASKS, AND GAVE DAILY MEDICAL BRIEFINGS TO THE PUBLIC.
· VICE PRESIDENT AND EPIDEMIOLOGIST CHEN CHIEN-JEN WAS CALLED TAIWAN'S WEAPON AGAINST CORONAVIRUS.*
· TAIWAN MOBILIZED ITS ROBUST DIGITAL HEALTH INFRASTRUCTURE TO MANAGE THE PANDEMIC.
*THE NEW YORK TIMES, MAY 9, 2020

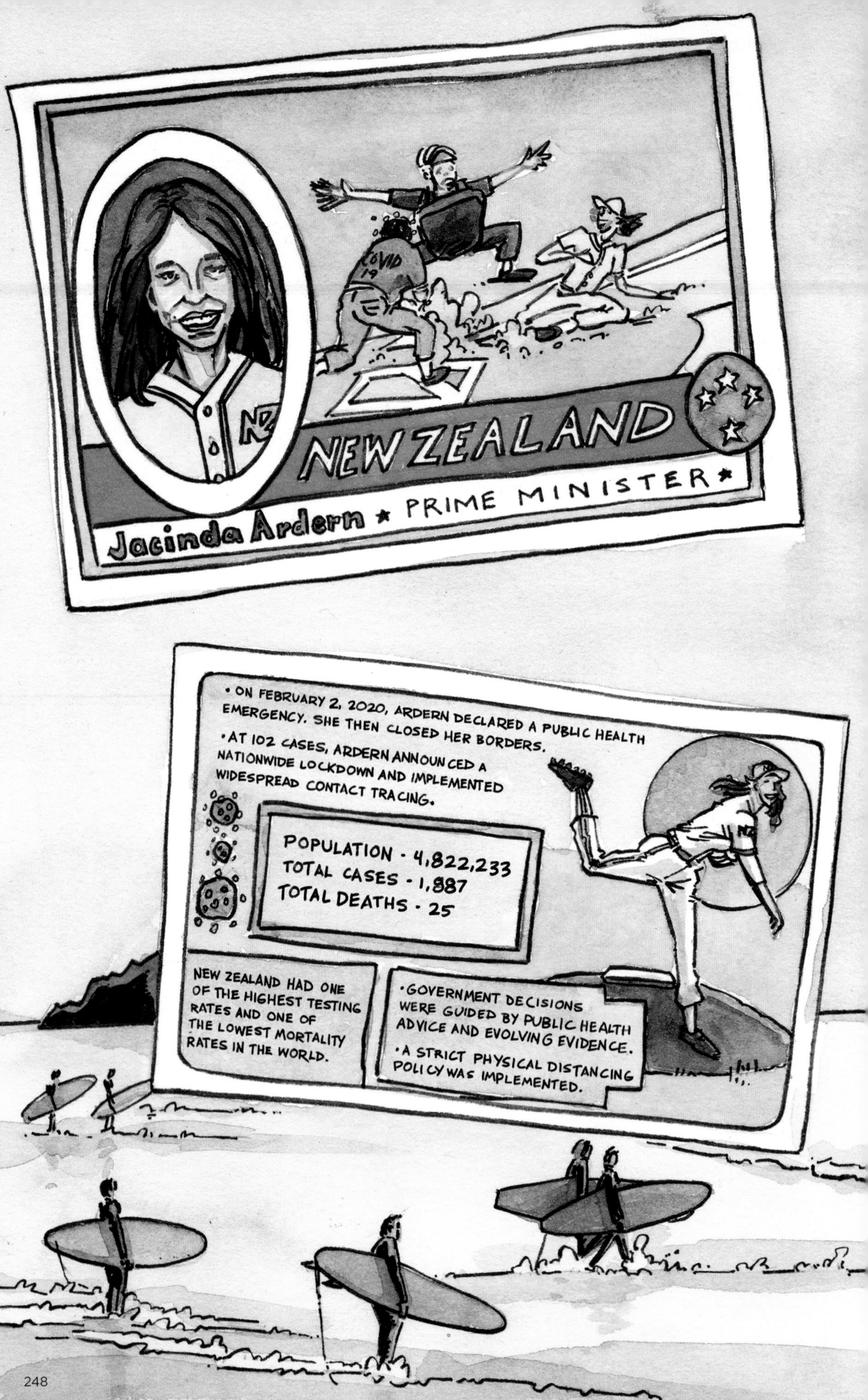
COVID 19
NEW ZEALAND
Jacinda Ardern ★ PRIME MINISTER ★
• ON FEBRUARY 2, 2020, ARDERN DECLARED A PUBLIC HEALTH EMERGENCY. SHE THEN CLOSED HER BORDERS.
• AT 102 CASES, ARDERN ANNOUNCED A NATIONWIDE LOCKDOWN AND IMPLEMENTED WIDESPREAD CONTACT TRACING.
POPULATION - 4,822,233
TOTAL CASES - 1,887
TOTAL DEATHS - 25
NEW ZEALAND HAD ONE OF THE HIGHEST TESTING RATES AND ONE OF THE LOWEST MORTALITY RATES IN THE WORLD.
• GOVERNMENT DECISIONS WERE GUIDED BY PUBLIC HEALTH ADVICE AND EVOLVING EVIDENCE.
• A STRICT PHYSICAL DISTANCING POLICY WAS IMPLEMENTED.

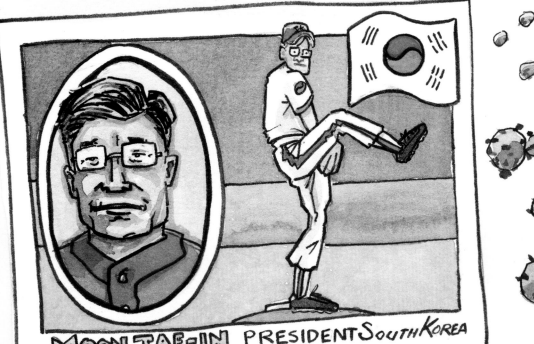

MOON JAE-IN PRESIDENT SOUTH KOREA

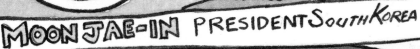

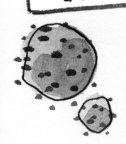

LESSONS LEARNED FROM THE 2015 MERS OUTBREAK PREPARED SOUTH KOREA FOR SUCCESSFULLY MANAGING COVID-19.

POPULATION · 51,171,706
TOTAL CASES · 25 333
TOTAL DEATHS · 447

MOON JAE-IN PRESIDENT

·PUBLIC BRIEFINGS OCCURRED TWICE DAILY.
·MASKING WAS NEARLY UNIVERSAL.
·ALL CONFIRMED CASES WERE ISOLATED.
·MEDICAL TREATMENT WAS FREE.

SOUTH KOREA HAS "BLENDED TECHNOLOGY AND TESTING LIKE NO OTHER," RESULTING IN THE CAPACITY FOR MORE THAN 50,000 TESTS PER DAY, WITH 24-HOUR RESULTS.*

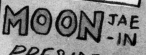

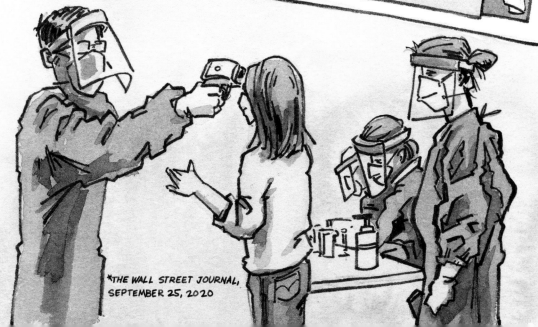

*THE WALL STREET JOURNAL, SEPTEMBER 25, 2020

249

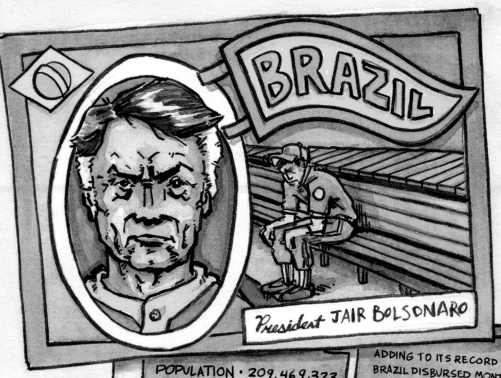

BRAZIL

President *JAIR BOLSONARO*

POPULATION · 209,469,323
TOTAL CASES · 5,250,727
TOTAL DEATHS · 154,176

ADDING TO ITS RECORD DEBT, BRAZIL DISBURSED MONTHLY STIMULUS CHECKS OVER THE COURSE OF THE SUMMER TO 32% OF ITS POPULATION. BY SEPTEMBER, BOLSONARO'S APPROVAL RATINGS WERE UP BY 32%.

• BOLSONARO CALLED COVID-19 "A MEASLY COLD" AND SAID THAT "SOME WILL DIE FROM IT BECAUSE SUCH IS LIFE."*

• BOLSONARO FIRED HIS HEALTH MINISTER FOR PRESCRIBING ISOLATION AND SOCIAL DISTANCING, AND HE RELAXED SHUTDOWN MEASURES AS THE DEATH TOLL CLIMBED.

BOLSONARO ENCOURAGED BRAZILIANS TO TAKE HYDROXYCHLOROQUINE.

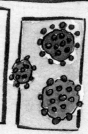

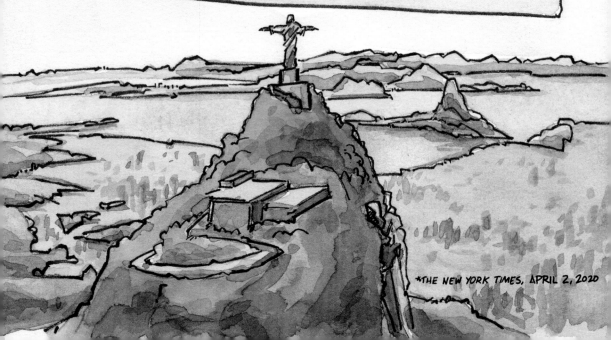

*THE NEW YORK TIMES, APRIL 2, 2020

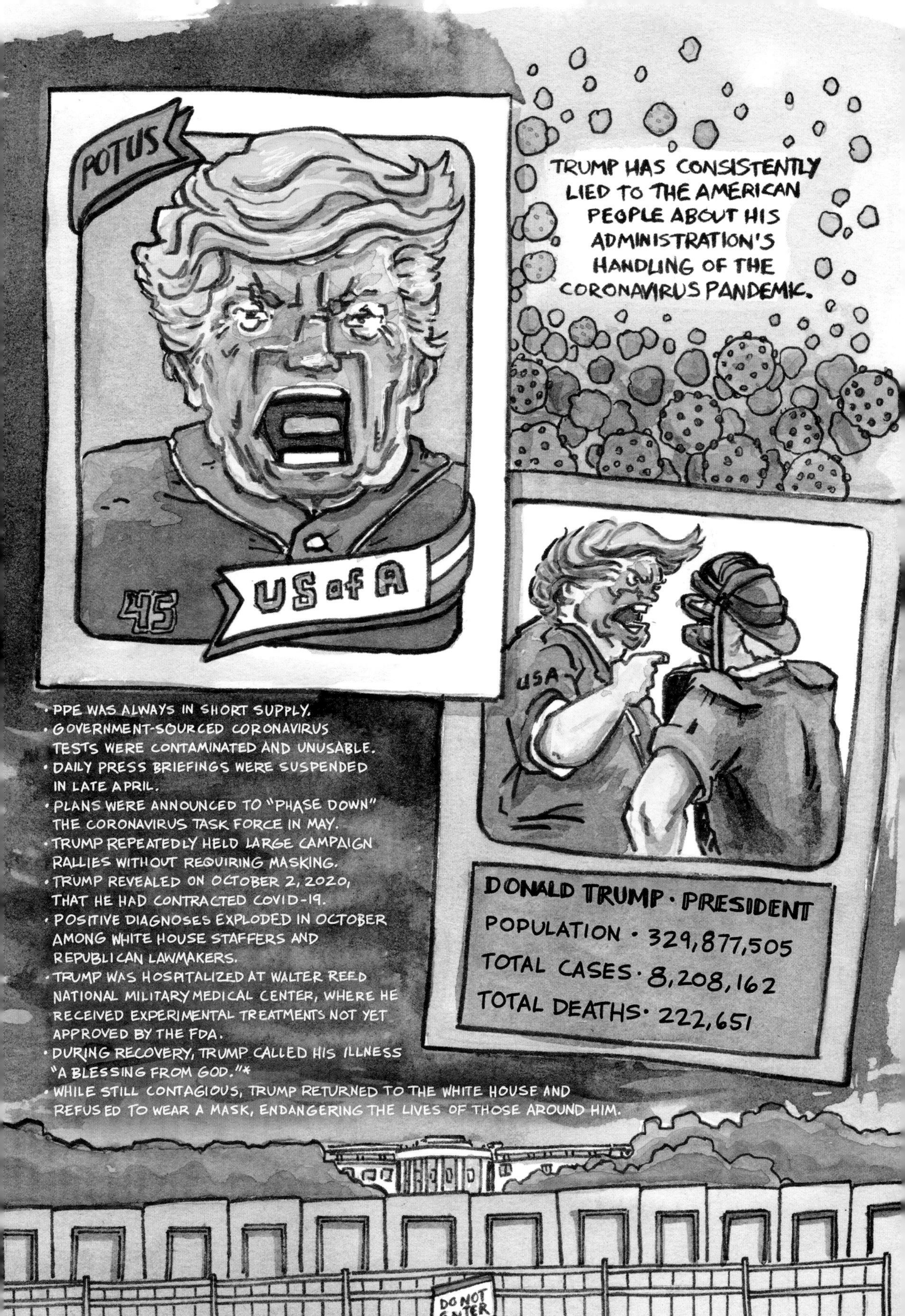
POTUS
45
US of A
TRUMP HAS CONSISTENTLY LIED TO THE AMERICAN PEOPLE ABOUT HIS ADMINISTRATION'S HANDLING OF THE CORONAVIRUS PANDEMIC.
USA
DONALD TRUMP · PRESIDENT
POPULATION · 329,877,505
TOTAL CASES · 8,208,162
TOTAL DEATHS · 222,651
· PPE WAS ALWAYS IN SHORT SUPPLY.
· GOVERNMENT-SOURCED CORONAVIRUS TESTS WERE CONTAMINATED AND UNUSABLE.
· DAILY PRESS BRIEFINGS WERE SUSPENDED IN LATE APRIL.
· PLANS WERE ANNOUNCED TO "PHASE DOWN" THE CORONAVIRUS TASK FORCE IN MAY.
· TRUMP REPEATEDLY HELD LARGE CAMPAIGN RALLIES WITHOUT REQUIRING MASKING.
· TRUMP REVEALED ON OCTOBER 2, 2020, THAT HE HAD CONTRACTED COVID-19.
· POSITIVE DIAGNOSES EXPLODED IN OCTOBER AMONG WHITE HOUSE STAFFERS AND REPUBLICAN LAWMAKERS.
· TRUMP WAS HOSPITALIZED AT WALTER REED NATIONAL MILITARY MEDICAL CENTER, WHERE HE RECEIVED EXPERIMENTAL TREATMENTS NOT YET APPROVED BY THE FDA.
· DURING RECOVERY, TRUMP CALLED HIS ILLNESS "A BLESSING FROM GOD."*
· WHILE STILL CONTAGIOUS, TRUMP RETURNED TO THE WHITE HOUSE AND REFUSED TO WEAR A MASK, ENDANGERING THE LIVES OF THOSE AROUND HIM.
DO NOT ENTER

* TRUMP, DONALD J. [@REALDONALDTRUMP]. (2020, OCTOBER 7) "A MESSAGE FROM THE PRESIDENT"! TWITTER. HTTPS://TWITTER.COM/REALDONALDTRUMP/STATUS/1313959702104023047

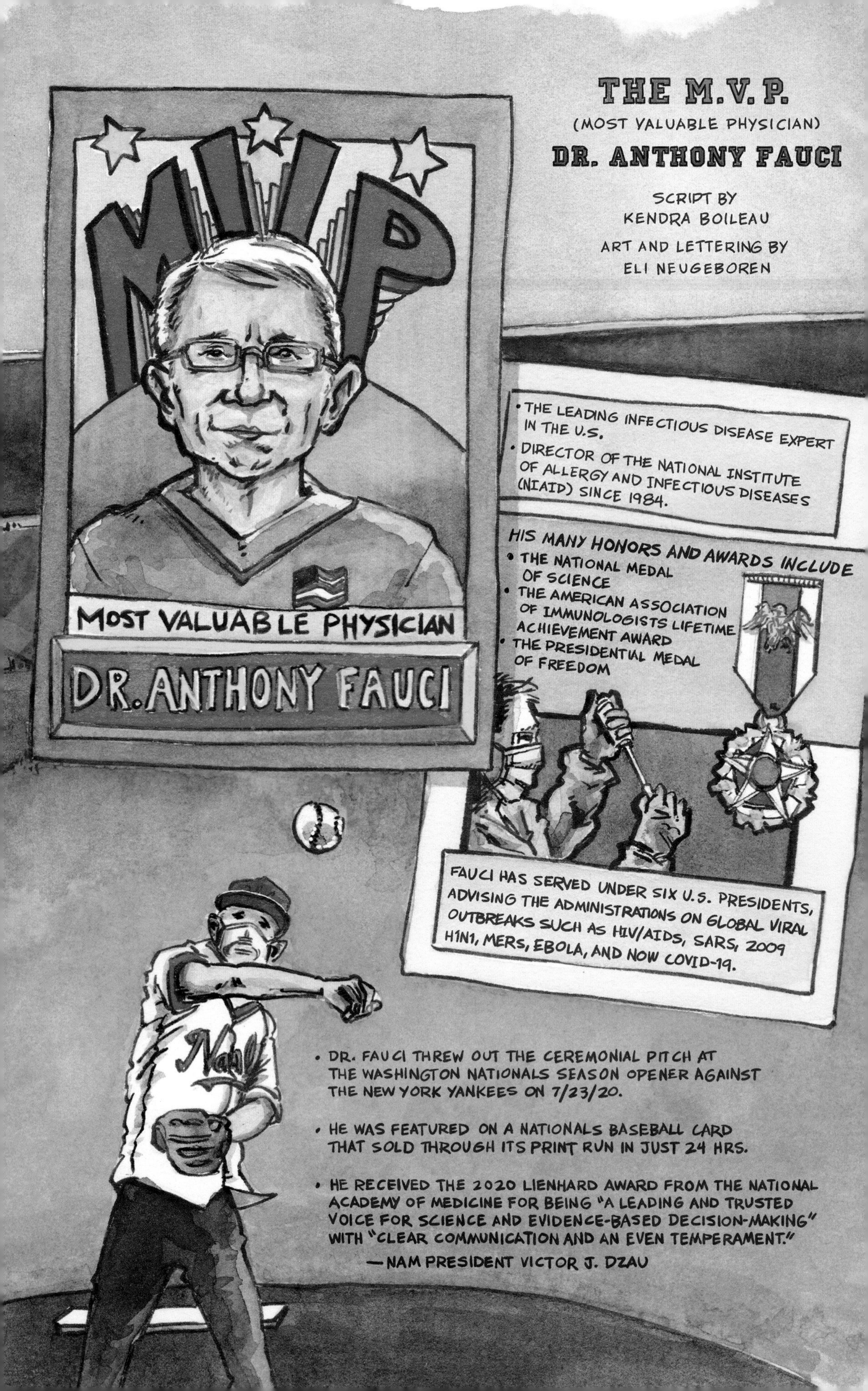
THE M.V.P.
(MOST VALUABLE PHYSICIAN)
DR. ANTHONY FAUCI
SCRIPT BY
KENDRA BOILEAU
ART AND LETTERING BY
ELI NEUGEBOREN
MVP
MOST VALUABLE PHYSICIAN
DR. ANTHONY FAUCI
• THE LEADING INFECTIOUS DISEASE EXPERT IN THE U.S.
• DIRECTOR OF THE NATIONAL INSTITUTE OF ALLERGY AND INFECTIOUS DISEASES (NIAID) SINCE 1984.
HIS MANY HONORS AND AWARDS INCLUDE
• THE NATIONAL MEDAL OF SCIENCE
• THE AMERICAN ASSOCIATION OF IMMUNOLOGISTS LIFETIME ACHIEVEMENT AWARD
• THE PRESIDENTIAL MEDAL OF FREEDOM
FAUCI HAS SERVED UNDER SIX U.S. PRESIDENTS, ADVISING THE ADMINISTRATIONS ON GLOBAL VIRAL OUTBREAKS SUCH AS HIV/AIDS, SARS, 2009 H1N1, MERS, EBOLA, AND NOW COVID-19.
Nat
• DR. FAUCI THREW OUT THE CEREMONIAL PITCH AT THE WASHINGTON NATIONALS SEASON OPENER AGAINST THE NEW YORK YANKEES ON 7/23/20.
• HE WAS FEATURED ON A NATIONALS BASEBALL CARD THAT SOLD THROUGH ITS PRINT RUN IN JUST 24 HRS.
• HE RECEIVED THE 2020 LIENHARD AWARD FROM THE NATIONAL ACADEMY OF MEDICINE FOR BEING "A LEADING AND TRUSTED VOICE FOR SCIENCE AND EVIDENCE-BASED DECISION-MAKING" WITH "CLEAR COMMUNICATION AND AN EVEN TEMPERAMENT."
—NAM PRESIDENT VICTOR J. DZAU

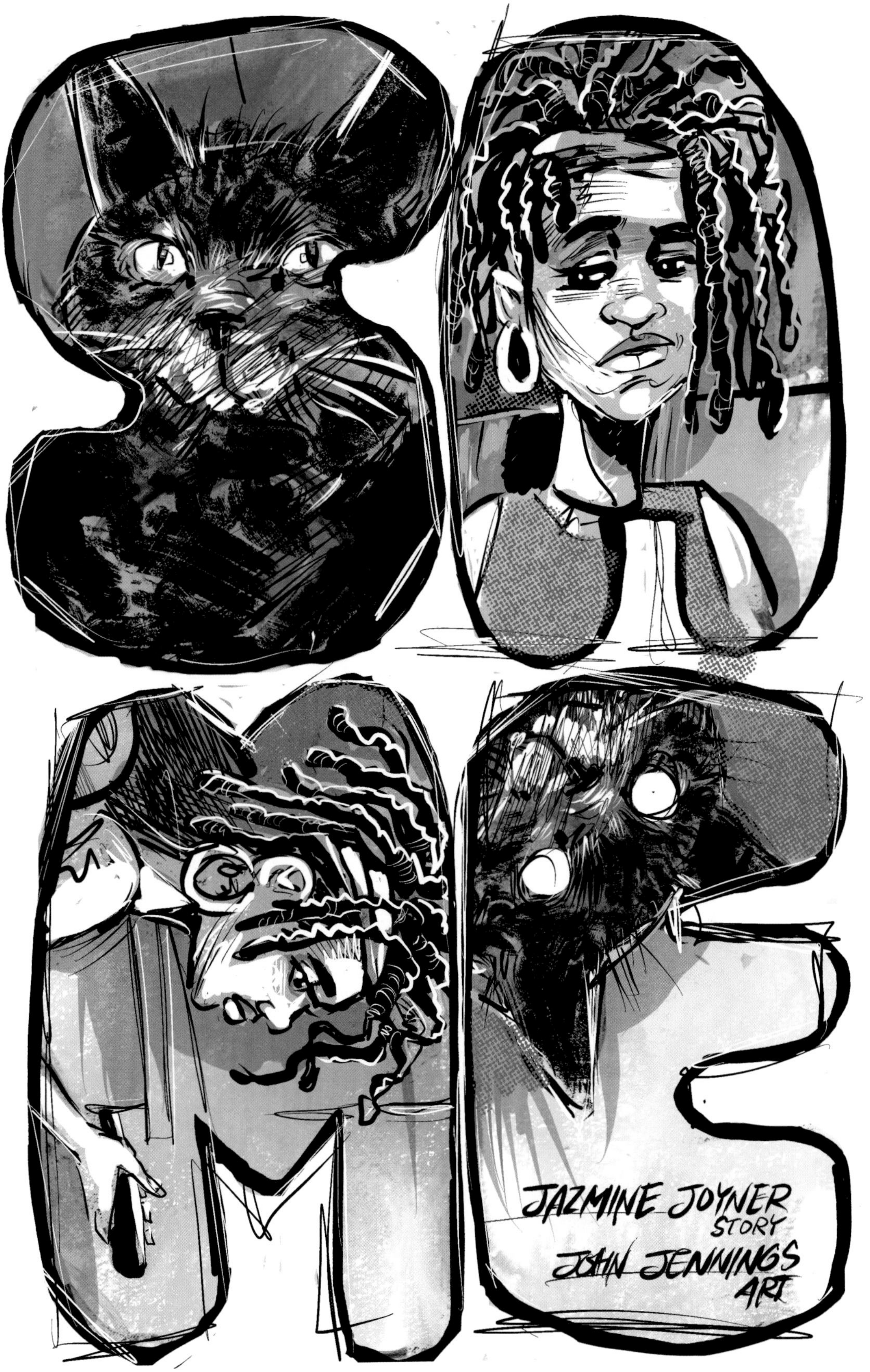
JAZMINE JOYNER
STORY
JOHN JENNINGS
ART

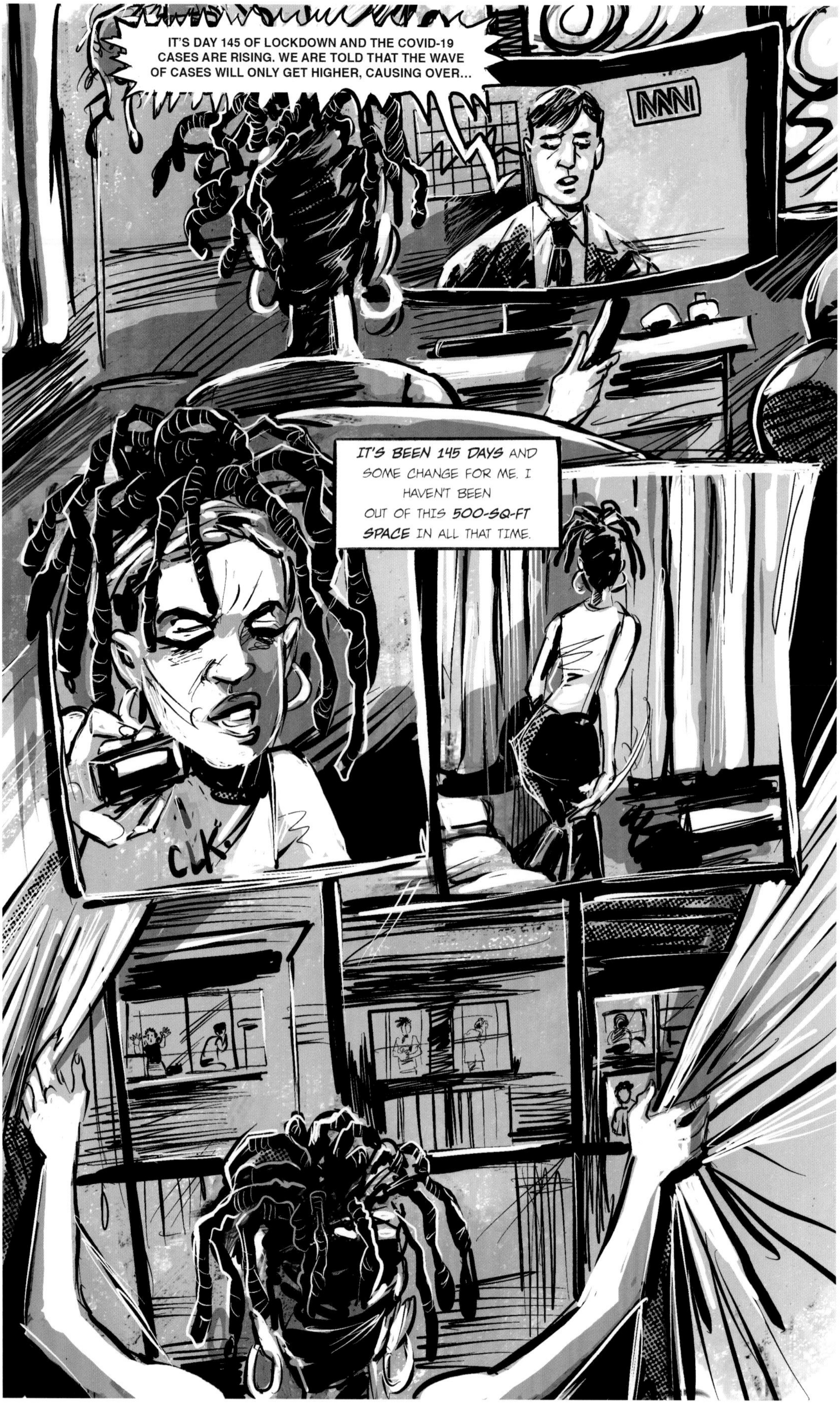
IT'S DAY 145 OF LOCKDOWN AND THE COVID-19 CASES ARE RISING. WE ARE TOLD THAT THE WAVE OF CASES WILL ONLY GET HIGHER, CAUSING OVER...
IT'S BEEN 145 DAYS AND SOME CHANGE FOR ME. I HAVEN'T BEEN OUT OF THIS 500-SQ-FT SPACE IN ALL THAT TIME.
CLK.

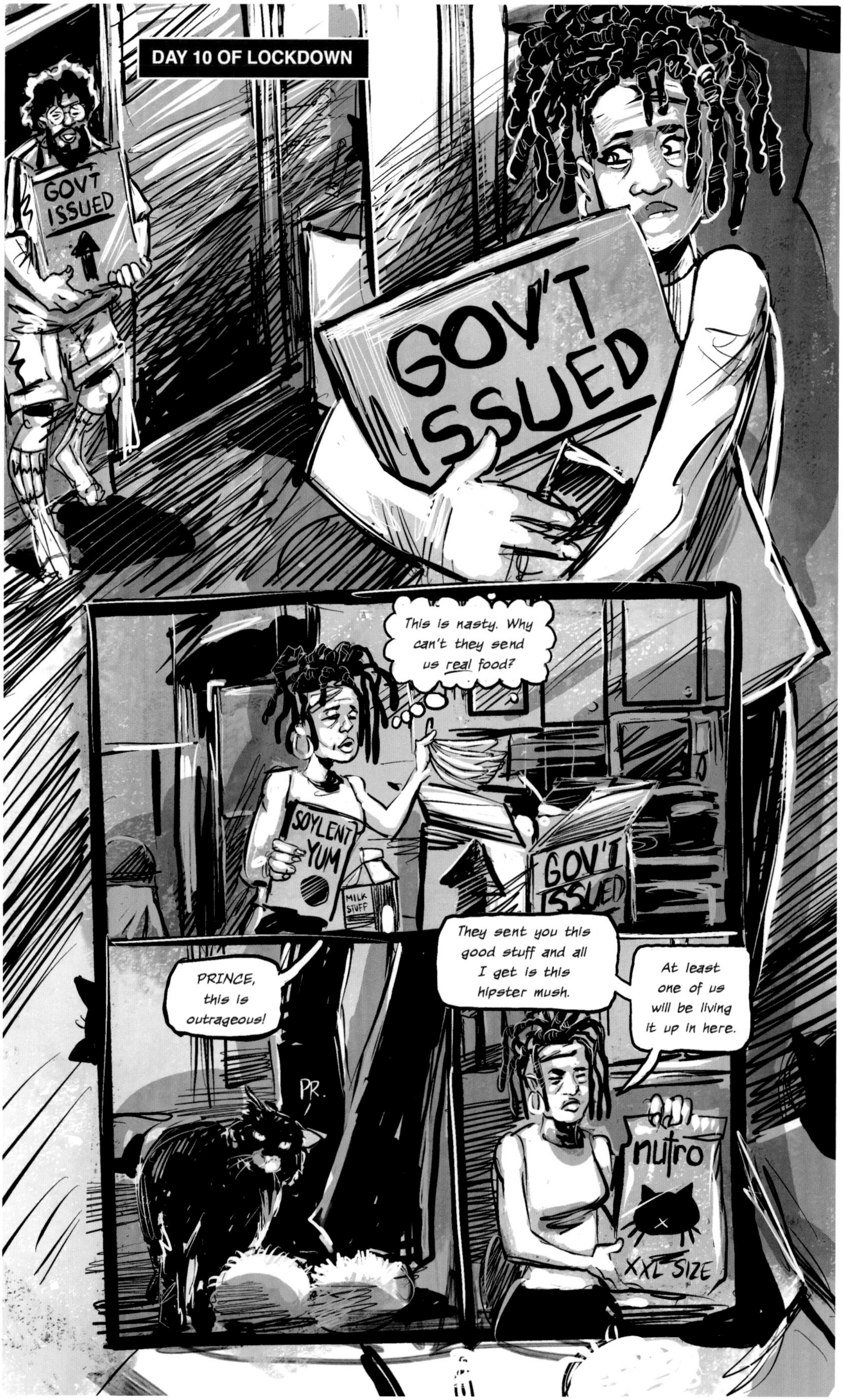
DAY 10 OF LOCKDOWN
GOV'T ISSUED
GOV'T ISSUED
This is nasty. Why can't they send us real food?
SOYLENT YUM
MILK STUFF
GOV'T ISSUED
PRINCE, this is outrageous!
PR.
They sent you this good stuff and all I get is this hipster mush.
At least one of us will be living it up in here.
nutro
XXL SIZE

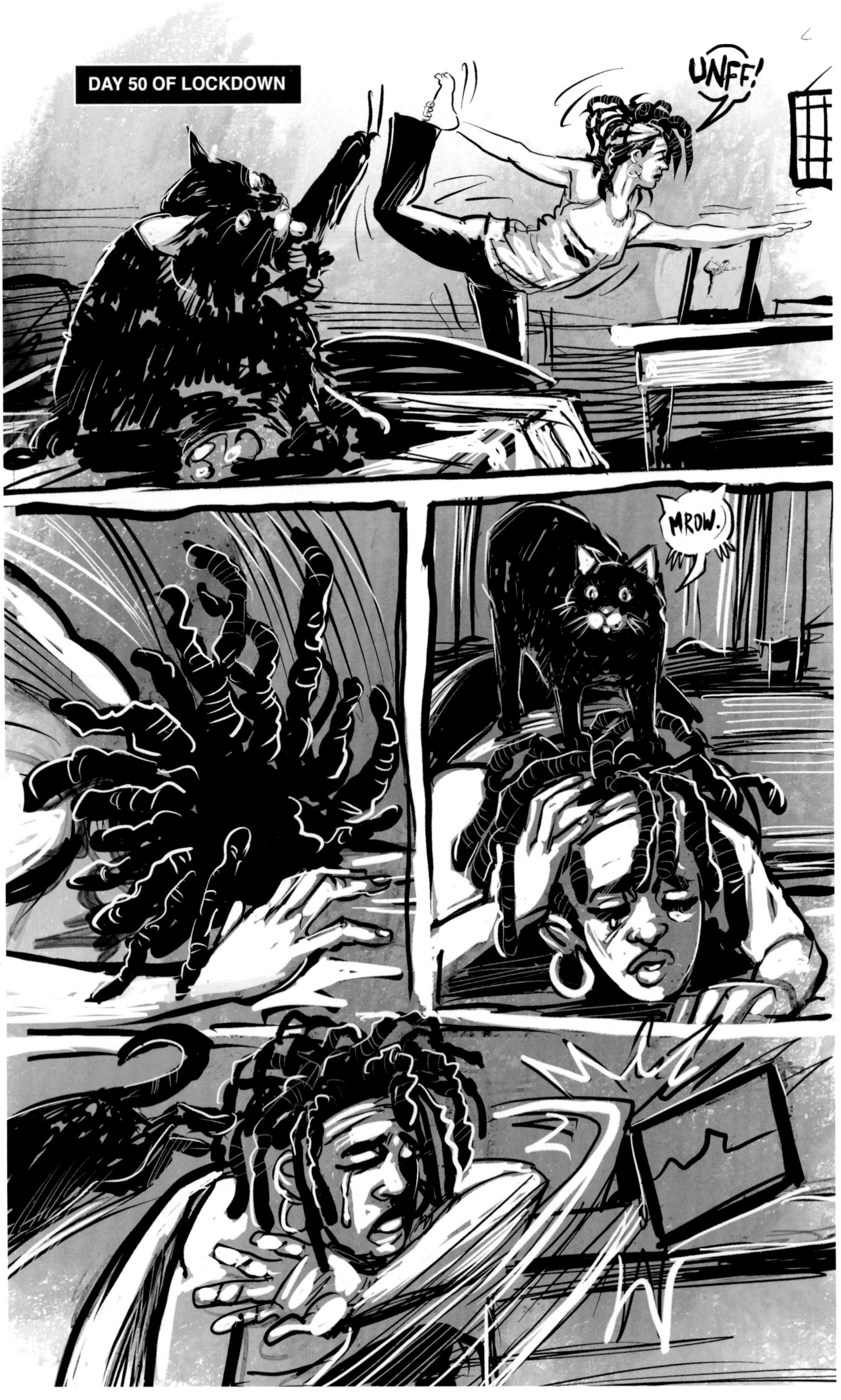
DAY 50 OF LOCKDOWN
UNFF!
MROW.

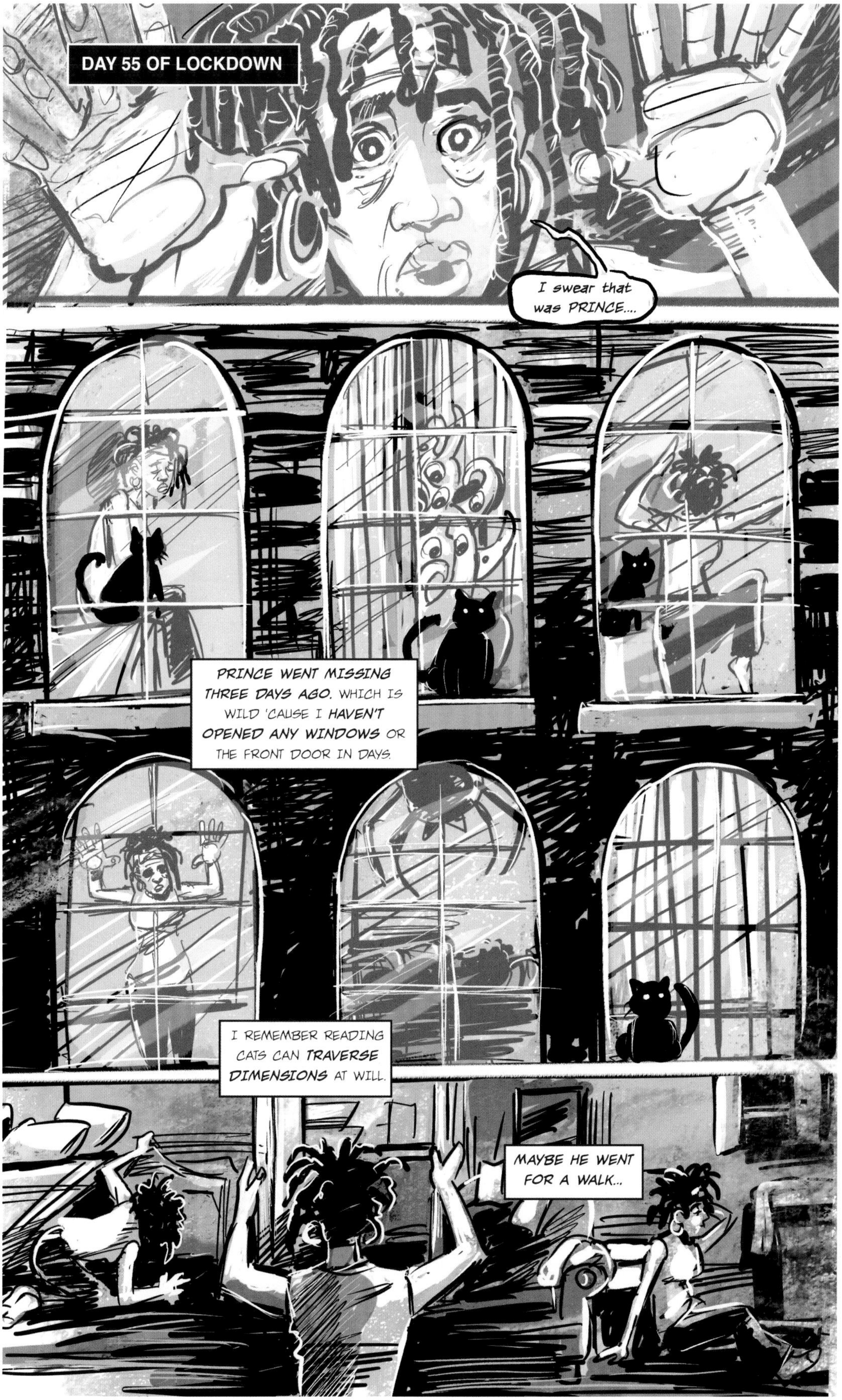
DAY 55 OF LOCKDOWN
I swear that was PRINCE....
PRINCE WENT MISSING THREE DAYS AGO. WHICH IS WILD 'CAUSE I HAVEN'T OPENED ANY WINDOWS OR THE FRONT DOOR IN DAYS.
I REMEMBER READING CATS CAN TRAVERSE DIMENSIONS AT WILL.
MAYBE HE WENT FOR A WALK...

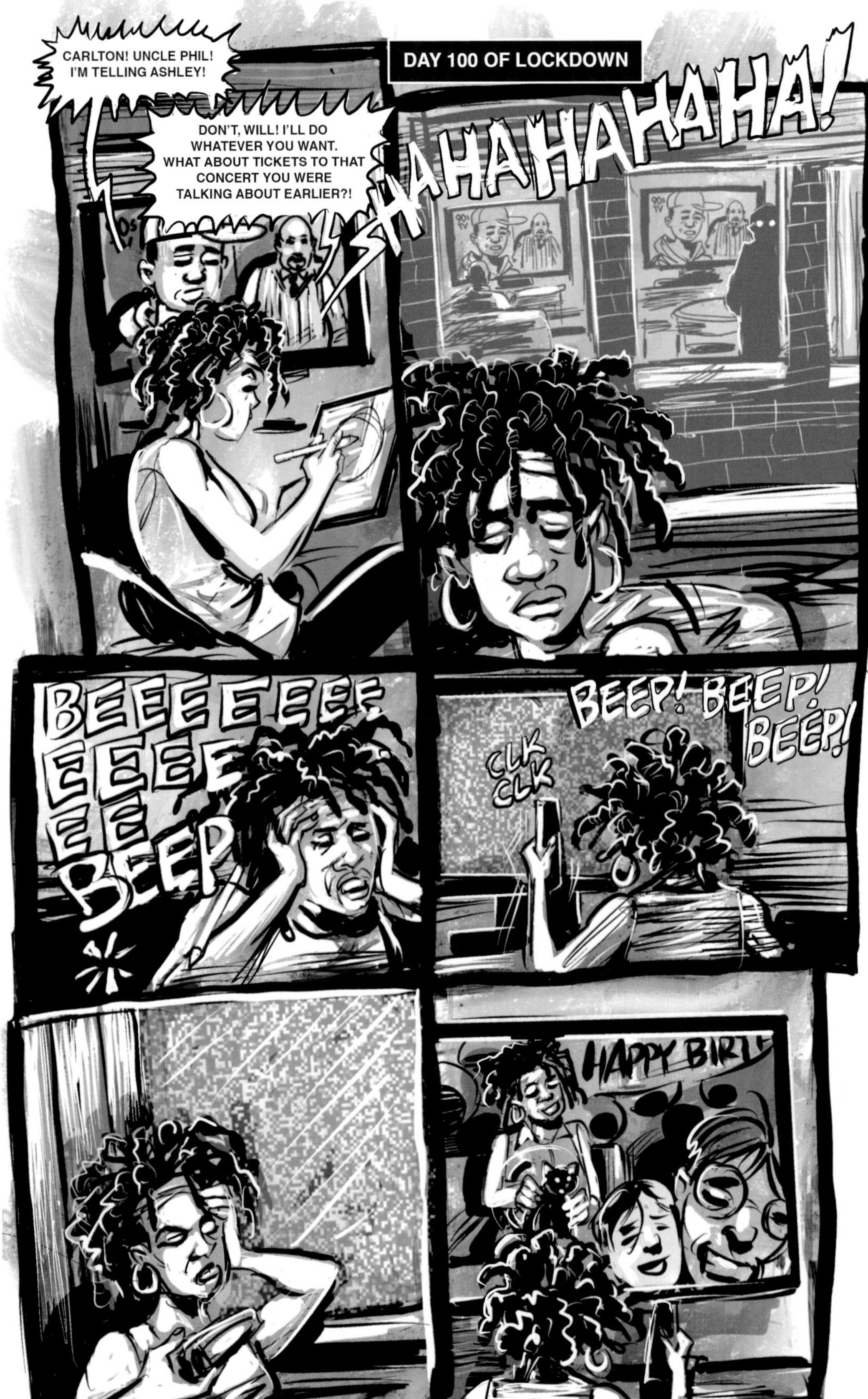
DAY 100 OF LOCKDOWN
CARLTON! UNCLE PHIL! I'M TELLING ASHLEY!
DON'T, WILL! I'LL DO WHATEVER YOU WANT. WHAT ABOUT TICKETS TO THAT CONCERT YOU WERE TALKING ABOUT EARLIER?!
HAHAHAHAHAHA!
BEEEEEEEEEEEEEEEEEP
BEEP! BEEP! BEEP!
CLK CLK
HAPPY BIR

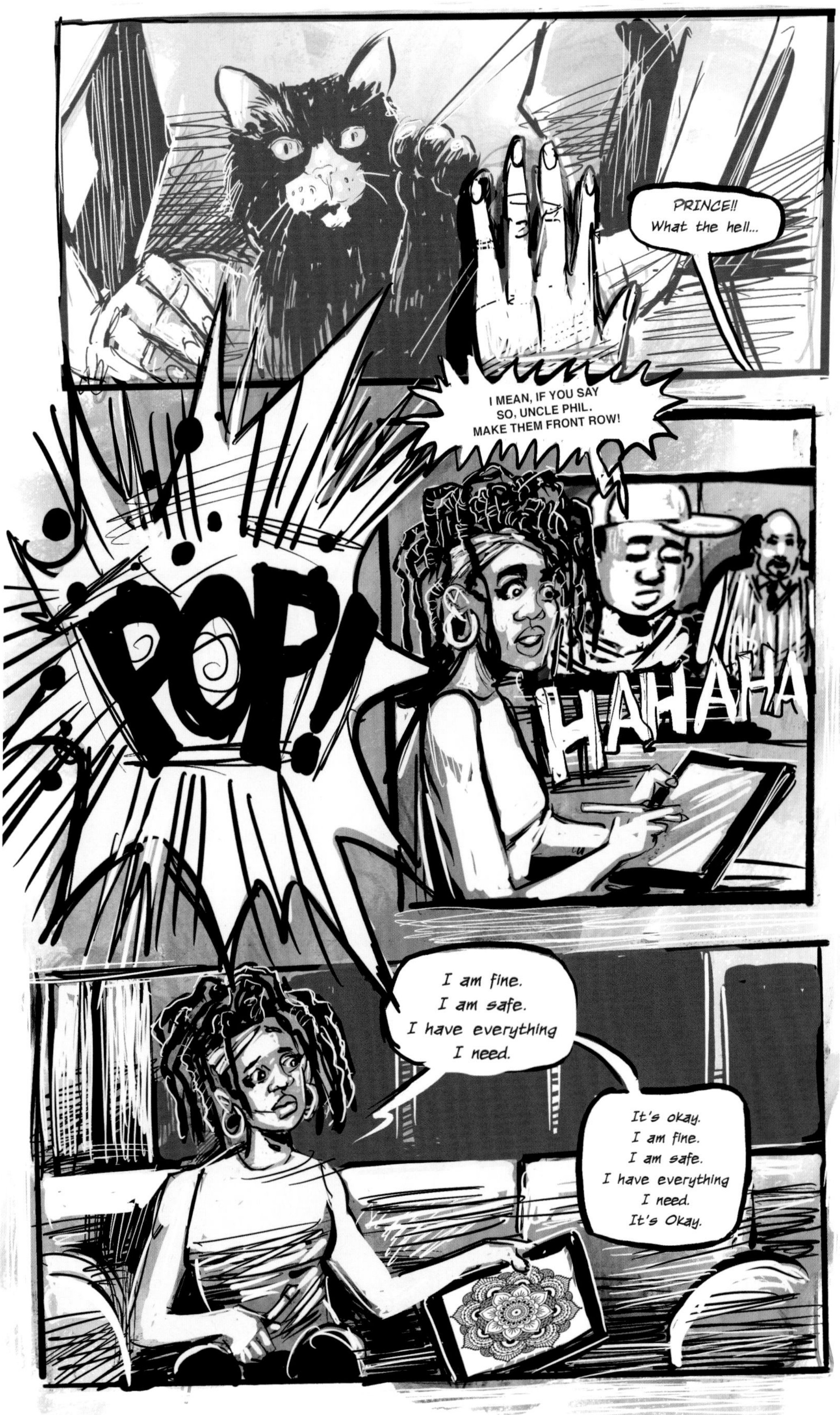
PRINCE!! What the hell...
I MEAN, IF YOU SAY SO, UNCLE PHIL. MAKE THEM FRONT ROW!
POP!
HAHAHA
I am fine. I am safe. I have everything I need.
It's okay. I am fine. I am safe. I have everything I need. It's Okay.

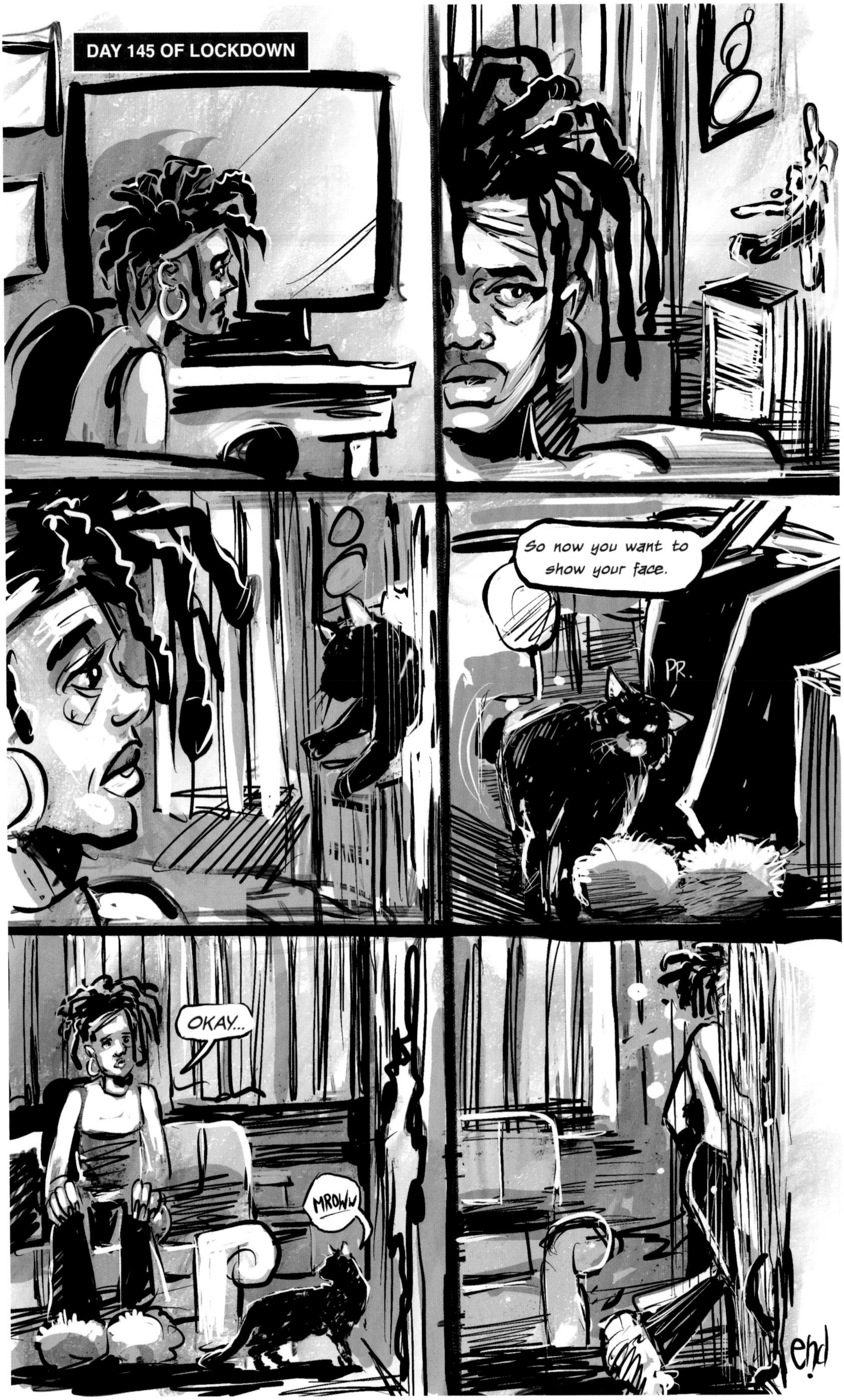
DAY 145 OF LOCKDOWN
So now you want to show your face.
PR.
OKAY...
MROWW
end

Corona Diary by Hatiye Garip

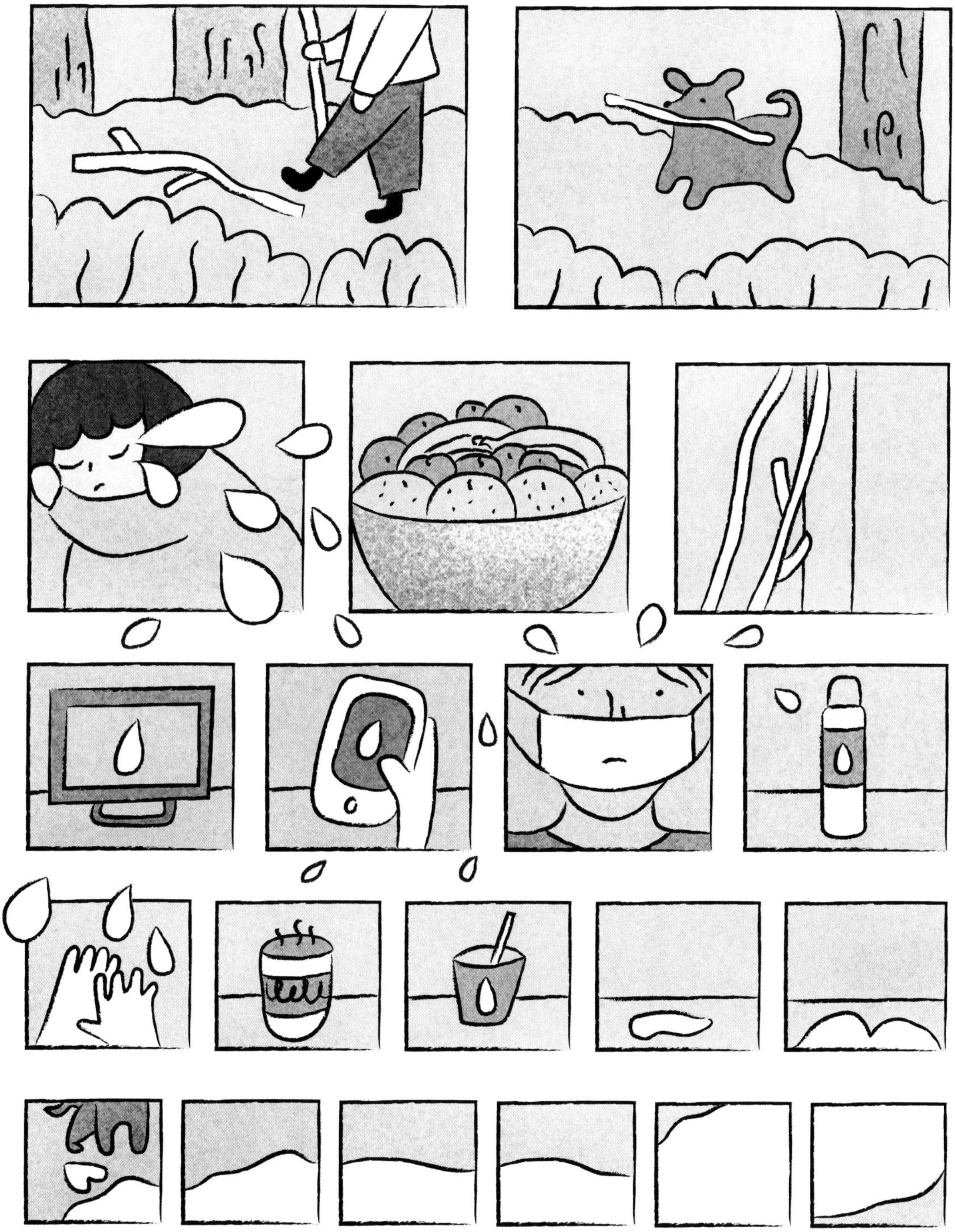

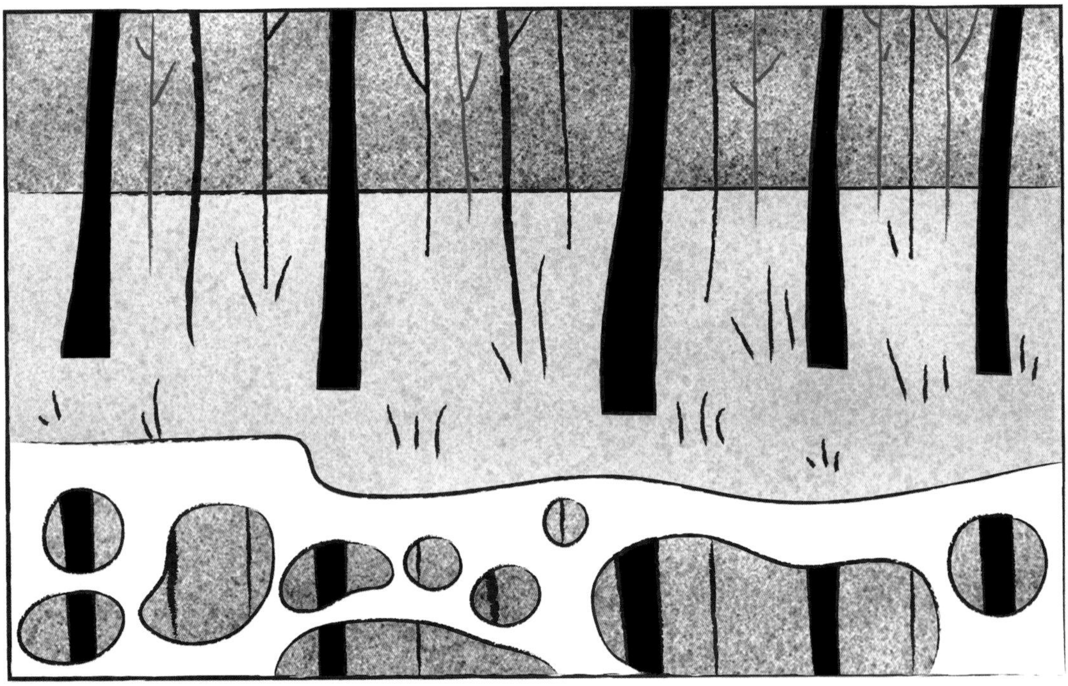

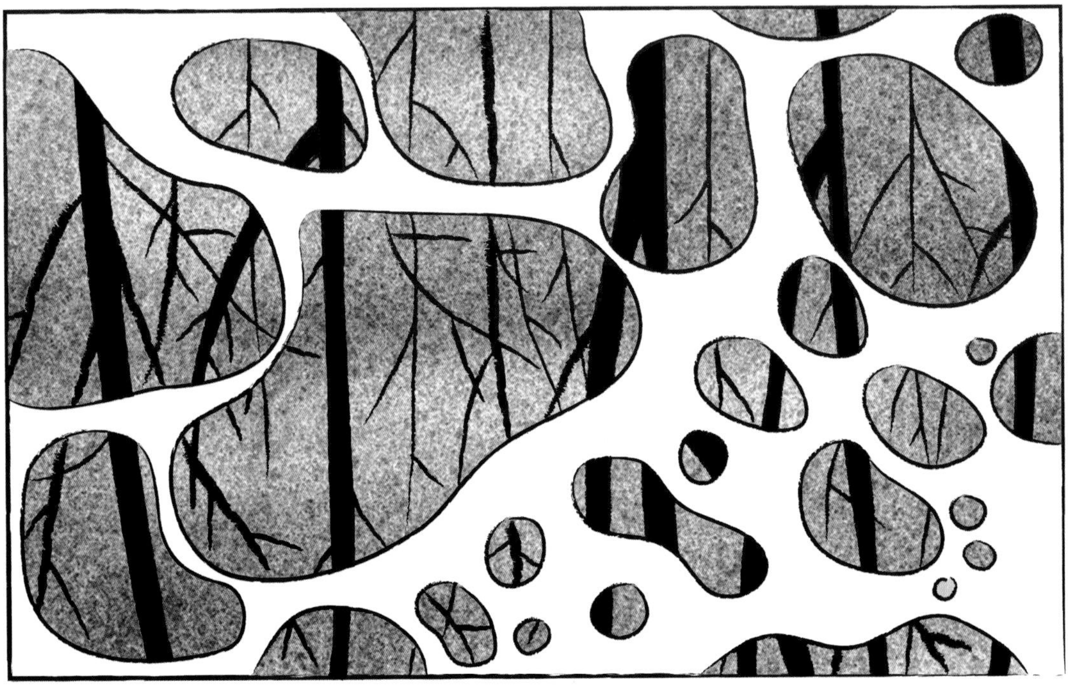

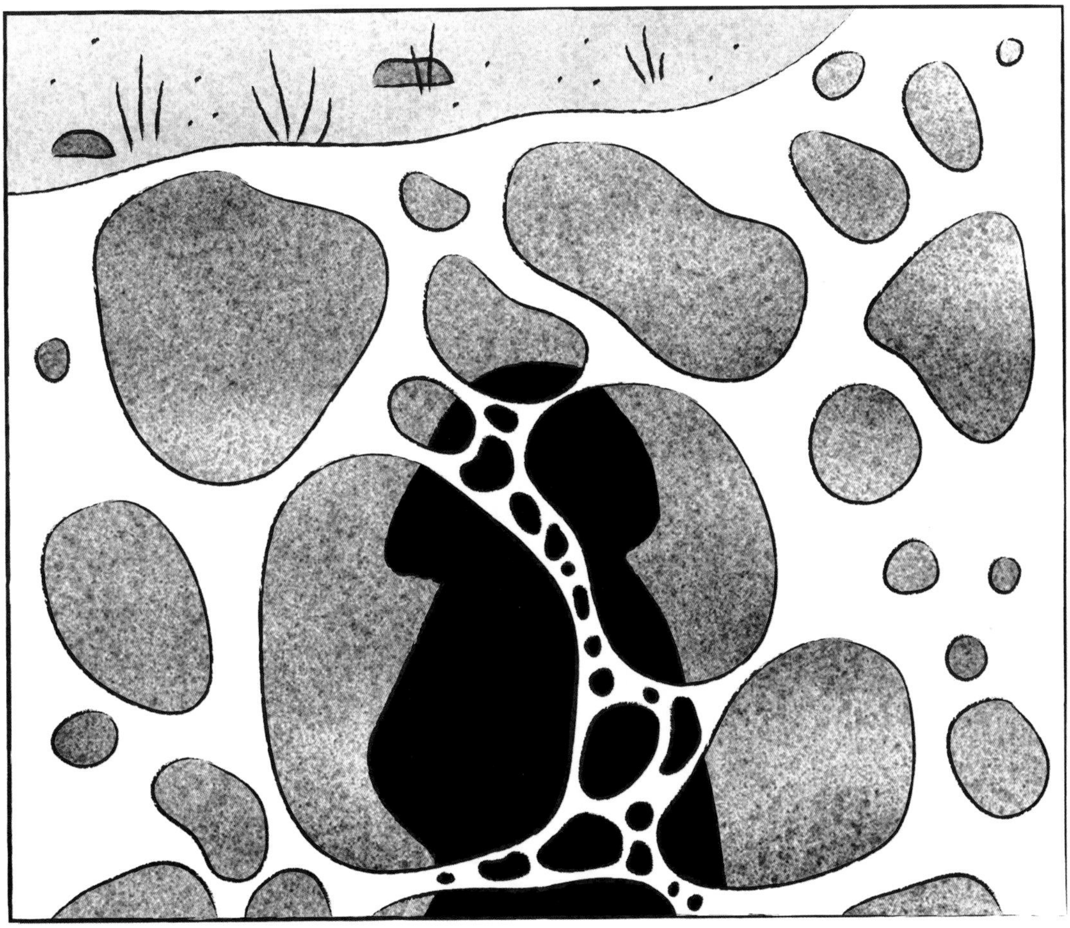

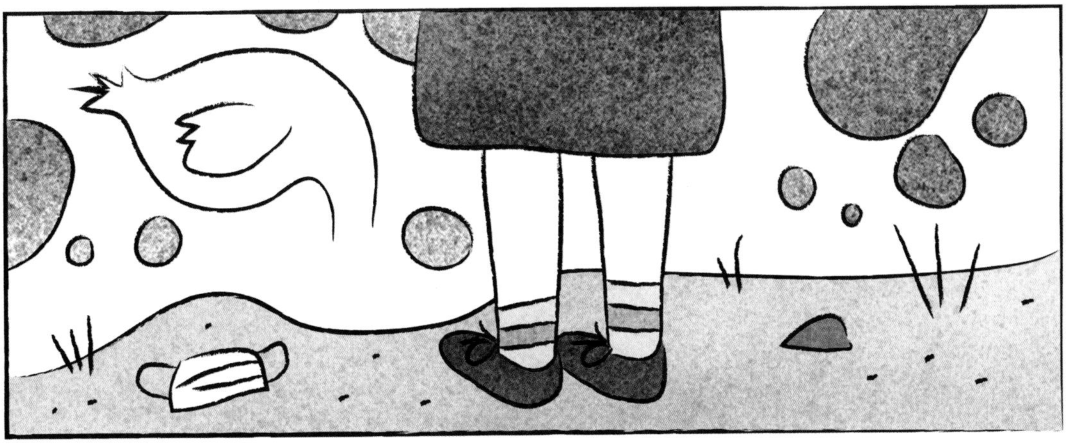

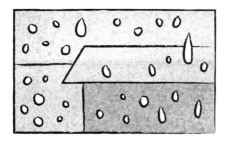
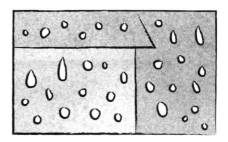
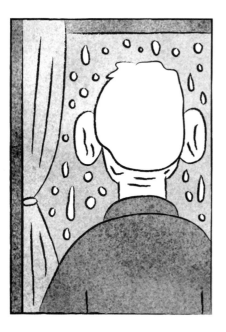
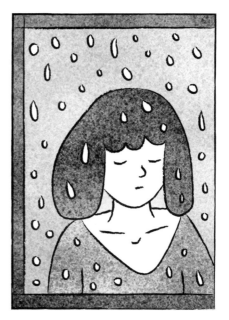
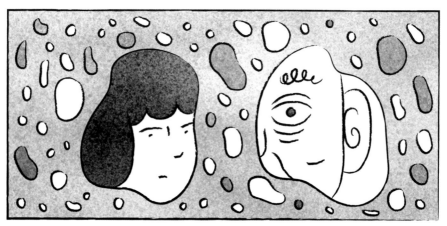

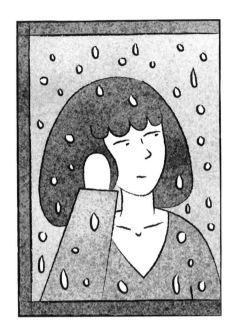
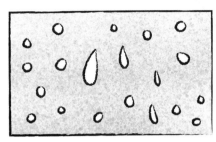
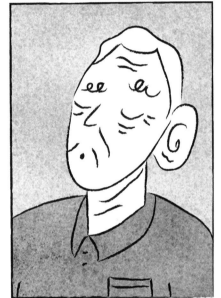
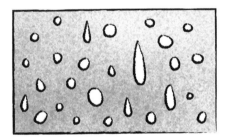
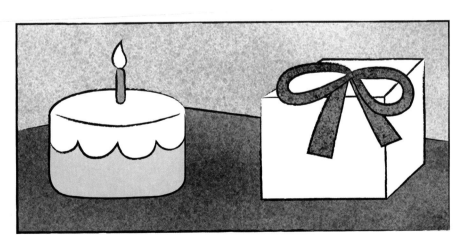

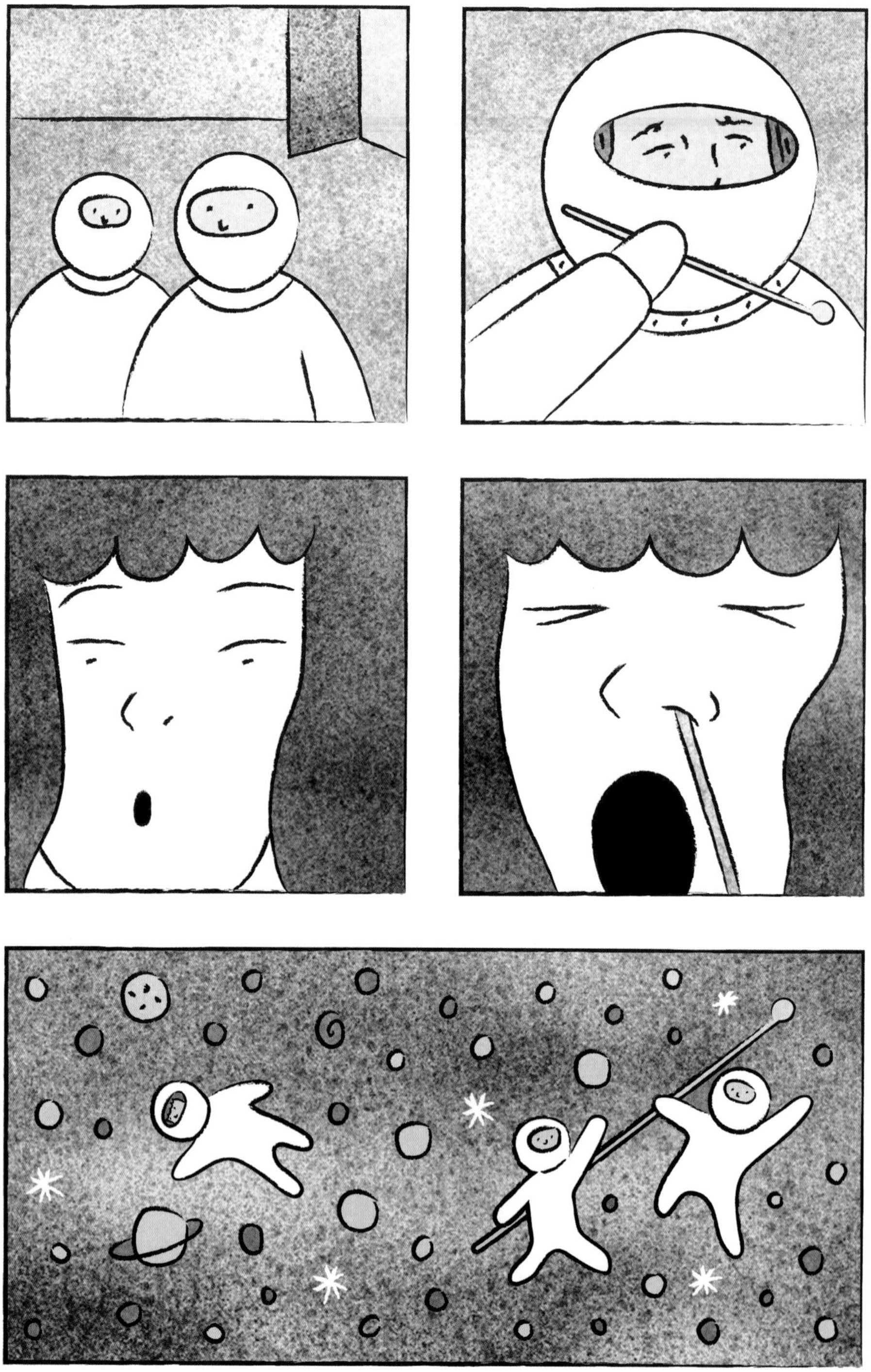

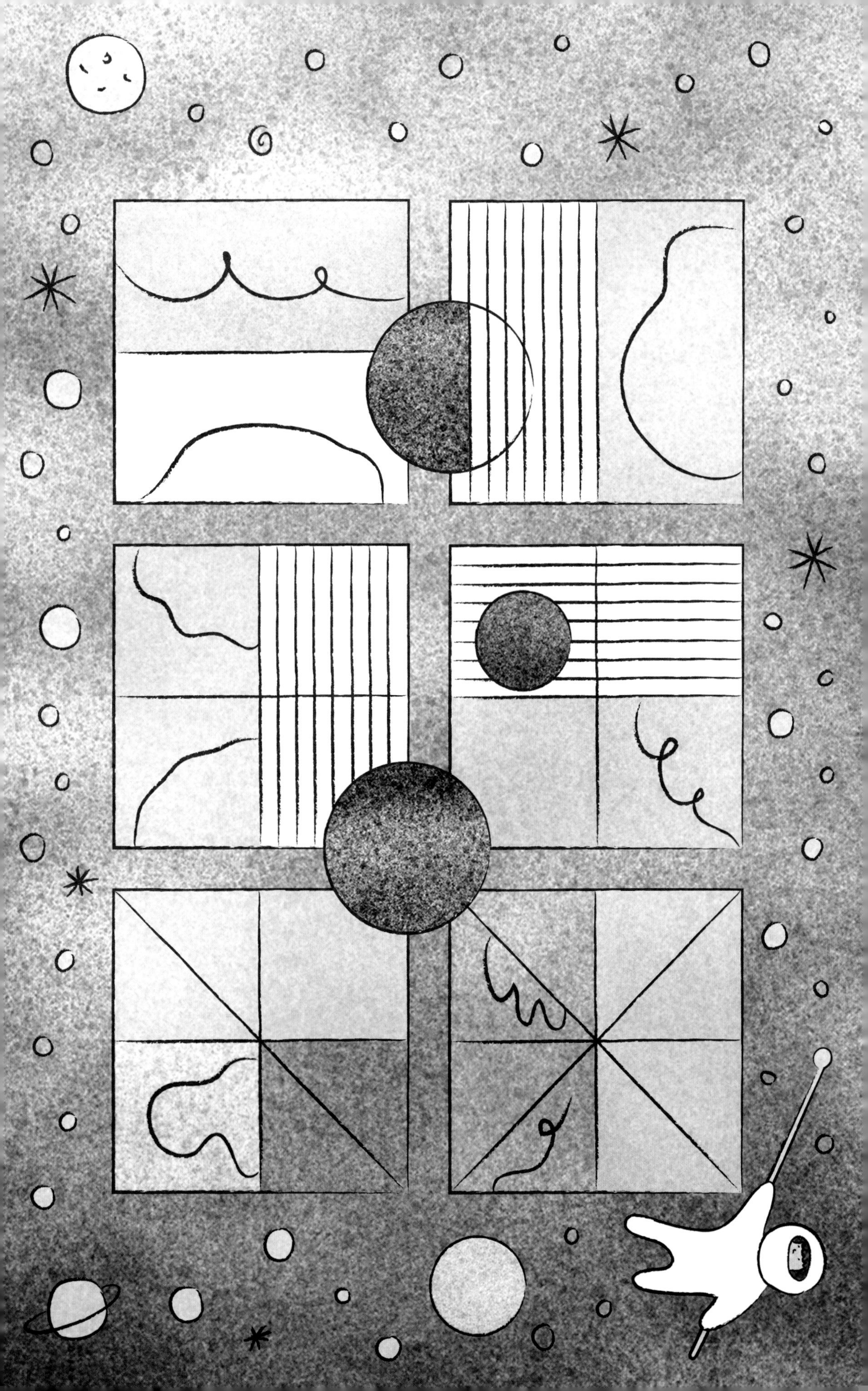

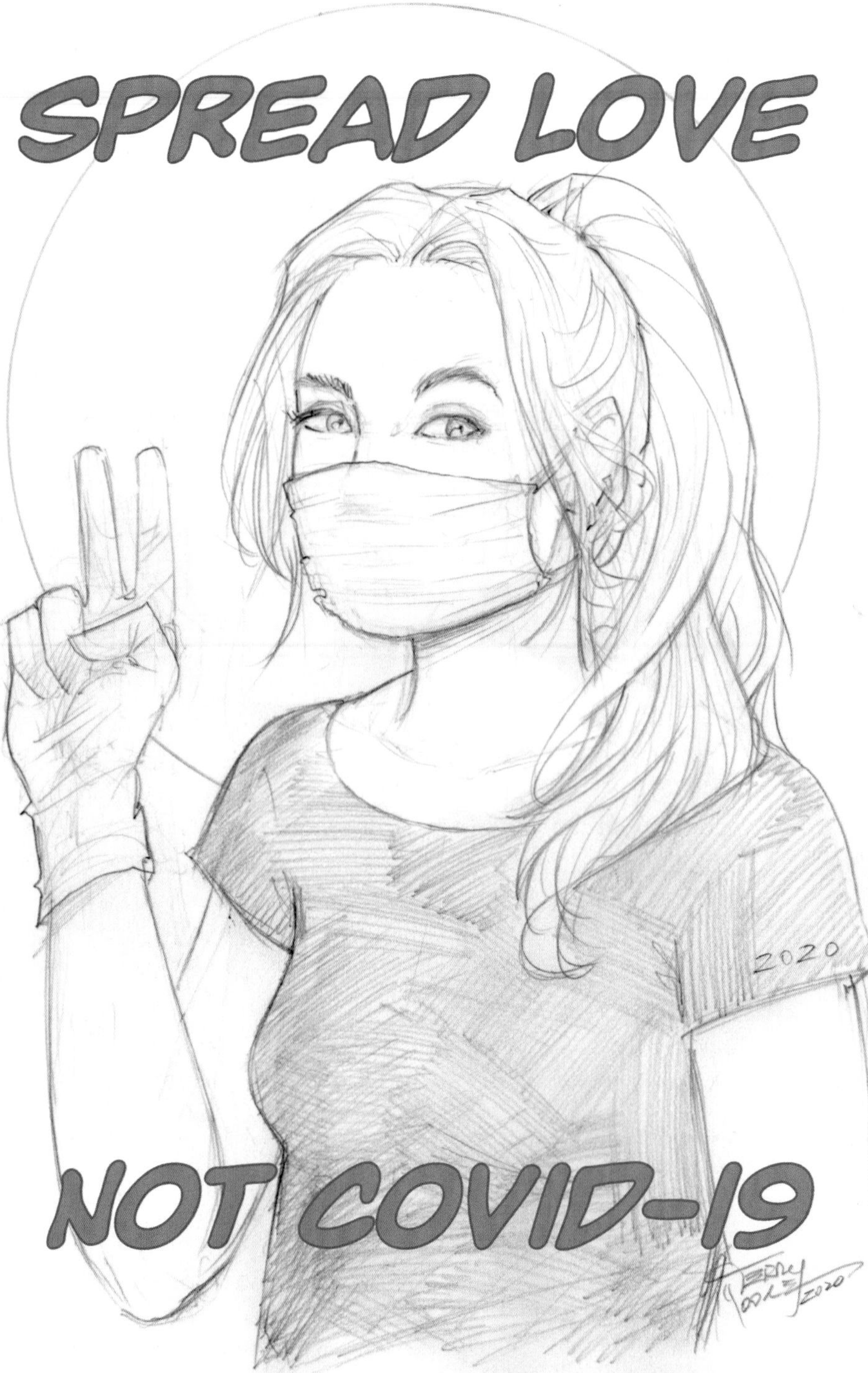
SPREAD LOVE
NOT COVID-19
2020

CONTRIBUTORS

Gene Ambaum is a Seattle-based librarian. He reads lots of comics, drinks unpeated Scotch, and loves teaching tricks to his cat, Soup. Gene co-created the comic about a library, *Unshelved*, and his current ongoing project with artist Willow Payne is *Library Comic*. Online at http://www.librarycomic.com. (129-33)

Julio Anta is a Latinx writer, based in New York City, writing about Latinx identity in America. His debut comic book series, *Home,* will be released by Image Comics this fall. *Frontera,* his debut YA graphic novel with artist Jacoby Salcedo, will be published by Harper Alley in 2023. In addition to writing, Anta runs The Native Sound, a DIY record label. (190-95)

Ned Barnett makes comics about heroes, health, and history. His work includes the self-published graphic memoirs *Dreamers of the Day* and *Hallo Spaceboy* and appears in comics anthologies published by A Wave Blue World and Boston Comics Roundtable. His internet homes are https://thenedbarnett.com and on Twitter as @TheNedBarnett. Ned's favorite dinosaur is the *Compsognathus*. (40-45)

Ken Best is a comic book artist and writer based in Queensland, Australia. He has done work for local, UK, and US comic anthologies and is the creator of the *Xtinct* comic book series. (184-89)

Kendra Boileau is the publisher of Graphic Mundi and the assistant director and editor-in-chief of Penn State University Press. She developed the Graphic Medicine line of graphic novels for the Press and went on to launch the Graphic Mundi imprint in 2021. Boileau has been a judge for the annual Lynd Ward Prize for the Best Graphic Novel of the Year, and she serves on the Lynd Ward Prize Advisory Board. Boileau is also a translator of French graphic novels. (ix-xi; 252)

Armond Boudreaux is an associate professor of English at East Georgia State College. He has previously published a novel and a book of popular philosophy. His sci-fi thriller *Forbidden Minds: The Way Out* will be published in August by Uproar Books. His short comic "Saint Raguel" (with art by J. Paul Schiek) will appear at http://www.HyperEpics.com soon. (140-45)

Eiri J. Brown is a freelance illustrator with experience in character creation and zines. Some examples of zines she has created are *How to Be a Pastel Greaser* (2019), *Moons of Neptune* (2019), and *Regrets Zine* (2017). Brown has done work for the charity zine *From Ashes* (2020), and she is currently a part of the Brisbane art collective TV Totem Pole. (221-25)

Thi Bui is the author of the bestselling graphic memoir *The Best We Could Do* (Abrams ComicArts, 2017). She is the Caldecott Honor–winning illustrator of *A Different Pond,* by Bao Phi, and the co-illustrator of *Chicken of the Sea* by Viet Thanh Nguyen and his son. She is currently researching and drawing *NOWHERELAND,* a work of graphic nonfiction about immigrant detention and deportation, to be published by One World, Random House. (218–19)

Maureen Burdock is a maker and scholar of comics. Born in the Black Forest in Germany in 1970, she grew up during the Cold War era in Germany and the United States. Her creative and scholarly work examines topics of displacement, gender, memory, and trauma. Burdock is currently working on *The Baroness of Have-Nothing*, a graphic memoir that is her dissertation in the cultural studies PhD program at the University of California, Davis. Before working toward her PhD, she earned an MFA in studio art and an MA in visual and critical studies from the California College of the Arts in San Francisco. Burdock is the creator of *Feminist Fables for the Twenty-First Century: The F Word Project*, a series of graphic fables that address forms of gender-based violence in several cultures, published by McFarland Books in 2015. (203–10)

Roland Burkart studied illustration at the Lucerne School of Art and Design in Switzerland. He lives with his wife in the old town center of Lucerne, near the Lion Monument. On May 17, 2020, they welcomed a daughter, Julie, into the world. Burkart's debut graphic novel, *Wirbelsturm,* was published by Edition Moderne in 2017 and will be published in English as *Twister* by Graphic Mundi in 2021. (238–43)

Brian Canini is a cartoonist in Columbus, Ohio, who has been making comics all his life, typically using the traditional media of pens, brushes, and Bristol board. His approach to creating art means using an art style that works well with its story, and this has led him to harness a vast array of styles and techniques in an ever-growing number of genres. Canini is married to a nurse and has two children, aged 4 and 12. (150–53)

Jason Chatfield is an Australian cartoonist and illustrator based in New York. His work has appeared in magazines, online, and in books published by Penguin Random House and HarperCollins. He is the current president of the National Cartoonists Society. Chatfield is an internationally syndicated cartoonist, writing and drawing the iconic comic strip *Ginger Meggs,* launched in 1921, which is published in thirty-four countries daily by Andrews McMeel Syndication. (1–17)

Lili Chin was born in Malaysia and lived in Sydney for twenty years before moving to Hollywood in the early 2000s to work on *Mucha Lucha*, a Warner Bros. masked-wrestling animated TV series that she co-created. These days, Chin's Doggie Drawings brand is best known for all things dog-related. When Chin is not making stylized prints and gift products for sale, she creates infographics for animal care professionals and licenses her designs for paper goods, puzzles, and pet blankets. Her author debut, *Doggie Language*, was published in 2020. In her spare time, Lili enjoys collaborating with Yōkai Parade, listening to podcasts, and playing board games. She lives in Los Angeles with Boogie, her rescued senior blue-eyed Boston terrier. (100–104)

Gerry Chow is a comics writer and artist by night. He debuted his first two printed comics in 2018: "Exclusion," a story about the Chinese Exclusion Act, and "The Vanishing Monastery," a dystopian political drama set in the American future. He has worked on a number of other comics projects, including a volunteer project about the Muslim Ban for the Asian Law Caucus, "We're Still Here," with award-winning cartoonists Raina Telgemeier and Thi Bui. Chow has been an active participant in Thi Bui's "Art Hack" group, a collective of artists who collaborate with progressive nonprofit organizations. By day, Chow is a nonprofit professional, and his current organization is working hard to raise funds and support the local public hospital in San Francisco as it responds to the COVID crisis. (75–82)

MK Czerwiec, RN, MA, is a nurse, cartoonist, and educator who has been making comics under the pseudonym Comic Nurse since 2000. She is the creator of *Taking Turns:*

Stories from HIV/AIDS Care Unit 371 (PSU Press, 2017), a co-author of *Graphic Medicine Manifesto* (PSU Press, 2014), and the editor of the comics anthology *Menopause: A Comic Treatment* (PSU Press, 2020). She co-manages the website, podcast, annual conferences, and online community of GraphicMedicine.org. Czerwiec regularly teaches graphic medicine at Northwestern Medical School, the School of the Art Institute of Chicago, the University of Illinois Medical School, and the University of Chicago. She has served as the Artist in Residence at Northwestern Medical School, a Senior Fellow of the George Washington School of Nursing Center for Health Policy and Media Engagement, and a Will Eisner Fellow in Applied Cartooning at the Center for Cartoon Studies in White River Junction, Vermont. (99)

Zack Davisson is an award-winning translator, writer, and folklorist. He is the author of *Yurei: The Japanese Ghost*, *Yokai Stories*, *Narrow Road*, *Amabie: Past and Present*, and *Kaibyo: The Supernatural Cats of Japan*. He is the translator of Shigeru Mizuki's multiple Eisner Award–winning *Showa: A History of Japan* and the famous folklore comic *Kitaro*, and he has translated globally renowned entertainment properties such as Go Nagai's Devilman and Cutie Honey, Leiji Matsumoto's Space Battleship Yamato and Captain Harlock, and Satoshi Kon's Opus. Davisson has lectured on manga, folklore, and translation at Duke University, Annapolis Naval Academy, UCLA, and the University of Washington, and he has contributed to exhibitions at the Henry Art Gallery, The Museum of International Folk Art, Wereldmuseum Rotterdam, and the Art Gallery of New South Wales. He lives in Seattle with his wife, Miyuki; dog, Mochi; cat, Shere Khan; and several ghosts. (100-104)

Joe Decie is a graphic novelist from the UK specializing in autobiography. His latest graphic novel, *Collecting Sticks,* was published by Jonathan Cape/Random House in 2017. (74; 232)

Zac Deloupy was born in Saint-Étienne, France, and holds a degree in comics from the European School of Visual Arts, Angoulême. He co-founded Jarjille Editions, where he published *Collisions, Comixland,* the series *L'Introuvable,* and his three-volume *Journal approximatif.* In 2016 he published the award-winning graphic novel *Love story à l'iranienne,* with Jane Deuxard (Delcourt), which will appear in an English translation for Graphic Mundi in 2021. And in 2018, he published *Pour la peau,* with Sandrine Saint-Marc (Delcourt), and *Algériennes,* with Swann Meralli (Marabulles). *Algériennes* was published by Penn State University Press in 2020 in its Graphic Medicine series. (cover art)

Ignacio Di Meglio has been a freelance cartoonist for more than a decade and has been drawing and telling stories for as long as he can remember. He has made comics, illustrations, and character designs for a variety of projects. You can find him on Twitter as @ignaciodimeglio or near the sea waiting for Cthulhu to wake up. (140-45)

Katy Doughty is an illustrator and healthcare administrator in Boston. After receiving her BFA in illustration from the Rhode Island School of Design, she has worked in design and communication with various nonprofits, driven by the idea that good storytelling can foster connection and action. (35-39)

Peter Dunlap-Shohl has retired from his over-twenty-five-year career as a prize-winning cartoonist for the *Anchorage Daily News.* He is the author of the graphic novel *My Degeneration: A Journey Through Parkinson's,* which relates his struggle with a diagnosis of Parkinson's at the age of 43. He has contributed to the online comics site The Nib and blogs for the Northwest Parkinson's Disease Foundation and for the website Health Union. He maintains two personal blogs: *Off and On, the Alaska Parkinson's Rag,* and *Frozen Grin.* He, his wife, Pam, and their two small yet mighty dogs divide their time between Alaska and Washington State. (173-76)

Sarah Firth is a Melbourne-based, Eisner Award–winning comic artist, author, and internationally renowned graphic recorder. Her work has been published by ABRAMS Books, ABC Arts, *frankie*, Penguin Random House, Picador, Allen & Unwin, The Nib, Black Inc, and Routledge. She is currently working on her debut graphic novel. (177-83)

Eduardo Garcia began his career as an illustrator thirty years ago. Since then, he has worked on many projects for Marvel, DC Comics, Zenescope Entertainment, Boom!, IDW, Capstone Publishing, and Simon & Schuster. (113-15)

Mike Garcia is a comic book artist based in Cancun, Mexico. He started working in educational, training, and entertainment comics after winning the Outlaw Entertainment International Artist Search in 2009. He enjoys projects where feelings and relationships are the main drivers of the story. (166-71)

Hatiye Garip is an illustrator, comic artist, and designer based in Istanbul, Turkey. She likes to draw birds, flowers, and ordinary moments. Her works have been exhibited and published in many countries, including Portugal, Lithuania, Bulgaria, the Czech Republic, South Korea, the US, and the UK. She is currently writing and illustrating her first picture book. You can see her work at https://hatiyegarip.com. (261-67)

Simon Gentry grew up in Lawrence, Kansas, and holds a BFA from Kansas University with a focus in painting. He co-founded Southseas Tattoo in Hilo, Hawaii, is the owner of Bitterroot Tattoo in Moscow, Idaho, and currently lives in Spokane, Washington, where he works at Anchored Art Tattoo. He enjoys gardening, bike riding, playing music, and being a father when he's not illustrating for fun. (88-89)

Aaron Guzman is a graphic artist born and raised within the concrete jungle of the island of Manhattan. He now creates full-time out of southern Connecticut, spending every waking moment drawing and building 3D construction models and web-based apps. Online at https://www.aaronguzman.com/sequential-art.html. (197-202)

Rivi Handler-Spitz is an associate professor in the department of Asian languages and cultures at Macalester College and a 2020–2021 fellow at the National Humanities Center. She is an author, editor, and translator, whose three books address classical Chinese and comparative literature. Her drawings have appeared in *Inside Higher Ed* and elsewhere. Handler-Spitz's comics in this collection come from the visual journal she has kept since the start of the pandemic. (34; 68; 112; 134; 160; 172; 196; 220; 228; 244)

Justin LaRocca Hansen grew up in the tiny town of Millis, Massachusetts, but spent most summers in a tinier village called Cataumet in Cape Cod, where he feels most at home. Comic books, cartoons, and toys captivated him as a child, and he would constantly create his own characters and stories. He got a BFA in illustration from Ringling College of Art and Design before moving to New York City to try to "make it" as an illustrator. It was a long journey with plenty of odd jobs, lots of rejections, and all the ups and downs that come with chasing a dream. He finally sold his first picture book, *Monster Hunter,* in 2012 to Sky Pony Press. The next few years would be consumed by a graphic novel trilogy called *Secondhand Heroes.* The first book of that trilogy, *Secondhand Heroes: Brothers Unite,* was published by Dial Books for Young Readers in 2016. Part 2, *Secondhand Heroes: In the Trenches,* came out in 2017, and part 3, *Secondhand Heroes: The Last Battle,* came out in 2018. He lives in Brooklyn with his amazing wife and his collection of Springsteen records. (124-28)

Kurt Hathaway is a comics veteran with over 1,400 comics stories under his belt. His client list includes just about every comics publisher there is. Online at http://www.cartoon-bal loons.com/. (113-15)

Mark Heinrichs is a cartoonist from Toronto, Canada. He draws to pass the time. (96-98)

Natascha Hoffmeyer is a freelance translator who divides her time between State College, Pennsylvania, and Berlin, Germany. Her most recent graphic novel translation is Roland Burkart's *Twister* (Graphic Mundi, 2021). She is also the lead singer of the State College–based jazz band Natascha and the Spy Boys. (238-43)

Laura Holzman activates art, its history, and its institutions to strengthen communities and promote equity. She is an associate professor of art history and museum studies at Indiana University, IUPUI, where she is also appointed Public Scholar of Curatorial Practices and Visual Art. Her scholarship has manifested in exhibitions, academic journal articles, and the monograph, *Contested Image: Defining Philadelphia for the Twenty-First Century* (Temple University Press, 2019). Her current creative work intersects directly with public health advocacy and is included in the exhibition *FIX: Heartbreak and Hope Inside Our Opioid Crisis* at the Indiana State Museum. Online at https://lauraholzman.com. (48-53)

John Jennings is a professor of media and cultural studies at the University of California at Riverside. He is co-editor of the Eisner Award–winning collection *The Blacker the Ink: Constructions of the Black Identity in Comics and Sequential Art*. Jennings is also a 2016 Nasir Jones Hiphop Studies Fellow with the Hutchins Center at Harvard University. His current projects include the horror anthology *Box of Bones*, the coffee-table book *Black Comix Returns* (with Damian Duffy), and the Eisner-winning, Bram Stoker Award–winning, *New York Times* best-selling graphic novel adaptation of Octavia Butler's classic dark fantasy novel *Kindred*. Duffy and Jennings recently released their graphic novelization of Octavia Butler's prescient dystopian novel *Parable of the Sower* (Abrams ComicArts).

Jennings is also the founder and curator of the ABRAMS Megascope line of graphic novels. (253-60)

Rich Johnson is a publishing consultant and the founder of Brick Road Media, LLC. Previously, he held leadership positions at Lion Forge Comics and DC Comics, and he was the co-founder and co-publishing director of Yen Press. He created the sales and marketing strategy for Neil Gaiman's *Sandman: Endless Nights*, the first original graphic novel to hit the *New York Times* Best Sellers list. In 2011, Johnson was selected as a judge for the Eisner Awards, considered by many to be the Oscars of comics. (245-51)

Quincy Scott Jones's work has appeared in the *African American Review, The North American Review, Love Jawns: A Mixtape,* and *The Feminist Wire,* as well as in the anthologies *Resisting Arrest: Poems to Stretch the Sky, Let Loose on the World: Celebrating Amiri Baraka at 75,* and *Black Lives Have Always Mattered: A Collection of Essays, Poems, and Personal Narratives.* With Nina Sharma, he co-created the Nor'easter Exchange, a multicultural, multi-city reading series. His first book, *The T-Bone Series*, was published by Whirlwind Press in 2009. His first comic, *Black Nerd*, is coming soon. (184-89)

Scott J. Jones has been doing comics since he was sixteen. A graduate of the Art Institute of Pittsburgh, Jones spent a few years working on short comic stories for small businesses and corporate newsletters. He is currently a freelance graphic artist and is working on his first graphic novel. Jones lives with his wife and three kids in Altoona, Pennsylvania. (154-56)

Jazmine Joyner is a writer and editor based in Southern California. She is the assistant editor for the Megascope imprint at Abrams ComicArts, and she has written for *Women Write About Comics, The Comics MNT, Wear Your Voice Magazine,* and others. In 2018, she was awarded the Harpy Agenda Grant for her work in comics journalism. Joyner has a collection of short stories called *The Cosmic Egg* as well as an ongoing diary comic called *The Bleeding*. She is online @jazmine_joyner. (253–60)

Kang Jing, also known as KJ, is a comic book creator from Singapore. In late 2019, KJ successfully published his debut comic series, *The World My Arena*, through Kickstarter. The martial arts-based series has since been featured on local media (justsaying.ASIA, CNA Lifestyle) and adapted into animated videos (ComicVid by VividThree Productions). It also led to a spin-off bilingual webcomic series, *The World My Arena Q—Save Me From Chloe*, in 2020. In addition, KJ has also worked on projects with both local and international comic book publishers, such as CS Comics and Arcane Inkdustries. (90–91)

Rob Kirby is a cartoonist and writer currently living in St. Paul, Minnesota. His books include *Curbside Boys* and the anthologies *The Book of Boy Trouble* (co-edited with David Kelly), the Ignatz-nominated *THREE*, the Ignatz-winning *QU33R*, and *The Shirley Jackson Project: Comics Inspired by Her Life and Work*. He is currently working on *Marry Me a Little,* a graphic memoir about getting (gay) married in middle age. Online at http://www.robkirby comics.com; Twitter & Instagram: @robkirby comics. (161–65)

Rob Kraneveldt is a Canadian writer of graphic novels and comic books. He is best known for his creative works under "Diver-sity Comics." He was awarded Writer of the Year and Best Story Award by the Amateur Creator's Union for his story *Lifer.* He is currently working on his newest graphic novel, *Unnatural.* Online at http://www.some thingwriteous.com. (166–71)

Jesse Lambert is an artist who has recently turned to making nonfiction comics. He is currently working on a graphic novel memoir about growing up in a communist psychotherapy cult, for which he was a final-ist for the Creative Capital Awards of 2020. His short graphic memoir, "That's Not What We're Called," will be included in the anthol-ogy, *American Cult*, to be published by Paper Rocket Comics. Lambert has contributed to *Clayton: Godfather of the Lower East Side—A Documentary*, a collaborative graphic novel biography of Clayton Patterson, artist, photog-rapher, anti–police brutality activist, and documenter of NYC's Lower East Side in the late '70s and '80s. (18–21)

Kelly Latham holds an MFA degree in sequen-tial art from the Savannah College of Art and Design, and a BFA in illustration from the University of Kansas. She is constantly curious, which leads to a lot of adventures, reading, and playing with mixed media. She is fond of lively color palettes, fun stories, and deep environments. In addition to creating, Kelly loves traveling, mismatched socks, fuzzy blankets, and collecting rubber ducks. (146–49)

Janet K. Lee is an illustrator best known for her Eisner Award–winning graphic novel *Return of the Dapper Men.* Her diverse body of work includes Jane Austen adaptations for Marvel and horror for DC Comics, as well as *Sea Sirens* and *Sky Island,* middle-grade comics from Viking. In March 2020, just before the nation locked down for a pandemic, Lee's neighborhood in Nashville was struck by an F4 tornado. Her story was inspired by this event. This is her first foray into writing. (69–73)

Ajuan Mance is a professor of English and ethnic studies at Mills College and a life-long artist and writer. She holds a BA from Brown University and an MA and PhD from the University of Michigan. In both her schol-arly writing and her visual art, Ajuan explores issues of race, gender, and the people and places in which they intersect. Her comics include the *Gender Studies* series and the web-based comic strip *Check All That Apply*. Her comics have also appeared in several anthologies, including *Alphabet* and *We're Still*

Here, both from Stacked Decked Press; *Drawing Power,* from Abrams Press; the *How to Wait* anthology, edited by Sage Persing; and *Menopause: A Comic Treatment,* from Penn State University Press. Her work has appeared in a number of digital and print media outlets, including, most recently, Blavity.com, BET.com, *Transition Magazine,* Buzzfeed.com, NPR.org, the *San Francisco Chronicle,* KPIX TV, Pen.org, PublishersWeekly.com, NewYork Times.com, and NewYorker.com. (31–33)

Luis Manriquez is a family physician who works as a hospitalist for the Spokane Family Medicine residency. On September 11, 2001, he had just begun film school at NYU. The events of that day led him to refocus on medicine as a means to be directly helpful. Dr. Manriquez is also a clinical assistant professor for the WSU Elson S. Floyd College of Medicine, where he oversees the health equity curriculum, street medicine team, and mobile medical unit. He is writing a dark comedy graphic novel on life in medical training, the universe, and everything else and is looking for a publisher. (88–89)

Lee Marrs was the first woman to work for DC Comics *and* Marvel simultaneously and one of the founding mommies of Wimmen's Comix. A 2016 Eisner Award nominee and a 1982 Inkpot Award winner, Lee has a wide spectrum of art styles that have ranged from illustrative (*Heavy Metal* magazine, *Epic Illustrated, Star*Reach, Prince Valiant, Lil' Orphan Annie*) to humorous (DC's *Plop, Weird Mystery, House of Secrets,* Marvel's "Crazy Lady"). She's best known for her book *Pudge, Girl Blimp,* with a blurb from Alison Bechdel and a foreword by Gloria Steinem. Her most recent work is in *Drawing Power,* edited by Diane Noomin (Abrams ComicArts). Most of Marrs's mainstream comics work as a writer for DC: *Wonder Woman: Annual* (1989), *Viking Glory: The Viking Prince* (1991), *Zatanna: Come Together* (1993), *Faultlines* (1997), and *Batman: Legends of the Dark Knight: Stalking* (1998), and

for Dark Horse: *Indiana Jones and the Arms of Gold* (1994) and *Indiana Jones and the Iron Phoenix* (1995). (119–23)

Seth Martel is a former EMT/emergency room tech. He now works as an illustrator and graphic designer in the Hudson Valley. He is humbled by the strength of the medical professionals putting in tireless effort during the uphill battle of the pandemic. (135–39)

Tom K. Mason is one of the founders of Malibu Comics. He now toils as an Emmy Award–winning television writer from his home on an island off the coast of Canada. He also writes comics and children's books in his spare time. (113–15)

Sean Seamus McWhinny has a background in game illustration and art direction. He publishes a web comic called "Your Moment of Duck" and self-published his graphic memoir, *Bunny Man: My Life in the Easter Charade,* about his work as the Easter Bunny in a dying mall after getting laid off in 2002. For the past six years, he has been caretaker and advocate for his mother during her final years, until her recent passing from COVID-19. Online at https://www.seanseamus.com. (54–59)

Ben Mitchell is an illustrator, cartoonist, and academic from Newcastle, NSW, Australia. He is currently producing a long-form comic book series called *Storm Clouds* and a thesis called *Losing Control of Comics: New Narrative Function in Comic Book Design.* He lives in a two-bedroom apartment in Newcastle West with a bodybuilder named Jeremy. (157–59)

Terry Moore is an indie powerhouse who began his career in comics with the critically acclaimed epic series *Strangers in Paradise,* the compelling love story of three unlikely friends who find themselves bound together by their pasts. The long-running series garnered many awards, including the coveted Eisner Award for Best Serialized Story and the National Cartoonists Society Comic Book Division

Reuben Award. *Strangers in Paradise* has been translated into nineteen languages and is as popular today as when it was first published in 1993. Moore has created other award-winning series, including *Motor Girl*, *Rachel Rising*, and *ECHO*, a science fiction thriller. In 2020 Terry concludes the exciting series *FIVE YEARS*, which brings together characters from all of his series in one heart-stopping story. Moore is the recipient of numerous industry awards worldwide. In addition to publishing work under his own label, Abstract Studio, Moore has worked for Marvel, DC, Dark Horse, Boom!, and other major publishers throughout his career. (268)

Eli Neugeboren is an award-winning illustrator, writer, and professor living and working in Brooklyn. He has been drawing ever since he could hold a crayon and does his best to draw every single day. His work, which is primarily a figurative and humanist approach to storytelling both in single editorial images and in sequential work, has been included in the *American Illustration* and *American Photography* annuals. He has worked as an illustrator at a product development company creating licensed goods, as a designer in the exhibition department at the American Museum of Natural History, and as a digital retoucher for clients such as Maybelline, Redken, and *SPIN Magazine*. When he was a kid he spent so much time at his local comic store, Moondance Comics, that his father told him he should ask them for a job. He did, and he was hired to organize their back room a few hours a week. At the shop, he got to meet the creators of TMNT, Kevin Eastman and Peter Laird, and the rest of the Mirage Studios crew, whose generosity and respect toward him influences his teaching philosophy to this day. (245–51; 252)

Tim E. Ogline is a Greater Philadelphia–based illustrator and writer as well as design professional. Ogline is the author/illustrator of the acclaimed *Ben Franklin for Beginners* (called

"beguiling" by Pulitzer Prize winner Joseph J. Ellis and "absolutely brilliant" by Geekadelphia). He is currently working on a graphic novel, *Benjamin Franklin's* The Way to Wealth *and Other Words of Wisdom*. Ogline's illustrations have appeared in *The Wall Street Journal*, *Institutional Investor*, *The Philadelphia Inquirer*, the *Utne Reader*, *Outdoor Life*, *Philadelphia Style*, *Loyola Lawyer*, and *How Magazine*, among others. Online at http://www.timog line.com. (92–95)

Hassan Otsmane-Elhaou is a comic book letterer and the editor of the Eisner Award–winning digital magazine *Panel X Panel*. His work as a letterer has appeared in titles published at Image, Oni Press, Aftershock, Vault, and more. (190–95)

Pavith C. is an aspiring comic colorist from Singapore with pages published both locally and internationally. As a colorist, his true aim is to elevate a narrative through the use of expressive colors that best reflect a story's emotions and atmosphere. (90–91)

Willow Payne is the current artist and co-writer of *Library Comic*. She loves cats, hates COVID-19, and is impartial to brussels sprouts. Originally wanting to be a cartoonist when she grew up, Payne now realizes that becoming a Ninja Turtle would have been a more stable career path. More of her work can be seen online at http://www.Willow Payne.com. (129–33)

Stephanie Nina Pitsirilos, MPH, is a writer, public health advocate, and volunteer librarian in a public elementary school in NYC. Comic book realism and the heavy hand of history are recurring themes of her writing. Her work can be found in the digital anthology *Insider Art*, a benefit anthology for the comic book industry; in *Heroes Need Masks*, a benefit anthology for #GetUsPPE; in the Webtoon short story *DR163*; and in *Speculative Fiction for Dreamers: A Latinx Anthology* (Ohio State University Press, 2020), which paneled at the 2020 AWP conference and book fair. (135–39; 197–202)

Joanna Regulska is a professor of gender, sexuality, and women's studies and Vice Provost and Associate Chancellor of Global Affairs at the University of California, Davis. Her scholarly and policy work has focused on decentralization, democracy, women's political participation, women's agency, and political identity as well as on changing gender roles under conditions of regime transformations. She is the author and co-author of seven books and the author of more than one hundred articles and chapters. Regulska earned her master's degree from the University of Warsaw, Poland, and her PhD from the University of Colorado, Boulder. She received a Doctor Honoris Causa from Tbilisi State University, Georgia (2011). (203–10)

S.I. Rosenbaum is a writer and artist based in Providence. (105–11)

Jacoby Salcedo is a Mexican American comic book artist based in Olympia, Washington. A graduate of the School of Visual Arts in New York, he has self-published three books. *Frontera,* his debut YA graphic novel, with writer Julio Anta, will be published by Harper Alley in 2023. (190–95)

Kay Sohini is a South Asian immigrant, comics maker, and PhD candidate in New York City originally from Calcutta, India. In her creative and academic work, she focuses on how comics can be utilized by scholars and artists alike to amplify marginalized voices. Her work has been published in *Assay: A Journal of Nonfiction Studies* and *Sequentials,* and will be published in the *Handbook of Comics and Graphic Narratives* by de Gruyter in 2020–21. (211–17)

Arigon Starr is an enrolled member of the Kickapoo Tribe of Oklahoma. She grew up on the road as part of a military family. Her parents, Ken Wahpecome (Kickapoo) and Ruth (Creek-Cherokee-Seneca), supported her artistic expressions, encouraging her to learn as much as possible about music, composition, art, and drama. Starr relocated to Los Angeles to work for entertainment companies like Viacom Productions and Showtime Networks, and in 1996, she left her corporate job to become an award-winning musician and actor. Also an accomplished artist, Starr used her drawing skills in pencils, inks, color, and letters, to bring *Super Indian* to life. *Super Indian* began as a weekly webcomic and has been published as two graphic novels, gaining a diverse audience among comic fans, hipsters, and academics. Her artwork has been featured at the Heard Museum in Phoenix, Museum of the American Indian in Santa Fe, and the Philbrook Museum in Tulsa. She has been featured at many comic conventions across the US, including the San Diego Comic-Con. Starr's comic work also resulted in the award-winning comic anthology *Tales of the Mighty Code Talkers, Volume One. Super Indian Volume Three* will be published in 2020, and her work will be on display at a future exhibit at the National Museum of the American Indian in New York City. A Tulsa Artist Fellow alumna, Starr continues to write, act, and perform. Based in Los Angeles, she is a member of the Screen Actors Guild and Actors' Equity. (105–11)

Emily Steinberg is a Philadelphia-based painter and visual narrative artist. She earned her MFA from the University of Pennsylvania and has exhibited work in the US and Europe. Most recently, her first cartoon was accepted into *The New Yorker* magazine. Her visual narratives have been regularly published in *Cleaver Magazine* since 2013. Her autobiographic novel, *Graphic Therapy*, was published serially at *Smith Magazine* (2008–10). She is a lecturer in fine art at Penn State University, Abington College, and Artist in Residence at Drexel College of Medicine in Philadelphia, where she works with medical students to translate their medical school experiences into words and images. (22–30)

Jay Stephens is a veteran illustrator on the small-press comics scene, solely responsible for *The Land of Nod, Atomic City Tales, SIN,* the *Jetcat Clubhouse* comic book series, the alternative weekly comic strip *Oddville!, Chick & Dee, Arrowhead* comics for OWL, and the daily newspaper strip *Oh, Brother!* (with Bob Weber Jr.). He has authored several drawing books for kids. Stephens has illustrated film, horror, brewery, and music event posters, and has participated in live art events. He is probably best known, however, for his animated television series *Tutenstein* and *The Secret Saturdays.* (281)

Sage Stossel is a contributing editor for the *Atlantic* and a cartoonist for the *Boston Globe,* TheAtlantic.com, and the *Provincetown Banner* (for which she received a New England Press Association Award). Her cartoons have been featured by the *New York Times* Week in Review*, The Washington Post, Politico, CNN Headline News,* and *Best Editorial Cartoons of the Year.* She is the author/illustrator of the children's books *On the Loose in Boston, On the Loose in Washington D.C., On the Loose in Philadelphia,* and *On the Loose in New York City,* and of the graphic novel *Starling.* (116-18)

Chris Summers is an artist from Texas and has been working professionally in art and comics for almost twenty years. As a professional comic artist / digital painter / colorist, his credits include *Evil Dead 2, GI Joe, Dungeons & Dragons, Superman, Nightwing, The Perhapanauts, Eternal Descent, Spartacus: Blood & Sand Comic Book, Motion Comic,* and many more. He also regularly serves as a guest lecturer in the art department at Hardin-Simmons University as well as doing freelance art and design. (113-15)

Brenna Thummler grew up writing and illustrating her own stories, primarily in genres such as early reader horror and autobiographical fairytale. These storytelling roots have proven useful in her career as a graphic

novelist. After illustrating the adaptation of *Anne of Green Gables,* she went on to create *Sheets* (2018) and the sequel, *Delicates* (2021), original works that feature ghosts and laundry. When she's not making books, you might find her tap dancing, baking cakes, or lost in the woods somewhere. (60-67)

Seth Tobocman is a comic book artist whose work often deals with political issues from a radical and independent point of view. He founded the magazine *World War 3 Illustrated* with Peter Kuper in 1979 and has been part of the editorial collective ever since. His work has appeared in *The New York Times, The Village Voice, Heavy Metal,* and many other magazines. He is the author of a number of graphic books, including *You Don't Have to Fuck People Over to Survive, War in the Neighborhood, Portraits of Israelis and Palestinians, Disaster and Resistance, Understanding the Crash, Len: A Lawyer in History,* and *The Face of Struggle.*

Tobocman's books have been translated into French, Italian, Korean, Spanish, and Greek, and his art has exhibited at The Museum of Modern Art, The New Museum of Contemporary Art, The Museum of The City of Ravenna, Exit Art, and ABC No Rio. His images have been used as posters, murals, banners, and tattoos by people's movements from squatting in New York's Lower East Side to the African National Congress in South Africa. (46-47; 226-27)

Tamara Tornado was born in Los Angeles, California, but has lived in New York City all her adult life. She is a painter and a technical illustrator. She is especially alarmed about climate change. She enjoys inking Seth Tobocman's drawings. (46-47; 226-27)

Shelley Wall is an artist and an associate professor in the biomedical communications graduate program at the University of Toronto, where graphic medicine is her primary area of research and creation. As of this writing, she is teaching online from her living room and trying to imagine what the future will look like. (83–87)

Ian Williams, aka The Bad Doctor, is a comics artist, writer, and doctor who lives in Brighton, UK. His critcally acclaimed graphic novels, *The Bad Doctor* and *The Lady Doctor,* were published in 2014 and 2019, respectively; he is working on a third, for the same publishers, provisionally titled *The Sick Doctor,* to be published in 2022. He studied fine art after medical school and then became involved in the medical humanities movement. He named the area of study called "graphic medicine," building the eponymous website in 2007, which he currently co-edits. He is the founder of the not-for-profit Graphic Medicine International Cooperative and co-author of the Eisner-nominated *Graphic Medicine Manifesto.* Between May 2015 and January 2017, Williams drew a weekly comic strip, *Sick Notes*, for *The Guardian.* Online at https://www .graphicmedicine.org. (229–31)

Richard You Wu, MD, PhD, BHSc, is an internal medicine resident physician at the University of Toronto who is passionate about story-telling, arts, and scientific research. He completed an eight-year combined MD/ PhD training at Toronto from 2012 to 2020, where he studied how diet can impact human health. His scientific and medical research was featured in several high-impact academic journals, including *Nature Communication*

and *Microbiome.* In 2014, he was selected as Canada's Vanier Scholar for his contribution to science, and he is the recipient of University of Toronto's Malkin Top MD/PhD Scholar Award and the Dr. Ocana Memorial Award. In his spare time, Wu is an avid reader and movie fanatic. (233–37)

Zen has been the staff letterer for *Aspen Comics* since 2016. He was the editor of the sold-out horror miniseries *The Circle* from Action Lab Entertainment. He also runs *H.C.M.P. High Concept Media Properties*, a comic book graphic design production company that utilizes his experience in a variety of roles to help clients make their ideas into comic books. Online at http://www.hicon media.com. (184–89)

Annie Zhu, MD, BHSc, is a neurology resident physician at the University of Toronto with a strong interest in sequential art and exploring narratives in medicine, especially those of physician and patient experiences. Her work has been featured in journals and conferences including *Annals of Internal Medicine* and the *White Coat Warm heART* exhibit. In her spare time, she enjoys reading comics and has also contributed works for the show *Doctor Who.* Online at https://cazezhu.carbonmade.com. (233–37)